Comprehensive Approach

Series Editors

Bernardo Carpiniello
Department for Medical Sciences, Public Health
University of Cagliari
Cagliari, Italy

Antonio Vita
Department of Clinical and Experimental Science
University of Brescia
Brescia, Italy

Claudio Mencacci
Department of Neuroscience
Azienda Ospedaliera Fatebenefratelli e O
Milano, Italy

This book series will cover a broad range of topics with each volume providing an up-to-date overview of subject matters of particular interest for psychiatrists and other professionals in the field of mental health, through a comprehensive approach, including clinical, therapeutical, forensic and psychosocial points of view.

The topics addressed will be selected in collaboration with the Italian Society of Psychiatry.

The book series is aimed at psychiatrists, psychotherapists, psychologists, social workers, nurses, psychiatric rehabilitation technicians, students and researchers.

This book series is published in partnership with the Italian Society of Psychiatry (SIP)

More information about this series at https://link.springer.com/bookseries/16231

Bernardo Carpiniello • Antonio Vita
Claudio Mencacci
Editors

Recovery and Major Mental Disorders

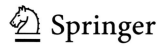
Springer

Editors
Bernardo Carpiniello
Department for Medical
Sciences, Public Health
University of Cagliari
Cagliari, Italy

Antonio Vita
Department of Clinical and Experimental
Sciences
University of Brescia
Brescia, Italy

Claudio Mencacci
Department of Neuroscience
Azienda Ospedaliera Fatebenefratelli e O
Milano, Italy

ISSN 2524-8405 ISSN 2524-8413 (electronic)
Comprehensive Approach to Psychiatry 2
ISBN 978-3-030-98303-1 ISBN 978-3-030-98301-7 (eBook)
https://doi.org/10.1007/978-3-030-98301-7

© The Editor(s) (if applicable) and The Author(s), under exclusive license to Springer Nature Switzerland AG 2022

This work is subject to copyright. All rights are solely and exclusively licensed by the Publisher, whether the whole or part of the material is concerned, specifically the rights of translation, reprinting, reuse of illustrations, recitation, broadcasting, reproduction on microfilms or in any other physical way, and transmission or information storage and retrieval, electronic adaptation, computer software, or by similar or dissimilar methodology now known or hereafter developed.

The use of general descriptive names, registered names, trademarks, service marks, etc. in this publication does not imply, even in the absence of a specific statement, that such names are exempt from the relevant protective laws and regulations and therefore free for general use.

The publisher, the authors and the editors are safe to assume that the advice and information in this book are believed to be true and accurate at the date of publication. Neither the publisher nor the authors or the editors give a warranty, expressed or implied, with respect to the material contained herein or for any errors or omissions that may have been made. The publisher remains neutral with regard to jurisdictional claims in published maps and institutional affiliations.

This Springer imprint is published by the registered company Springer Nature Switzerland AG
The registered company address is: Gewerbestrasse 11, 6330 Cham, Switzerland

Foreword

We are delighted to present the second volume of the series "Comprehensive Approach to Psychiatry", devoted to "Recovery and Severe Mental Disorders", edited by the Italian Society of Psychiatry (SIP) in collaboration with Springer. The volume is published in the context of the efforts of our association to contribute to the dissemination of scientific knowledge in the field of psychiatry and mental health. The topic discussed focuses on recovery from severe mental illness, a process based less on relief from symptoms than on the possibility of overcoming the trauma of the illness and its consequences, and the loss of abilities and opportunities providing access to social life. The concept of recovery itself is clearly in contrast with one of the most widespread stigmatizing prejudices associated with mental illness, i.e. its unavoidable chronic and highly disabling nature.

A large body of methodologically sound clinical studies indicates how an increasing number of patients with mental disorders who undergo appropriate pharmacological and psychosocial treatments are able to achieve sustained remission together with a satisfactory level of personal and social functioning, attaining a quality of working and relational life that allows them to attain social autonomy. Even major psychiatric disorders such as schizophrenia or bipolar disorder, when adequately treated through targeted interventions which take into account the personal needs, aspirations, and values of those affected may, in the same way as for other lifelong medical conditions, elicit equally positive outcomes. The latter indeed is particularly relevant when addressing the highly important issue of recovery from mental illness and dissemination of the findings reported, particularly in studies adopting a personalized approach to treatment based on scientific evidence. Numerous other lifelong conditions, including obsessive compulsive or anxiety disorders, may require equally effective interventions throughout the patient's lifespan. However, the impact of severe mental illness on the patient's life is significantly higher, increasing progressively as symptoms persist, and modifying the life trajectories of those affected, complicating interpersonal relationships and the acquisition or maintenance of satisfying social roles, frequently resulting in overt social exclusion. These aspects are widely acknowledged by staff working in the Italian mental health services, the majority of which have adopted a recovery-oriented approach to care.

Therefore, the decision to place particular focus in this volume on the issue of recovery in schizophrenia and mood disorders is coherent in view of the severe burden frequently affecting both the affected subjects and their families. The portrayal of recovery as a tangible target conveys a highly significant message to mental health workers, as well as to those who are suffering and their caregivers, fostering an urge to seek treatment as early as possible, particularly as recovery depends largely on intervention as soon as possible after onset of the illness.

Contributions to the volume have been provided by Italian and foreign experts in the field to convey the most updated and in-depth knowledge relating to numerous aspects of this composite, and often controversial, issue.

We are confident that the volume will provide readers with a series of theoretical and practical elements which will prove valuable in enhancing the recovery of patients in their care and thus allow them to make full benefit of their civil rights and dignities.

Turin, Italy   Enrico Zanalda
Chieti, Italy   Massimo Di Giannantonio

Introductory Remarks. The Recovery Model in Mental Health

From an etymological viewpoint, the term recovery in its medical connotation generally indicates the act or process of returning to health following injury or sickness [1]. In this sense, recovery may be considered the goal of healing process [2]. However, although commonly used, this commonly accepted medical understanding of the concept has been criticized as being inadequate, too general, and somewhat inaccurate, taking into account the different conceptions of "malady" as intended by diverse groups of people: *disease,* in the opinion of medical and health-care professionals, *illness*, according to the first-person perspective, and *sickness*, as decreed by the social institutions [3]. Indeed, each of the above groups will decide whether or not the person in question has recovered according to his or her own perspective; moreover, a patient may be considered recovered from one perspective (e.g. biomedical), whilst having failed to do so from another perspective (e.g. first-person) [3]. In the field of psychiatry, these different perspectives are reflected in at least two divergent, and seemingly incompatible, means of conceptualizing recovery. The first is focused on recovery as a clinical construct in which objective dimensions are considered as a comprehensive and reliable measure of outcome; the other relates to recovery as a personal process of living with a mental disorder, described through a series of subjective experiences. The first approach was developed in clinical contexts and the second within the user movement. Both approaches to recovery are progressively contributing towards changing paradigms both in mental health care and clinical research, as attested to by the increasing number of citations over the last 20 years detected by means of a simple PubMed search for the keywords "recovery" and "mental disorders", yielding more than 23,000 bibliographic citations, corresponding to approximately 2000 per year in both 2019 and 2020. This notwithstanding, all that glitters is not gold. As authoritatively quoted, although "many mental health services would declare themselves *recovery-oriented*, it is not common that a focus on empowerment, identity, meaning and resilience is ensured in ordinary practice" [4]. Moreover, although the concept of recovery as applied to mental health is undoubtedly "appealing", a persistent lack of knowledge, together with a series of controversies, shortcomings, and difficulties of a conceptual and methodological nature should be acknowledged.

In recent years, a growing interest in clinical and personal recovery has also emerged in relation to bipolar disorder and major depression. In view of the significantly lower amount of research conducted to investigate recovery in major affective disorders, finding that in this context unresolved questions and issues are even more pronounced than in primary psychoses should not be surprising.

This volume, published under the aegis of the Italian Society of Psychiatry thanks to the cooperation of some of the leading researchers and clinicians working in the field, intends to contribute towards improving knowledge of recovery with regard to severe mental disorders, based upon both evidence/convergences and knowledge gaps and divergences.

The first part of the volume, devoted to schizophrenia and related disorders, is introduced by a contribution from Carpiniello and collaborators [5] addressing the issue of clinical recovery as a dimensional construct, together with a critical approach to a series of controversial issues such as the large variability in prevalence rates, the instability of clinical recovery, and its fleeting correlations with personal recovery. Functioning is a fundamental dimension of clinical recovery. The contribution by Giordano el al. [6] deals with factors related to both the disease and personal resources or social context that may have a significant impact on functional outcome, such as social and non-social cognition, functional capacity, negative symptoms, resilience, and access to family and social incentives, all involved as predictors or mediators of outcome, showing how the identification of these factors is crucial for an integration and personalization of recovery-oriented treatments. Rossi et al. [7] address the issue of "personal recovery" as a deeply personal, unique process of changing one's attitudes, values, feelings, goals, skills, and roles, highlighting how recovery-oriented interventions should support people with severe mental illness in pursuing their goals, achieving subjective well-being, promoting resilience, personal skills and hope, facilitating self-determination, enhancing individual strengths, preferences, and aspirations, to allow those concerned to live a fulfilling and productive life despite disability [7]. The process of personal recovery for patients who commit illegal acts is addressed by Shepherd [8], who considers personal recovery a complex process of individual identity work, complicated by the experience of criminal offending and care within forensic settings. The authors illustrate how recovery in forensic settings can be seen as a sequential process of developing a sense of safety and security, expression and understanding of personal trauma, and of developing a sense of personal identity and competence, final individuation, and self-expression. It is commonly assumed that recovery-oriented treatments require a real sharing of the "personal recovery paradigm" by mental health professionals. This would signify, amongst other things, freedom from stigmatizing attitudes. Roncone and co-workers [9] explore barriers such as stigma and orientation, investigating their influence on recovery-oriented interventions, examining studies conducted in a series of Italian facilities which reveal somewhat contradictory attitudes towards the mentally ill, with professionals having less than 15 years of experience and students displaying more favourable attitudes and knowledge than more experienced professionals with regard to expectations of recovery. Hence, the existing practices of the Italian Departments of Mental Health, aimed at inclusion and citizenship of the mentally ill and their rights to live a satisfying life, may be further improved through a more widespread adoption of a "personal recovery paradigm". Psychosocial interventions are univocally considered as an essential component of recovery-oriented treatments. Vita and colleagues [10] focus on evidence-based psychosocial practices to achieve recovery in schizophrenia, including psychoeducation, cognitive behavioural therapy for psychosis, cognitive remediation, and interventions which have fostered potential benefits in this population, such as healthy lifestyle interventions, physical exercise, and integrated treatments for co-occurring substance use disorder. The authors underline how, despite the recommendations established by international guidelines, to date, only a minority of patients have received a person-centred, evidence-based psychiatric rehabilitation intervention. Contrary to long-standing views, data deriving both from clinical experience and the literature reveal how people diagnosed with very significant forms of psychosis may over time achieve a substantial and meaningful recovery. Indeed, evidence from literature illustrate that recovery is a tangible outcome and how specific psychotherapeutic interventions may play a crucial role. Starting from these premises, Lysaker and co-workers [11] illustrate research on metacognition as a construct for the understanding of more subjective aspects of recovery from psychosis, describing a series of emerging forms of recovery-oriented treatment such as Open Dialogue, Cognitive Behaviour Therapy for Psychosis, Metacognitive Reflection and Insight Therapy, and Narrative Enhancement Cognitive Therapy. Working is contextually viewed as both a desired outcome of recovery-oriented treatments and a means of achieving recovery. Mencacci and collaborators [12] delineate how by encouraging dialogue between different sectors and fostering a more nuanced view of disabled job applicants—intended as citizens, patients, and workers—a culture of inclusion can be fostered and appropriate models of intervention disseminated, including at an organizational level. Starting from a comprehensive review of the most widespread models of inclusion for people with mental disorders in Italy, the authors outline a clinical and organizational model for the inclusion of those affected by mental disorders developed in a Mental Health Department in the Metropolitan City of Milan. A shift towards recovery-oriented psychopharmacological treatment has emerged in recent years, with clinical stabilization indicated as a recognized prerequisite for the achievement of clinical recovery. Gorwood and colleagues [13] illustrate the role of psychopharmacological interventions in recovery, the importance of adherence and of minimizing the impact of side effects on adherence itself and well-being, showing how different pharmacological approaches may be of use in diminishing the side effects and how the use of long-acting injectable antipsychotics may enhance the potential for recovery in the context of a shared decision-making approach to improve adherence and empowerment.

The paradigm of recovery, originally established in relation to primary psychosis, little by little has also taken hold in the scientific literature focusing on major affective disorders. Vieta and colleagues [14] illustrate the concept of clinical recovery in bipolar disorders, underlining how symptomatic remission does not necessarily lead to an acceptable level of functioning, necessary to define a condition of full recovery. The authors show how recovery in bipolar disorder is largely hampered by cognitive impairment and subclinical depressive symptoms, defined as residual symptoms, and illustrate not only available treatment strategies but also a wider spectrum of new opportunities in the management of bipolar disorders from a recovery-oriented perspective. The group of Carla Torrent [15] starts from the premise that over the last decade the treatment target in clinical and research settings has focused not only on clinical remission, but also on functional recovery and, more recently, personal recovery, taking into account patients' well-being and quality of life. Hence, the trend in psychiatry and psychology is to treat bipolar disorder in an integrative and holistic manner, using psychosocial therapies with proven efficacy to enhance functional outcomes or prevent functional decline and to improve patients' well-being, quality of life, and personal recovery. Fagiolini and collaborators [16] dispute the idea that pharmacological therapy is only a partially effective tool used to eliminate severe symptoms alone, without providing a concrete prolonged benefit to the patient. The authors underline the essential role of personalized treatment in achieving the resolution of acute symptoms and preventing future pathological episodes, highlighting the need to amalgamate data acquired, thanks to research and clinical practice with a recovery-oriented approach.

Over the course of recent years, the main focus of clinicians and individuals living with MDD has shifted from merely achieving symptomatic remission to clinical recovery, functional recovery, and ultimately personal recovery. Based on these assumptions, Albert and co-workers [17] note that living well despite residual depressive symptoms and the scars of an often chronic, recurrent, long-lasting condition such as MDD (e.g cognitive scars, social scars, physical scars) is not only possible, but should become the main objective in the management of MDD, as recently acknowledged by international clinical guidelines. Thus, the "journey" towards personal recovery in MDD may be viewed as a sequential, multi-dimensional route in which several individuals contribute to the final outcome. This journey commences by adopting strategies aimed at fostering clinical recovery, to then allow a rapid progression towards implementing strategies aimed at promoting existential, functional, physical, and social recovery. In this process, healthcare providers, individuals living with the condition, peers and family members/caregivers can each contribute in their own way to this final outcome. Addressing the issue of treatments, Fiorillo and colleagues [18] reiterate how nowadays the ultimate goal in the treatment of MDD should be to achieve a complete and long-term clinical, functional, and personal recovery of patients. The authors further emphasize that, in order to personalize treatment in line with the recovery-oriented model, it is essential that the symptom complexity of depression be acknowledged and patients provided with a tailored and integrated approach to include pharmacological, psychological, and psychosocial interventions in the context of a shared decision-making approach.

Cagliari, Italy	Bernardo Carpiniello
Milano, Italy	Claudio Mencacci
Brescia, Italy	Antonio Vita

References

1. Merriam Webster Dictionary. https://www.merriam-webster.com/dictionary/recovery#synonyms. Accessed 29 Sept 2021.
2. Both Hsu C, Phillips WR, Sherman KJ, et al. Healing in primary care: a vision shared by patients, physicians, nurses, and clinical staff. Ann Fam Med. 2008;6:307–14. https://doi.org/10.1370/afm.838.
3. Friedman Y. On recovery: re-directing the concept by differentiation of its meanings. Med Health Care Philos. 2021;24:389–99.
4. Maj M, van Os J, Hert M, et al. The clinical characterization of the patient with primary psychosis aimed at personalization of management. World Psychiatry. 2021;20(1):4–33.
5. Carpiniello B, Pinna F, Manchia M, Tusconi M. Dimensions and course of clinical recovery in schizophrenia and related disorders. In: Carpiniello B, Mencacci C, Vita A, editors. Recovery and major mental disorders. Springer; 2021.
6. Giordano GM, Galderisi S, Pezzella P, Perrottelli A, Bucci. P. Determinants of clinical recovery in schizophrenia. In: Carpiniello B, Mencacci C, Vita A, editors. Recovery and major mental disorders. Springer; 2021.
7. Rossi R, Socci V, Rossi A. Personal recovery in Schizophrenia: a narrative review. In: Carpiniello B, Mencacci C, Vita A, editors. Recovery and major mental disorders. Springer; 2021.
8. Shepherd A. Personal Recovery within forensic settings. In: Carpiniello B, Mencacci C, Vita A, editors. Recovery and major mental disorders. Springer; 2021.
9. Roncone R, Giusti L, Bianchini V, Salza A, Casacchia M. Stigma and attitude towards personal recovery from mental illness among Italian mental health professionals. In: Carpiniello B, Mencacci C, Vita A, editors. Recovery and major mental disorders. Springer; 2021.
10. BarlatI S, regina V, Deste G, Galluzzo A, Turrina C, Valsecchi P, Vita A. Psychosocial recovery-oriented intervention in schizophrenia. In: Carpiniello B, Mencacci C, Vita A, editors. Recovery and major mental disorders. Springer; 2021.
11. Lysaker PH, Wiesepape CN, Hamm JA, Cheli S, Leonhardt BL. Recovery from psychosis: emerging definitions, research and select clinical application. In: Carpiniello B, Mencacci C, Vita A, editors. Recovery and major mental disorders. Springer; 2021.
12. Mazzardis S, Quarenghi A, Rubelli P, Sanna B, Mencacci C. Treatments and recovery to enhance employment outcomes for people with schizophrenia and other major mental disorders. An innovative clinical and organizational model of work inclusion in Milan and surrounding area, in Schizophrenia. In: Carpiniello B, Mencacci C, Vita A, editors. Recovery and major mental disorders. Springer; 2021.
13. Mallet J, Le Strat Y, Dubertret C, Gorwood P. Recovery oriented psychopharmacological interventions in Schizophrenia. In: Carpiniello B, Mencacci C, Vita A, editors. Recovery and major mental disorders. Springer; 2021.

14. Fico G, Anmella G, Murru A, Vieta E. Predictors of clinical recovery in bipolar disorders. In: Carpiniello B, Mencacci C, Vita A, editors. Recovery and major mental disorders. Springer; 2021.
15. del Mar Bonnin C, Montejo L, Martinez-Aran A, Solé B, Comes M, Torrent C. Psychosocial recovery-oriented treatments in Bipolar Disorders. In: Carpiniello B, Mencacci C, Vita A, editors. Recovery and major mental disorders. Springer; 2021.
16. Fagiolini A, et al. Psychopharmacological recovery-oriented treatments in Bipolar Disorders. In: Carpiniello B, Mencacci C, Vita A, editors. Recovery and major mental disorders. Springer; 2021.
17. Luciano M, Carmassi C, Albert U. Dimensions and predictors of personal recovery in Major Depression. In: Carpiniello B, Mencacci C, Vita A, editors. Recovery and major mental disorders. Springer; 2021.
18. Sampogna G, Fiorillo A, et al. Recovery oriented treatments in MD. In: Carpiniello B, Mencacci C, Vita A, editors. Recovery and major mental disorders. Springer; 2021.

Contents

Part I   Recovery in Schizophrenia and Related Disorders

1   Dimensions and Course of Clinical Recovery in Schizophrenia and Related Disorders 3
Bernardo Carpiniello, Federica Pinna, Mirko Manchia, and Massimo Tusconi

2   Determinants of Clinical Recovery in Schizophrenia 23
Giulia M. Giordano, Silvana Galderisi, Pasquale Pezzella, Andrea Perrottelli, and Paola Bucci

3   Personal Recovery in Schizophrenia: A Narrative Review 45
Rodolfo Rossi, Valentina Socci, and Alessandro Rossi

4   Personal Recovery Within Forensic Settings 57
Andrew Shepherd

5   Stigma and Attitude Towards Personal Recovery from Mental Illness Among Italian Mental Health Professionals 65
Rita Roncone, Laura Giusti, Valeria Bianchini, Anna Salza, and Massimo Casacchia

6   Psychosocial Recovery-Oriented Interventions in Schizophrenia 77
Stefano Barlati, Valentina Regina, Giacomo Deste, Alessandro Galluzzo, Cesare Turrina, Paolo Valsecchi, and Antonio Vita

7   Recovery from Psychosis: Emerging Definitions, Research and Select Clinical Application 99
Paul H. Lysaker, Courtney N. Wiesepape, Jay A. Hamm, and Bethany L. Leonhardt

8   Treatments and Recovery to Enhance Employment Outcomes for People with Schizophrenia and Other Major Mental Disorders: An Innovative Clinical and Organisational Model of Work Inclusion in Milan and Surrounding Area 117
Sonia Mazzardis, Andrea Quarenghi, Paola Fiorenza Rubelli, Barbara Sanna, and Claudio Mencacci

xiii

9 Recovery-Oriented Psychopharmacological Interventions in Schizophrenia ... 131
Jasmina Mallet, Yann Le Strat, Caroline Dubertret, and Philip Gorwood

Part II Recovery in Mood Disorders

10 Predictors of Clinical Recovery in Bipolar Disorders ... 155
Giovanna Fico, Gerard Anmella, Andrea Murru, and Eduard Vieta

11 Psychosocial Recovery-Oriented Treatments in Bipolar Disorders ... 173
Caterina del Mar Bonnin, Laura Montejo, Anabel Martinez-Aran, Brisa Solé, Mercè Comes, and Carla Torrent

12 Psychopharmacological Recovery-Oriented Treatments in Bipolar Disorders ... 199
Alessandro Cuomo, Alessandro Spiti, Marco Chioccioli, Despoina Koukouna, Arianna Goracci, Simone Bolognesi, and Andrea Fagiolini

13 Dimensions and Predictors of Personal Recovery in Major Depression ... 225
Mario Luciano, Claudia Carmassi, and Umberto Albert

14 Recovery-Oriented Treatments in Major Depressive Disorder ... 245
Gaia Sampogna, Matteo Di Vincenzo, Vincenzo Giallonardo, Mario Luciano, and Andrea Fiorillo

Part I
Recovery in Schizophrenia and Related Disorders

Dimensions and Course of Clinical Recovery in Schizophrenia and Related Disorders

Bernardo Carpiniello, Federica Pinna, Mirko Manchia, and Massimo Tusconi

1.1 Introduction

Since the inception of Kraepelin's point of view relating to unavoidable "deterioration" [1], schizophrenia has traditionally been viewed as a chronic condition characterized by an extremely negative outcome. Bleuler himself seemed to share a pessimistic view of the disorder; indeed, when describing patients with an apparent return to normal functioning, he referred to "recovery with defect" or "healing with scarring" [2]. Subsequently, this view was confuted in part on the basis of the findings of a series of long-term studies carried out over the twentieth century, demonstrating a more complex picture of the course and outcome of the disorder, with a large heterogeneity in results [3] explained, at least in part, by differences in study methods and samples. Indeed, despite the overall relatively poor outcome of schizophrenia reported in follow-up studies, evidence of subgroups of patients affected by schizophrenia emerged, highlighting extended periods of recovery, at times even in the absence of intensive mental health treatments [4]. Thus, little by little a new paradigm, consisting in a less negative view of the disorder, has developed, based largely on the findings of long-term outcome studies of schizophrenia that provide evidence in favor of the potential for recovery. Indeed, in many cases symptom remission and improvement of functioning early in the course of the disease was

B. Carpiniello (✉)
Department for Medical Sciences, Public Health, University of Cagliari, Cagliari, Italy
e-mail: bcarpini@iol.it

F. Pinna · M. Manchia · M. Tusconi
Department of Medical Science and Public Health, Unit of Psychiatry, University of Cagliari, Cagliari, Italy
e-mail: bcarpini@iol.it; fedepinna@inwind.it; mirkomanchia@unica.it; massimotusconi@yahoo.com

© The Author(s), under exclusive license to Springer Nature Switzerland AG 2022
B. Carpiniello et al. (eds.), *Recovery and Major Mental Disorders*, Comprehensive Approach to Psychiatry 2,
https://doi.org/10.1007/978-3-030-98301-7_1

deemed feasible, together with a more or less sustained improvement in later life. Based on these findings, two ways of conceptualizing schizophrenia, the so-called "broken brain" and the "recovery model," have been confronted in recent years [5]. Some authors have contested the "myth of schizophrenia as a progressive brain disease" [6], in consideration of the fact that the progressive deterioration in functioning may not be intrinsically linked to the disorder, being interpreted rather as the consequence of a series of additional factors (e.g., poor access and adherence to treatments, concurrent external conditions, social and financial impoverishment). Indeed, nowadays recovery is deemed possible and represents the therapeutic goal for people with schizophrenia; it is however acknowledged that not all those affected by this disorder will succeed in achieving recovery [7]. The concept of the "recovery model" was encouraged by a growing influence of "user/consumer" movements geared towards fostering a role of subjective experiences, empowerment, and interpersonal support, which ultimately led to the implementation worldwide of services focused on a collaborative approach to treatments [8]. Indeed, the vision of recovery as a personal experience has triggered a change in mental health policies in many countries, generating an at times profound transformation in mental health systems [9]. Accordingly, two clear-cut parallel visions of recovery have developed, one adhered to by clinicians and the other based on the personal, subjective experience of people suffering from schizophrenia. The two visions represent completely separate and distinct concepts, each with their own specific dimensions, although at the same time interconnected and reciprocally influencing [10].

1.2 Clinical Recovery

1.2.1 Conceptual Heterogeneity of Clinical Recovery

In the wake of the advancement of pharmacological and psychosocial treatment options [10, 11], clinical recovery is currently seen as the ultimate treatment goal in schizophrenia, beyond the achievement of symptom reduction, remission and prevention of recurrences, and functional improvement. However, although intuitive and appealing, the concept of clinical recovery continues to lack a univocal definition, unlike the concept of clinical remission, for which an operative definition was reached years ago [12], gaining broad consensus from both researchers and clinicians [13], although not devoid of criticism [14].

Indeed, on analyzing how clinical recovery is conceived, we are clearly faced with a series of significantly different components put forward by different authors. The heterogeneity of the concept emerges from the depiction of recovery yielded by the definitions afforded by some of the most eminent clinical researchers in the field. Based on these definitions, recovery may encompass symptom remission and functional elements such as cognition, social functioning and quality of life [15], be inclusive of freedom from distressing psychotic symptoms and relapses, satisfaction with life and daily activities and appropriate functioning in everyday life [7], or may comprise remission of symptoms together with engagement in productive activity (work, school), independent management of day-to-day needs, cordial family relations, recreational activities, and satisfying peer relationships [16]. Given the "protean" definitions and lack of precision in the meaning of the word "recovery," which promotes "ambiguity and confusion" with a consequent "potential for miscommunication," several years ago Lieberman proposed the use of "qualifying terms" for recovery as a possible solution. For instance, he suggested referring to "recovery of cognitive functioning" or "recovery of vocational functioning," etc. to indicate significant improvements in specific areas [17]. To summarize the state of the art, recovery is at times conceived as a "*unidimensional*" construct, simply indicating a more or less sustained remission [18], or, more frequently, as a "*bidimensional*" construct, including both clinical remission and functional remission as aspects to be concurrently considered [10, 13, 19, 20]. Indeed, although a positive correlation is generally present between remission and functioning, a large proportion of poorly functioning subjects may still be detected among remitted patients [21], with a significant influence of more or less stringent remission criteria on rates of functional remission [14]. Finally, clinical recovery may be represented by a "*multidimensional*" construct, including not only "objective" dimensions such as symptom remission and functioning, but also "subjective" aspects including self-evaluated well-being and/or quality of life [22].

1.2.2 Prevalence of Clinical Recovery

1.2.2.1 Methodological Issues

One of the main issues arising with regard to recovery relates to the number of patients that actually succeed in attaining the same. Unfortunately, a series of factors make it difficult to provide a reliable answer to this question. Firstly, the conceptual heterogeneity of clinical recovery and the methodological differences present in the instruments and criteria of evaluation used to assess the different dimensions of recovery should be taken into account. Indeed, with regard to remission, a considerably relevant difference in criteria and instruments for evaluation has characterized the scientific literature [23, 24], at least prior to the introduction of the above-cited "consensus criteria" [12]. However, a different application of these criteria, with particular focus on the duration of remission, continues to represent a source of heterogeneity. Taking into consideration the evaluation of functioning, the situation does not seem to have changed compared to 2007 when Burn and Patrick affirmed that "scales varied greatly in terms of measurement approach, number and types of domains covered and scoring systems" [25]. Indeed, a "reference" scale for the evaluation of personal and social functioning, similar to the PANSS or BPRS scales with regard to symptomatology, is still lacking, with a similar or even worse situation existing for the evaluation of quality of life or subjective well-being. Indeed, a series of other sources of methodological heterogeneity should be considered together with all the previously mentioned aspects, including how clinical recovery is measured (i.e., how many "dimensions" are taken into account as previously described), the characteristics of the sample considered in the study (e.g., incident cases, prevalent cases or mixed samples; patients with schizophrenia or with schizophrenia spectrum psychoses or simply with "psychosis"), the study design (e.g., cross-sectional or longitudinal studies), to mention solely the main sources of variance. Bearing these issues in mind, the finding of a wide variability of data emerging from some of the most representative studies on clinical recovery conducted in recent years, as described below, should not be surprising.

1.2.2.2 Data from Studies Based on Prevalent Cases

A large body of data derives from studies based on prevalent cases, i.e., including patients of different ages who were at different stages of their illness. In a 1-year follow-up study conducted in Spain on 452 remitted outpatients with schizophrenia, in which symptomatic remission (SR) was defined according to the "consensus" criteria and remission in functioning (RF) was indicated as a Global Assessment of Functioning scale score of at least 80, 22.8% patients fulfilled the recovery definition (SR + RF) at baseline, a proportion that was found to have increased to 27.1% after 1 year [26, 27]. However, taking into account the entire sample initially recruited (n = 1010), the rates of recovery were, respectively, 10.1% at baseline (102/1010) and 10.2% 1 year later (103/110). The 3-year international, prospective, observational study on antipsychotic treatment named "Schizophrenia Outpatients Health Outcomes (SOHO)" study adopted a stringent definition of recovery, including both long-lasting symptomatic and functional remission as well as an adequate quality of life for a minimum of 24 months and up until the 36-month visit; during the 3-year follow-up period the prevalence of recovered subjects among the 6642 patients analyzed was only 4% [28]. In the Italian Network for Research on Psychoses follow-up study, 616 of the original cohort of 921 patients affected by schizophrenia were available for re-assessment 4 years after first evaluation. Patients were deemed as being recovered at follow-up when two criteria were met: the presence of symptomatic remission based upon the "consensus" criteria (limited to severity without the duration criterion), and the presence of functional recovery, defined as a weighted score of at least 76.2 on SLOF "interpersonal relationships," "work skills," and "everyday life skills" scales; according to these criteria, 20.1% of the sample (124/616) were found to have attained recovery [29]. The Chicago Follow-up Study conducted on 64 schizophrenic patients who were compared with samples of patients with other psychoses (12 schizophreniform patients, 81 other psychotic patients) and 117 nonpsychotic patients, all recruited at the time of hospital admission, were re-evaluated five times over a 15-year period; recovery was defined by outcome status achieved during the follow-up period of 1 year on the basis of operational criteria requiring the absence of major symptoms throughout the follow-up year (absence of psychotic activity and absence of negative symptoms), adequate psychosocial functioning, including instrumental (or paid) work half-time or more during the follow-up year and no psychiatric rehospitalizations during the follow-up year; according to these criteria, 41% of patients were found to have recovered during the 15-year follow-up period [30]. These studies show a large variation in recovery rates, ranging from 4% to approx. 40%, with lower rates more evident in studies focused on multiple dimensions and/or linked to the requirement of longer duration of periods prior to deeming patients recovered.

1.2.2.3 Data from Studies Based on Incident Cases

It may be of interest to review studies based on the investigation of incident cases, generally defined as "first-episode studies," to verify whether outcome in terms of recovery is better in younger cohorts of patients who are at the initial stage of the disorder. A follow-up study of 70 out of 143 antipsychotic-naïve patients with first-episode schizophrenia or schizoaffective disorder, selected on the basis of nationwide Danish registers, and re-evaluated after 4–18 years, found 23% fully recovered (i.e., showing symptomatic plus functional remission) subjects, a proportion which fell to 17% when vocational status was added to the recovery criteria [31]. A post hoc analysis of a German cohort of 392 young previously untreated patients with schizophrenia followed over 36 months in the context of the European SOHO study found a 23.6% rate of recovery in terms of symptomatic plus functional remission, but when a third criterion was also considered (subjective well-being), recovery rate fell to 17.1% [32]. A Dutch follow-up study examined prospectively a sample of first-episode patients ($N = 125$), evaluating recovery during the last 9 months of a 2-year follow-up period, revealing how the rate of recovery, considered as a combination of symptomatic and functional remission, related to approx. one-fifth (19.2%) of patients [33]. The 2-year follow-up of the Danish prospective Opus Study assessed the "full recovery" of a cohort of first-episode patients ($n = 547$), linked to patients meeting criteria for both symptom remission and social and (or)vocational recovery, together with the absence of hospitalization during the preceding year; this study reported that 17% of patients had "fully recovered" [34]. The fifth year follow-up of the OPUS study showed a rate of recovery of 18% ($N = 265$ subjects), defined as absence of psychotic or negative symptoms in subjects living independently, GAF (f) > 59, and who either worked or studied [35]. At the 10-year follow-up of the same study, conducted on a total of 304 patients, 14% met the criteria for symptomatic and psychosocial recovery [36]. In the Early Psychosis Prevention and Intervention Centre (EPPIC) study, a naturalistic, prospective follow-up study of an epidemiologic sample of 723 consecutive first-episode patients, 651 of the baseline cohort of 723 participants were re-evaluated at a median of 7.4 years after initial presentation, with 66.9% ($n = 484$) re-interviewed; approximately a quarter of these patients achieved both symptomatic remission and social/vocational recovery [37]. A study conducted in Hong Kong on a sample of 107 patients (70% of the original sample) with a diagnosis of schizophrenia-spectrum disorder who received an early intervention service in 2001–2002 were re-interviewed at a 10-year follow-up; the study found that 25% of patients were recovered in terms of both symptomatic and functional recovery [38]. A prospective follow-up study of 118 first-episode patients affected by schizophrenia or schizoaffective disorder conducted in the USA adopting composite criteria for full recovery (concurrent remission of positive and negative symptoms and adequate social/vocational functioning in terms of fulfillment of age-appropriate role expectations, performance of daily living tasks without supervision, and engagement in social interactions) found that after 5 years only 13.7% of subjects met full recovery criteria for 2 years or longer; the following rates were achieved for each single follow-up: 9% at the third year, 11% at the fourth year, and 12% at the fifth year [39]. In a 7-year follow-up of a 2-year open randomized clinical trial comparing a dose reduction/discontinuation (DR) vs maintenance treatment (MT) in a cohort of 128 first-episode, remitted patients, Wunderink et al. [40] found that the recovery rates of the 108 patients re-evaluated at the final follow-up were, respectively, 40.4% and 17.6% in the DR and MT groups. The overall picture emerging from these studies on incident cases tends to indicate a certain variability of recovery rates, with somewhat higher rates in studies using less stringent criteria and/or lower duration required for recovery, and lower rates in studies where recovery included more stringent criteria in terms of recovery dimensions and duration.

1.2.2.4 Data from Meta-analytical Studies

The only meta-analytic study on clinical recovery was published years ago by Jääskeläinen et al. [41]. Given the methodological heterogeneity of recovery studies, the authors decided to include in their meta-analysis only observational, noninterventistic studies focusing on schizophrenia and related psychoses based upon a bidimensional concept of recovery, in terms of both symptom and social domains for defining recovery. In particular, the authors chose to include in their meta-analysis only studies providing evidence that improvements in at least one of the two domains included in the concept of recovery had persisted for at least 2 years based on a retrospective or prospective design. In other words, cases were viewed as recovered when the improvement threshold had been reached in both the symptom and functioning domain during follow-up, but not necessarily for a 2-year duration for both domains. It should also be taken into account that this meta-analytic study includes mainly studies published before 2010, and a considerably limited number of studies investigating first-episode patients. The authors selected 50 studies and found a median proportion of cases meeting recovery criteria of 13.5% (range 8.1–20.0%). This finding is largely below the recovery rates reported by Warner [42] who considered 114 follow-up studies relating to "complete recovery" (loss of psychotic symptoms and return to pre-illness level of functioning) and/or "social recovery" (economic and residential independence and low social disruption). Based on these criteria, Warner found a rate ranging from 11 to 33% of fully recovered patients and from 22 to 53% of socially recovered subjects. The evident differences between the data published by Jääskeläinen et al. and the findings of Warner may be largely due to the differences in defining recovery, including the fact that Warner did not include in his definition any criterion relating to the persistence of recovery, and the time periods considered, as Jääskeläinen et al. considered studies published mostly from 1940 onwards, while Warner also included studies published between 1904 and 2000. Another important finding emerging from the meta-analysis was the lack of any evidence of a greater proportion of women with schizophrenia meeting recovery criteria compared to men. This evidence is in contrast with the better outcome of schizophrenia traditionally attributed in general to women [43] and with findings from several follow-up studies, showing clearly higher recovery rates among females [44–46]. In interpreting this discrepancy, it should be taken into account that the prevalence of recovery rates (and of both

1 Dimensions and Course of Clinical Recovery in Schizophrenia and Related Disorders

symptom and functional remission considered singly) among females is largely focused on European countries, particularly Southern and Northern Europe, with opposite data reported for Latin America, and lacking any clear differences for other areas of the world [47]. Jääskeläinen et al. also reported a lack of evidence to confirm that the proportion of cases that recover changes significantly over time, a finding which is consistent with the findings of Warner [42]. Moreover, the authors indicate that recovery rates do not change as a function of the diagnostic criteria adopted in the study, given that no difference in prevalence rates was detected between studies using non-Kraepelinian vs Kraepelinian diagnostic systems, a finding in contrast with the largely cited metanalysis on outcome studies in schizophrenia by Hegarty et al. [48] which showed that the more stringent or Kraepelinian criteria were correlated with worse outcomes. The meta-analysis of Jääskeläinen et al. moreover failed to detect evidence that recovery is less prevalent in the presence of increasingly stringent criteria, specifically in terms of both symptom and functioning remission lasting 2 years, and that recovery is more prevalent in first-episode samples compared with general samples. The only significant difference found in the meta-analysis related to the finding of significantly higher median recovery rates among patients living in lower-middle income (36.4%) than among patients of upper-middle (12.1%) and high-income countries (13.0%), a finding which is in line with literature data showing better outcomes in developing countries [49, 50], but in contrast with other studies which refute this common assumption [51, 52].

1.2.3 Time Course of Recovery

One of the most intriguing questions relates to the potential degree of stability of recovery. Medium-long term studies conducted at different times using different methodologies have reported how recovery seems to assume a relatively stable course over time. Harrow et al. [30] in their 15-year multi-follow-up study reported a proportion of recovered patients corresponding to 19% after 4.5 years of follow-up, 22% after 7.5 years, and 19% both at the 10th and 15th year. Grossman et al. [46] in their 20-year follow-up study reported separate data for males and females (Table 1.1), with more prevalent cases for women and a fluctuation of recovery rates in general. However, more recent data have been published from first-episode follow-up studies. For example, the Opus study [35] has reported a recovery rate of, respectively, 22%, 29%, and 25% at 2.5, 5, and 10 years. According to the metanalysis by Jääskeläinen et al. [41], the chances of recovery in studies with a duration of recovery lower than or exceeding 5 years were similar (respectively 13.2% and 14.5%). The finding of

Table 1.1 Recovery rates by time and gender according to Grossman et al. [47]

	2 years	4.5 years	7.5 years	10 years	15 years	20 years
Males	7%	16%	19%	10%	23%	25%
Females	31%	21%	21%	39%	25%	32%

recovery rates that remained more or less stable over the years emerging in several studies may be misleading, as almost all follow-up studies tend to indicate solely the proportion of subjects who were recovered at the time of each follow-up, failing to indicate how many patients had continued to be deemed recovered and for how long throughout follow-up. However, a limited number of studies may shed further light on this issue. In the context of the Opus Study, an interesting paper by Albert et al. [53] investigating predictors and trajectories of recovery of a cohort (n = 225) of patients affected by a first episode of non-affective psychosis found rates of recovery (remission of positive and negative symptoms, working or studying and having a GAF score of 60 or above. not living in supported housing or being hospitalized during the last 2 years of the follow-up) of 9% at the first year, 16% at the second year, and 15.7% at the fifth year; in particular the study identified three groups featuring different trajectories among the 40 recovered patients: (1) the "early stable" recovery group (4% of the total sample), comprising subjects who met recovery criteria at the first, second, and fifth year; (2) the "early unstable" group, including subjects who met recovery criteria at the last follow-up as well as at either the first or the second follow-up (5.8% of the total sample); (3) the "late recovery" group, comprising those who met recovery criteria only at the 5-year follow-up (8% of the total sample). In other terms, the findings underline how recovery is largely a fluctuating, unstable condition, given that: (a) only a minority of patients maintain recovery for 3 consecutive years; (b) a substantial part of the cohort fluctuated from illness to recovery over time; and (c) subjects who were identified as recovered after 5 years are a mixed group, made up in a limited proportion by early recovered patients who remained stable throughout the entire follow-up (22.5% in the cited study) and in a more consistent proportion by patients who achieved recovery status over one of the subsequent years (32.5% in the cited study), with the most consistent proportion represented by those who achieved recovery later (45% in the cited study). The naturalistic, prospective 3-year follow-up study of first-episode patients affected by non-affective psychoses carried out by Ayesa-Arriola et al. [54] was specifically devoted to describing patterns of recovery in a sample of 373 consecutive FEP patients. This study used recovery criteria based on both symptomatic remission according to the Remission Working Group and functional remission, in terms of a score 1 or less at the Disability Assessment Scale. Four patterns of recovery emerged from the study: (a) a "Good stable" course which characterized patients who maintained recovery status throughout the 3-year follow-up period (26% of the sample); (b) a "Good unstable" course, in which patients failed to recover by the first year but achieved recovery by the second or third year (21% of the sample); (c) a "Poor unstable" course, characterizing patients who recovered in the first year, but lost this status in subsequent years (10% of the sample); and (d) a "Poor stable" course, comprising patients who failed to recover throughout the 3-year period (43%). A total of 47% of patients had recovered by the third year of follow-up, while 53% failed to achieve recovery or achieved it only temporarily. Although the different methodologies used hinder any direct comparison of the results obtained, both studies converge to indicate that a discrete proportion of first-episode patients achieved persistent recovery lasting 3–5 years. The percentage of patients who maintained recovery over a longer time span (5 years) is significantly lower (4%) than the sample (26%) who achieved recovery of shorter-lasting duration (3 years). Unfortunately, no extended follow-up studies reporting patterns of recovery were identified in the literature, although the expectation of finding a relatively low proportion of subjects achieving persistent recovery lasting for more than 5 years is somewhat realistic. This is likely not surprising, considering that recovery implies the achievement of both a sustained clinical remission and functioning—a somewhat difficult goal to reach as demonstrated by data from research. Indeed, remission in schizophrenia can occur at any time, although the probability tends to decrease over the longitudinal course of the disease, with a persisting risk of relapse over time, even in presence of long-term maintenance treatment with antipsychotics [55]. Moreover, although symptomatic remission is by definition a prerequisite to recovery, taken alone it is not sufficient [56], particularly as not all patients displaying symptomatic remission are also functionally remitted. Indeed, research studies have demonstrated how functioning is a multi-determined dimension, in which symptomatology represents only one of a series of other determinants. To this regard, data from the study conducted by the Italian Network on Psychosis, one of the largest longitudinal studies conducted to date on schizophrenia, clearly indicates that real-life functioning of people with schizophrenia is correlated with a complex interplay of a multiplicity of clinical, contextual, and personal factors [29, 57–59].

1.2.4 Recovery Beyond Schizophrenia

Generally speaking, clinical recovery is viewed as the most comprehensive outcome target for psychotic disorders, thus raising the question as to whether more effective recovery is achieved in non-schizophrenic disorders than in schizophrenia. Findings obtained in a series of studies favor the latter hypothesis. The study conducted by Grossman et al. [45] found a cumulative rate of patients experiencing recovery throughout the 20-year follow-up of 61% in women and 41% in males, with regard to schizophrenia, and 85% in women and 64% in males for psychoses "other than schizophrenia." The study by Harrow et al. [30] revealed the distribution of patients who had attained recovery at any time during the 15-years follow-up, corresponding to 41% of patients with schizophrenia, 55% of those with schizophreniform psychoses, 67% of patients with "other psychoses" and 78% of nonpsychotic patients; rates of recovery in patients affected by schizophrenia were consistently lowest at each follow-up appointment (Table 1.2). Albert et al. [53] reported how after 5 years the rate of recovery in patients with a diagnosis of schizophrenia was 13.5% versus

Table 1.2 Recovery rates by time and diagnosis according to Harrow et al. [30]

	2 years	4.5 years	7.5 years	10 years	15 years
Schizophrenia	13%	19%	22%	19%	19%
Schizophreniform	18%	27%	33%	27%	25%
Other psychoses	20%	37%	40%	39%	43%
Non-psychotic	39%	46%	51%	51%	50%

23.6% of those with a non-schizophrenic psychotic disorder (F2 ICD 10 Category). In a study investigating the long-term outcome of non-affective psychoses, Pinna et al. [60] assessed a sample of DSM IV schizophrenia ($n = 46$) and schizoaffective ($n = 66$) patients with a comparable long-term illness (208.0 ± 119 and 187 ± 104 months, respectively); remission was cross-sectionally evaluated (no criteria of duration adopted) using criteria of the Remission Working Group, while functional remission was considered as having a PSP scale score of at least 70; patients were deemed recovered when in remission in terms of both symptomatology and functioning. According to these criteria, 43.5% of schizophrenics and 54.5% of schizoaffective patients were deemed symptomatically remitted, with, respectively, 3% and 25.8% being considered functionally remitted; in both cases differences were not statistically significant. On the contrary, 6.5% of schizophrenic and 22.7% of schizoaffective patients were judged as having achieved recovery, a highly significant difference. In a prospective longitudinal study of 56 patients recruited during the first adequate treatment for schizophrenia ($n = 35$) or other psychotic disorders ($n = 21$) (psychotic bipolar disorder, delusional disorder, psychotic disorder NOS) Svendsen et al. [61] used the Remission Working Group criteria to evaluate symptom remission, with functional remission defined as having an employment level equal to full-time work or studies, and social activities equivalent to at least weekly patient-initiated contact with family and/or friends. At 7-year follow-up, 14% of subjects with schizophrenia and 67% of those with other psychoses were found to have achieved recovery, in terms of both symptom and functional remission. In this study, irrespective of the evident variance in prevalence rates, once again attributable to methodological differences among studies, as expected, a significantly higher proportion of recovered subjects was detected among non-schizophrenic psychotic patients.

1.2.5   Recovery in the Elderly

The vast majority of studies focused on recovery in schizophrenia and other psychoses have been conducted on young adult or adult patients, thus raising the question as to whether recovery is achievable in elderly psychotic patients. The few studies that have addressed this issue may be of use in helping to provide an answer. Auslander and Jeste [62] compared a sample of 155 elderly patients affected by schizophrenia with a matched sample of community-dwelling elderly people; the criteria applied required patients to have been in full symptomatic remission for the past 2 years (Sustained remission), over the same period of time been living independently without caretaker supervision, they should not have undergone psychiatric hospitalization over the last 5 years, with a current caregiver-reported status of psychosocial functioning within "normal range," and should either not have been taking antipsychotic medications or taking no more than one-half of the highest daily dose since enrollment. The authors reported that twelve (8%) of the 155 elderly patients met the criteria for sustained remission, and were living independently, and could therefore be considered "recovered." The same authors explained that the relatively low rate of recovery detected might be explained, at least in part, by the strict criteria adopted in defining sustained remission and in the selection of subjects. Cohen et al. recruited a sample of 198 community-dwelling persons aged 55 and over who had developed schizophrenia before the age of 45, together with a community comparison group ($N = 113$) [63]; symptom remission was evaluated based on the criteria of the Remission Working Group, while functional remission was evaluated based on the ability to independently manage medications and money and having at least one confidant; recovery was deemed achieved once criteria for both symptom and functional remission had been met. Based on these criteria, remission and recovery criteria were met by 49% and 17%, respectively, of the Schizophrenia group, remarkably similar figures therefore to those observed in younger age groups. The same group [64], on analyzing data derived from their previous follow-up studies performed in New York City, reported how 26% of elderly patients attained concurrent clinical remission and high community integration at baseline, i.e., "objective recovery"; only 12% of the sample simultaneously attained clinical remission and high community integration at both time points; moreover, only 18% experienced no clinical remission and had low community integration at both assessments. To summarize, 7 out of 10 people featured some combination of the remission and community integration. More recently, Cohen et al. [65] published a study on early-onset schizophrenia spectrum disorder in which a subsample of 102 of 248 community-dwelling subjects over the age of 55 was reassessed at a mean of 52 months from first evaluation; clinical recovery was assumed when criteria for both symptom remission (evaluated by a modified version of the Schizophrenia Working group) and functioning, in terms of community integration (score of 9 or more on the Community Integration Scale), were met. The study reported that 12% of subjects remained persistently in clinical recovery at both baseline and follow-up (defined as Tier 1), while 18% failed to meet the criteria for clinical recovery (defined as Tier 5) at any time. The remaining subjects (approx. 70% of the sample) displayed a variable mix of components of clinical recovery during follow-up, namely: (a) a stable state group (named tiers 3), comprising 11% of the sample, characterized by persistent clinical remission but no community integration (6%) or persistent community integration without any clinical remission (5%); (b) a fluctuating group (defined as tiers 4), constituted by 37% of the sample, including subjects who had achieved clinical remission or community integration at only one point in time; and (c) a stable group (defined as tiers 5) including those who had never achieved recovery, as failing to attain either clinical remission or community integration at any point in time. Overall, the figures emerging from this study demonstrate the possibility of achieving recovery in the elderly at rates similar to or better than those detected in younger age groups, highlighting how different patterns of recovery may be observed for the elderly in the same way as for all other age groups. In an editorial on "Late life schizophrenia," commenting data on recovery in the elderly, Meersters [66] reminded us that "…it is clear that at present enduring recovery is too high a goal for the large majority of younger schizophrenia patients… most likely, the same holds true for old," and that "..if recovery is considered as an all-or-nothing goal, these findings are clearly discouraging. Such a dichotomous approach, however, does not do justice to the versatile reality of coping with everyday life that most clinicians who work with older schizophrenia patients will recognize. Although most patients do not attain complete recovery, many show significant improvements in psychosocial functioning and well-being as they age. Interestingly, this parallels the finding in successful aging research, that positive self-appraisal increases with age, even in the midst of physical and cognitive declinage…".

1.3 Clinical and Personal Recovery

As mentioned previously, although clinical and personal recovery are separate and distinct concepts, they are interconnected and reciprocally influencing, thus highlighting the appropriateness of fostering a deeper understanding of their relationships.

1.3.1 Personal Recovery; Definitions, Characteristics, Processes, Stages

The concept of personal recovery was developed from the point of view of users of mental health services with the aim of prioritizing more meaningful, personalized treatment goals. Personal recovery has often been compared with the traditional treatment targets of symptomatic remission or improvement in social and occupational functioning (functional remission) [67–69]. A widely used definition of personal recovery is "a deeply personal, unique process of changing one's attitudes, values, feelings, goals, skills and/or roles. It is a way of living a satisfying, hopeful, and contributing life even with limitations caused by the illness" [70]. Accordingly, it resembles a process or a "journey," as often described: "a journey of healing and transformation that enables a person to live a meaningful life in a community of his or her choice while striving to achieve maximum human potential" [71]. According to the latter definition developed by the USA Substance Abuse and Mental Health Services Administration (SAMHSA), recovery does not necessarily signify symptom remission or attainment of normal functioning [72], but rather refers to subjective experiences of optimism, empowerment, interpersonal support, peer support, and stigma reduction [8]. One of the major difficulties in studies investigating personal recovery has been represented by an uncertainty as to how to operationalize this process, given the relevant number of aspects that could potentially be included and evaluated within this concept (Table 1.3). Chiu et al. [73] attempted to empirically test the SAMHSA recovery model assuming subjective Quality of life as a proxy indicator of consumer-defined recovery. In their study, 204 patients aged 18–60 affected by schizophrenia spectrum disorder attending two participating outpatient clinics were interviewed using a number of inventories to assess the component dimensions included in the model and a measure of self-evaluated, health-related

1 Dimensions and Course of Clinical Recovery in Schizophrenia and Related Disorders

Table 1.3 Dimensions of personal recovery according to the SAMHSA model [73]

Perceived respect
Competence
Empowerment
Personal responsibility
Sense of self-determination
Hope
Person-centered treatment
Understanding of the recovery process
Peer support
Holistic (comprehensive) recovery: psychosocial symptoms, social support, spirituality)

quality of life; canonical correlation analysis was performed on two sets of variables, the SAMHSA recovery components and the QoL domain scores of the WHOQOL-BREF scale, revealing significant correlations between most of the recovery components proposed in the SAMHSA recovery model and the health-related quality of life measure.

In view of the acknowledged need for a greater conceptual clarity on the issue of personal recovery, Leamy et al. [74] developed a conceptual framework for personal recovery through a systematic review and a narrative synthesis. The resulting conceptual framework consists in a series of characteristics of the recovery journey (e.g., recovery as an active process, a unique process, a nonlinear process, a journey), five recovery processes comprising connectedness, hope and optimism about the future, identity, meaning in life and empowerment, and, finally, a recovery staging within a transtheoretical model of change which includes precontemplation, contemplation, preparation, action, maintenance, and growth.

1.3.2 Clinical vs. Personal Recovery

Van Eck et al. performed a meta-analysis to investigate the relationship between clinical and personal recovery in patients with schizophrenia spectrum disorders [75]. The majority of studies were conducted on chronic patients, with only one study specifically investigating early psychosis patients. The meta-analysis initially revealed a substantial heterogeneity across studies. Random effect meta-analysis of the relationship between overall symptom severity and personal recovery revealed a significant mean weighted correlation coefficient of $r = -0.21$ (95% CI = -0.27 to -0.14, $p < 0.001$), indicating that patients displaying a higher level of overall psychopathology reported a slightly lower personal recovery. The study also evaluated the association between personal recovery and different symptom domains (Table 1.4), again showing a high heterogeneity between studies and an inverse correlation between symptom dimensions and personal recovery measures. A small significant positive effect size was also found for the association with general

Table 1.4 Correlations between symptom dimensions and personal recovery according to van Eck et al. [75]

Symptom dimension	r	IC and significance
Positive symptoms	−0.20	95% CI = −0.27 to −0.12, $p < 0.001$
Negative symptoms	−0.24	95% CI = −0.33 to −0.15, $p < 0.001$
Affective symptoms	−0.34	95% CI = −0.44 to −0.24, $p < 0.001$)

Table 1.5 Correlations between symptom dimensions and hope according to van Eck et al. [75]

Symptom dimension	r	IC and significance
Positive symptoms	−0.14	95% CI = −0.23 to −0.05, $p = 0.004$
Negative symptoms	−0.26	95% CI = −0.32 to −0.19, $p < 0.001$
Affective symptoms	−0.43	95% CI = −0.51 to −0.35, $p < 0.001$

functioning ($r = 0.21$ (95% CI = −0.09 to 0.32, $P < 0.001$), indicating that the higher the degree of functioning, the higher the personal recovery reported by patients.

The study reports separately meta-analytic data relating to the relationship between symptomatology and hope (Table 1.5). All symptom dimensions show an inverse, significant correlation with hope measures, indicating that the lower the levels of positive, negative, and, above all, affective symptoms, the higher the level of hope among patients. As regard to empowerment, only the correlation with overall symptoms could be calculated, obtaining a mean weighted correlation coefficient of $r = −0.23$ (95% CI = −0.36 to −0.09, $P < 0.001$).

The relative importance of affective symptoms in boosting personal recovery and hope has been highlighted in particular by this meta-analytic study, raising the question of whether depression might contrast the achievement of personal recovery and hope or whether personal recovery and hope may be capable of preventing depression.

A study by Chang et al. [76] aimed at examining simultaneously how different recovery processes contribute to personal well-being, focused in particular on the additional contribution of personal recovery to well-being through a regression analysis after controlling for clinical and functional recovery. The results of this study demonstrated how personal recovery was not only positively associated with well-being, contributing to a 26.0% incremental variance in predicting the latter, but also that its effect on well-being was independent of clinical recovery. A recent contribution by Rossi et al. [77] in the context of the cited study of the Italian Network for Research on Psychoses was aimed at exploring the relationship between self-reported "personal recovery" (SRPR) and clinical recovery for the purpose of identifying variables capable of influencing outcome. Personal recovery measures were based on resilience, self-esteem, recovery style, coping strategies, and internalized stigma. By means of a cluster analysis of SRPR-related variables, three clusters were identified. The first cluster, characterized by highest scores on the recovery style scales, Self-Esteem Rating Scale and Problem Focused Coping Scale, and the lowest scores on the scale of Internalized Stigma, included subjects attaining the best clinical recovery measures. The third cluster was represented by those achieving the lowest scores at the majority of self-reported personal recovery scales and included subjects with the poorest clinical outcome. The second cluster was characterized by better insight, higher levels of self-stigma, lowest self-esteem and personal strength, and highest emotional coping, and included subjects with intermediate levels of clinical recovery, thus revealing a somewhat complex pattern, with a "paradoxical" mixture of positive and negative personal and clinical features of recovery.

1.4 Concluding Remarks

Despite the heterogeneity of data relating to the proportion of patients affected by schizophrenia and related disorders, it is feasible to maintain that by far the most extensively shared definition of recovery is the attainment of both sustained symptom and functional remission. At this point, an impellent need is perceived for a shared definition of the tools to be used in evaluating functioning and in setting threshold scores to be adopted for functional remission, particularly given the availability of a shared definition and criteria for clinical remission. Data from literature demonstrate how recovery, as above defined, is attainable in approximately 15% of patients, although this proportion may likely increase in first-episode patients subjected to an early intervention program, who seem to achieve an overall better outcome, at least in the short-medium term [78], including higher recovery rates [79], a result that might possibly be ascribed to better results in terms of functioning [80, 81]. However, it should be underlined how other authors have expressed their doubt with regard to the positive impact of early interventions, at least in terms of higher recovery rates [82, 83]. It has been reported that the median estimate of the annual recovery rate for schizophrenia is 1.4%., meaning that for every 100 individuals with schizophrenia, 1 or 2 per year would meet the recovery-related criteria; therefore, approximately 14% of subjects would be expected to recover over any 10-year period [41]. The main issue however is that we are not yet sure whether this progressive increase of recovery may extend beyond the 10-year period, nor how to ensure this annual rate increases further. The authors of the above-cited study have affirmed that some evidence has been obtained to suggest that recovery outcomes failed to improve over time. This was defined by the authors as a "sobering finding, in light of the advancements in the delivery of care for those who are affected from schizophrenia." The reasons underlying the persistent negative outcomes in schizophrenia are linked to a multiplicity of factors including lack of involvement and engagement in treatment, poor treatment response and adherence, presence of cognitive deficits and comorbidity with substance use disorders and concurrent medical illness, preexisting developmental problems and poor functioning prior to diagnosis, effects of medication, social determinants of health, and finally an adaptation to disability and shifting of expectations [84]. Moreover, the significant treatment gap for schizophrenia is highly relevant and should be duly investigated [85] with particular focus on the delay of treatments and difficulty in improving functioning of patients affected by schizophrenia, probably due to the ongoing failure to adequately apply psychosocial treatments in clinical settings [85–87] despite proof of their effectiveness [10]. The latter finding however may be partly justified by the observation that clinical trials on psychosocial interventions, upon which recommendations included in the main treatment guidelines are based, are frequently lacking a pragmatic design, ultimately leading to uncertainty over the applicability of recommendations in everyday clinical practice [88].

References

1. Jablensky A. Living in a Kraepelinian world: Kraepelin's impact on modern psychiatry. Hist Psychiatry. 2007;18:381–8.
2. Bleuler E. Dementia praecox or the group of schizophrenias. Joseph Zinkin, trans-ed. New York, NY: International Universities Press; 1950.
3. Huber G. The heterogeneous course of schizophrenia. Schizophr Res. 1997;28:177–85.
4. Jobe TH, Harrow M. Long-term outcome of patients with schizophrenia: a review. Can J Psychiatr. 2005;50(14)
5. Lieberman JA, Drake ER, Sederer LI, et al. Science and recovery in schizophrenia. Psych Serv. 2008;59:487–96.
6. Zipursky RB. The myth of schizophrenia as a progressive brain disease. Schizophr Bull. 2013;39(6):1363–72.
7. Harvey PD, Bellack AS. Toward a terminology for functional recovery in schizophrenia: is functional remission a viable concept? Schizophr Bull. 2009;35:300–6.
8. Warner R. Recovery from schizophrenia and the recovery model. Curr Opin Psychiatry. 2009;22:374–80.
9. Slade M, Amering M, Farkas S, et al. Uses and abuses of recovery: implementing recovery-oriented practices in mental health systems. World Psychiatry. 2014;13:12–20.
10. Vita A, Barlati S. Recovery from schizophrenia: is it possible? Curr Opin Psychiatry. 2018;31:246–55.
11. Kane JM, Correll CU. Pharmacologic treatment of schizophrenia. Dialogues Clin Neurosci. 2010;12:345–57.
12. Andreasen NC, Carpenter W, Kane JM, et al. Remission in schizophrenia: proposed criteria and rationale for consensus. Am J Psychiatry. 2005;162:441–4.
13. Emsley R, Chiliza R, Asmal L, Lehloenya K. The concepts of remission and recovery in schizophrenia. Curr Opin Psychiatry. 2011;24:114–21.
14. Pinna F, Tusconi M, Bosia M, Cavallaro R, Carpiniello B. Criteria for symptom remission revisited: a study of patients affected by schizophrenia and schizoaffective disorders. BMC Psychiatry. 2013;13:235.
15. Leucht S, Lasser R. The concept of remission and recovery in schizophrenia. Pharmacopsychiatry. 2005;39:161–70.
16. Liberman RP. Recovery from disability. Manual of psychiatric rehabilitation. Washington, DC: Am Psych Publishing; 2008.
17. Lieberman JA, Drake RE, Sederer LI, et al. Science and recovery in schizophrenia. Psychiatr Serv. 2008;59(5):487–96.
18. Salzer MS, Brusilovskiy E, Townley G. National estimates of recovery-remission from serious mental illness. Psychiatr Serv. 2018;69(5):523–8.
19. Leucht S. Measurements of response, remission, and recovery in schizophrenia and examples for their clinical application. J Clin Psychiatry. 2014;75(Suppl 1):8–14.
20. Slade M, Amering M, Oades L. Recovery: an international perspective. Epidemiol Psichiatr Soc. 2008;17(2):128–37.

21. Pinna F, Deriu L, Lepori T, Maccioni R, Milia P, Sarritzu E, Tusconi M, Carpiniello B, Cagliari Recovery Study Group. Is it true remission? A study of remitted patients affected by schizophrenia and schizoaffective disorders. Psychiatry Res. 2013;210(3):739–44.
22. Lambert M, Schimmelmann BG, Naber D, et al. Prediction of remission as a combination of symptomatic and functional remission and adequate subjective well-being in 2960 patients with schizophrenia. J Clin Psychiatry. 2006;67(11):1690–7.
23. Leucht S. Measuring outcomes in schizophrenia and examining their clinical application. J Clin Psychiatry. 2014;75(6):15.
24. Leucht S, Lasser R. The concepts of remission and recovery in schizophrenia. Pharmacopsychiatry. 2006;39(5):161–70.
25. Burns T, Patrick D. Social functioning as an outcome measure in schizophrenia studies. Acta Psychiatr Scand. 2007;116(6):403–18.
26. Ciudad A, Bobes J, Alvarez E, et al. Clinical meaningful outcomes in schizophrenia: remission and recovery. Rev Psiquiatr Salud Ment. 2011;4(1):53–65.
27. Bobes J, Ciudad A, Álvarez E, et al. Recovery from schizophrenia: results from a 1-year follow-up observational study of patients in symptomatic remission. Schizophr Res. 2009;115:58–66.
28. Novick D, Haro JM, Suarez D, et al. Recovery in the outpatient setting: 36-month results from the Schizophrenia Outpatients Health Outcomes (SOHO) study. Schizophr Res. 2009;108(223):230.
29. Galderisi S, Bucci P, Mucci A, et al. The interplay among psychopathology, personal resources, context-related factors and real-life functioning in schizophrenia: stability in relationships after 4 years and differences in network structure between recovered and non-recovered patients. World Psychiatry. 2020;19(1):81–91.
30. Harrow M, Grossman LS, Jobe TH, et al. Do patients with schizophrenia ever show periods of recovery? A 15-year multi-follow-up study. Schizophr Bull. 2005;31(3):723–34.
31. Klærkea LR, Baandrupa L, Fagerlunda B, et al. Diagnostic stability and long-term symptomatic and functional outcomes in first-episode antipsychotic-naïve patients with schizophrenia. Eur Psychiatry. 2019;62:130–7.
32. Lambert M, Naber D, Schacht A, et al. Rates and predictors of remission and recovery during 3 years in 392 never-treated patients with schizophrenia. Acta Psychiatr Scand. 2008;118(3):220–9.
33. Wunderink L, Sytema S, Nienhuis FJ, Wiersma D. Clinical recovery in first-episode psychosis. Schizophr Bull. 2009;35(2):362–9.
34. Petersen L, Thorup A, Øqhlenschlaeger J, et al. Predictors of remission and recovery in a first-episode schizophrenia spectrum disorder sample: 2-year follow-up of the OPUS trial. Can J Psychiatr. 2008;53(10):660–70.
35. Bertelsen M, Jeppesen P, Petersen L, et al. Course of illness in a sample of 265 patients with first-episode psychosis—five-year follow-up of the Danish OPUS trial. Schizophr Res. 2009;107(2–3):173–8.
36. Austin SF, Mors O, Secher RG, et al. Predictors of recovery in first episode psychosis: the OPUS cohort at 10 year follow-up. Schizophr Res. 2013;150(1):163–8.
37. Henry LP, Amminger GP, Harris MG, et al. The EPPIC follow-up study of first-episode psychosis: longer-term clinical and functional outcome 7 years after index admission. J Clin Psychiatry. 2010;71(6):716–28.
38. Chan SKW, Hui CLM, Chang WC, et al. Ten-year follow up of patients with first-episode schizophrenia spectrum disorder from an early intervention service: predictors of clinical remission and functional recovery. Schizophr Res. 2019;204:65–71.
39. Robinson DG, Woerner MG, McMeniman M, et al. Symptomatic and functional recovery from a first episode of schizophrenia or schizoaffective disorder. Am J Psychiatry. 2004;161(3):473–9.
40. Wunderink L, Nieboer RM, Wiersma D, et al. Recovery in remitted first-episode psychosis at 7 years of follow-up of an early dose reduction/discontinuation or maintenance treatment strategy: long-term follow-up of a 2-year randomized clinical trial. JAMA Psychiat. 2013;70(9):913–20.

41. Jääskeläinen E, Juola P, Hirvonen N, et al. A systematic review and meta-analysis of recovery in schizophrenia. Schizophr Bull. 2013;39(6):1296–306.
42. Warner R. Recovery of schizophrenia: psychiatry and political economy. London: Routledge; 2004.
43. Leung A, Chue P. Sex differences in schizophrenia, a review of the literature. Acta Psychiatr Scand Suppl. 2000;401:3–38.
44. Thorup A, Albert N, Bertelsen M, et al. Gender differences in first-episode psychosis at 5-year follow-up—two different courses of disease? Results from the OPUS study at 5-year follow-up. Eur Psychiatry. 2014;29(1):44–51.
45. Grossman LS, Harrow M, Rosen C, Faull R. Sex differences in outcome and recovery for schizophrenia and other psychotic and nonpsychotic disorders. Psychiatr Serv. 2006;57(6):844–50.
46. Grossman LS, Harrow M. Rosen C, et al. Sex differences in schizophrenia and other psychotic disorders: a 20-year longitudinal study of psychosis and recovery. Compr Psychiatry. 2008;49(6):523–9.
47. Novick D, Montgomery W, Treuer T, et al. Sex differences in the course of schizophrenia across diverse regions of the world. Neuropsychiatr Dis Treat. 2016;12:2927–39.
48. Hegarty JD, Baldessarini RJ, Tohen M, et al. One hundred years of schizophrenia: a meta-analysis of the outcome literature. Am J Psychiatry. 1994;151:1409–16.
49. Craig TJ, Siegel C, Hopper K, et al. Outcome in schizophrenia and related disorders compared between developing and developed countries. A recursive partitioning re-analysis of the WHO DOSMD data. Br J Psychiatry. 1997;170:229–33.
50. Kulhara P, Shah R, Grover S. Is the course and outcome of schizophrenia better in the 'developing' world? Asian J Psychiatry. 2009;2(2):55–62.
51. Esan OB, Ojagbemi A, Gureje J. Epidemiology of schizophrenia—an update with a focus on developing countries. Int Rev Psychiatry. 2012;24(5):387–92.
52. Burns J. Dispelling a myth: developing world poverty, inequality, violence and social fragmentation are not good for outcome in schizophrenia. Afr J Psychiatry. 2009;12(3):200–5.
53. Albert N, Bertelsen M, Thorup A, et al. Predictors of recovery from psychosis analyses of clinical and social factors associated with recovery among patients with first-episode psychosis after 5 years. Schizophr Res. 2011;125(2–3):257–66.
54. Ayesa-Arriola R, Pelayo Terán JM, Setién-Suero E. Patterns of recovery course in early intervention for FIRST episode non-affective psychosis patients: the role of timing. Schizophr Res. 2019;209:245–54.
55. Haro JM, Novick D, Suarez D, et al. Remission and relapse in the outpatient care of schizophrenia: three-year results from the Schizophrenia Outpatient Health Outcomes study. J Clin Psychopharmacol. 2006;26(6):571–8.
56. Wunderink L, Sytema S, Nienhuis FJ, Wiersma D. Clinical recovery in first-episode psychosis. Schizophrenia Bull. 2009,35(2):362–9.
57. Galderisi S, Rossi A, Rocca P, et al. The influence of illness-related variables, personal resources and context-related factors on real-life functioning of people with schizophrenia. World Psychiatry. 2014;13(3):275–87.
58. Galderisi S, Bucci P, Kirkpatrick B, et al. Interplay among psychopathologic variables, personal resources, context-related factors, and real-life functioning in individuals with schizophrenia: a network analysis. JAMA Psychiat. 2018;75(4):396–404.
59. Mucci A, Galderisi S, Gibertoni D, et al. Factors associated with real-life functioning in persons with schizophrenia in a 4-year follow-up study of the Italian network for research on psychoses. JAMA Psychiat. 2021;78(5):550–9. https://doi.org/10.1001/jamapsychiatry.2020.4614.
60. Pinna F, Sanna L, Perra V. Pisu Randaccio R, Diana E, Carpiniello B, Cagliari Recovery Study Group. Long-term outcome of schizoaffective disorder. Are there any differences with respect to schizophrenia? Riv Psichiatr. 2014;49(1):41–9.
61. Svendsen IH, Øie MG, Møller P, et al. Basic self-disturbances independently predict recovery in psychotic disorders: a seven year follow-up study. Schizophr Res. 2019;212:72–8.
62. Auslander LA, Jeste DV. Sustained remission of schizophrenia among community dwelling older outpatients. Am J Psychiatry. 2004;161:1490–3.

1 Dimensions and Course of Clinical Recovery in Schizophrenia and Related Disorders 21

63. Cohen CI, Pathak R, Ramirez PM, Vahia I. Outcome among community dwelling older adults with schizophrenia: results using five conceptual models. Community Ment Health J. 2009;45(2):151–6.
64. Cohen CI, Freeman K, Ghoneim D, et al. Advances in the conceptualization and study of schizophrenia in later life. Psychiatr Clin North Am. 2018;41(1):39–53.
65. Cohen CI, Reinhardt MM. Recovery and recovering in older adults with schizophrenia: a 5-tier model. Am J Geriatr Psychiatry. 2020;28(8):872–5.
66. Meesters PD. Late-life schizophrenia: remission, recovery, resilience. Am J Geriatr Psychiatry. 2014;22(5):423–6.
67. Bellack AS. Scientific and consumer models of recovery in schizophrenia: concordance, contrasts, and implications. Schizophr Bull. 2006;32:432–42.
68. Davidson L, Schmutte T, Dinzeo T, Andres-Hyman R. Remission and recovery in schizophrenia: practitioner and patient perspectives. Schizophr Bull. 2008;34:5–8.
69. Whitley R, Drake RE. Recovery: a dimensional approach. Psychiatr Serv. 2010;61(12):1248–50.
70. Anthony W. Recovery from mental illness: the guiding vision of the mental health system in the 1990s. Psychosoc Rehabil J. 1993;16:11–23.
71. Substance Abuse and Mental Health Services Administration. National census statement on mental health recovery. National Mental Health Information Center, US Government; 2006.
72. Schrank B, Slade M. Recovery in psychiatry. Psychiatr Bull. 2007;31:321–5.
73. Chiu MY, Ho WW, Lo WT, et al. Operationalization of the SAMHSA model of recovery: a quality of life perspective. Qual Life Res. 2010;19:1–13. https://doi.org/10.1007/s11136-009-9555-2.
74. Leamy M, Bird V, Le Boutillier C, et al. Conceptual framework for personal recovery in mental health: systematic review and narrative synthesis. Br J Psychiatry. 2011;199(6):445–52.
75. Van Eck RM, Burger TJ, Vellinga A, et al. The relationship between clinical and personal recovery in patients with schizophrenia spectrum disorders: a systematic review and meta-analysis. Schizophr Bull. 2018;44(3):631–42.
76. Chan RC, Mak WW, Chio FH, et al. Flourishing with psychosis: a prospective examination on the interactions between clinical, functional, and personal recovery processes on well-being among individuals with schizophrenia spectrum disorders. Schizophr Bull. 2018;44(4):778–86.
77. Rossi A, Amore M, Galderisi S, et al. The complex relationship between self-reported 'personal recovery' and clinical recovery in schizophrenia. Schizophr Res. 2018;192:108–12.
78. Correll CU, Galling B, Pawar A, et al. Comparison of early intervention services vs treatment as usual for early-phase psychosis: a systematic review, meta-analysis, and meta-regression. JAMA Psychiat. 2018;75(6):555–65.
79. Hegelstad WT, Larsen TK, Auestad B, et al. Long-term follow-up of the TIPS early detection in psychosis study: effects on 10-year outcome. Am J Psychiatry. 2012;169(4):374–80.
80. Puntis S, Minichino A, De Crescenzo F, et al. Specialised early intervention teams for recent-onset psychosis. Cochrane Database Syst Rev. 2020;11:CD013288. https://doi.org/10.1002/14651858.CD013288.pub2.
81. Santesteban-Echarri O, Paino M, Rice S, et al. Predictors of functional recovery in first-episode psychosis: a systematic review and meta-analysis of longitudinal studies. Clin Psychol Rev. 2017;58:59–75.
82. Chan SK, So HC, Hui CL, et al. 10-year outcome study of an early intervention program for psychosis compared with standard care service. Psychol Med. 2015;45(6):1181–93.
83. Chan SKW, Chan HYV, Devlin J, et al. A systematic review of long-term outcomes of patients with psychosis who received early intervention services. Int Rev Psychiatry. 2019;31(5–6):425–40.
84. Zipursky J. Why are the outcomes in patients with schizophrenia so poor? J Clin Psychiatry. 2014;75(suppl 2):20–4.
85. Kohn R, Saxena S, Levav I, Saraceno B. The treatment gap in mental health care. Bull World Health Organ. 2004;82(11):858–66.

86. Dixon LB, Dickerson F, Bellack AS, et al. Schizophrenia Patient Outcomes Research Team (PORT). The 2009 schizophrenia PORT psychosocial treatment recommendations and summary statements. Schizophr Bull. 2010;36(1):48–70.
87. Ince P, Haddock G, Tai S. A systematic review of the implementation of recommended psychological interventions for schizophrenia: rates, barriers, and improvement strategies. Psychol Psychother. 2016;89(3):324–50.
88. Gastaldon C, Mosler F, Toner S, et al. Are trials of psychological and psychosocial interventions for schizophrenia and psychosis included in the NICE guidelines pragmatic? A systematic review. PLoS One. 2019;14(9):e0222891. https://doi.org/10.1371/journal.pone.0222891.

Determinants of Clinical Recovery in Schizophrenia

2

Giulia M. Giordano, Silvana Galderisi, Pasquale Pezzella, Andrea Perrottelli, and Paola Bucci

2.1 Introduction

Schizophrenia is a severe mental disorder with a high heterogeneity in terms of risk factors, comorbidities, clinical presentation, course, response to treatment, and functional outcome [1, 2].

About 75% of people suffering from this disorder show a clinical course characterized by remission and relapse phases, and about one in seven people meet criteria for recovery [3–5].

Recovery, to date, seems to represent the end point of an historical, cultural, and scientific process that, for the care of people with schizophrenia, initially regarded as a target the improvement of symptom severity, then moved to symptomatic remission, and finally to recovery [3, 6–9].

Actually, this reflects the development in the conceptualization of schizophrenia. In the first descriptions it was named "dementia praecox" and regarded as a progressive and irreversible disorder with an unfavorable course [10]. This pessimistic view began to change with the discovery of antipsychotic medications in 1950s, which led to the discharge to the community of the vast majority of people institutionalized due their disorder [6]. Therefore, with the advent of antipsychotics, the main target to achieve was the improvement of severity of schizophrenia symptoms and, consequently, the prognosis was based primarily on the response to treatment. Although a clear agreement on the definition of response to treatment was never reached, "response" is a relative term, which defines an overall improvement of patient's signs and symptoms [11]. Conversely, "remission" is an absolute term,

---

G. M. Giordano · S. Galderisi (✉) · P. Pezzella · A. Perrottelli · P. Bucci
Department of Psychiatry, University of Campania "Luigi Vanvitelli", Naples, Italy
e-mail: giuliamgiordano@gmail.com; silvana.galderisi@gmail.com;
pezzella.pasquale3@gmail.com; andreaperrottelli@gmail.com; paolabucci456@gmail.com

© The Author(s), under exclusive license to Springer Nature
Switzerland AG 2022
B. Carpiniello et al. (eds.), *Recovery and Major Mental Disorders*,
Comprehensive Approach to Psychiatry 2,
https://doi.org/10.1007/978-3-030-98301-7_2

defined by a specific threshold of severity of core symptoms (delusions, hallucinations, disorganized speech, disorganized or catatonic behavior, negative symptoms). In particular, according to the Remission in Schizophrenia Working Group, a patient is in remission when schizophrenia core symptoms are scored as mild or less on psychopathological rating scales (e.g., the Positive and Negative Syndrome Scale-PANSS, The Scale for the Assessment of Negative Symptoms and Positive Symptoms, or the Brief Psychiatric Rating Scale) for at least 6 months [12].

However, it became evident that the symptomatic remission concept did not cover all the dimensions of schizophrenia, which include not only core symptoms, but also depressive symptoms, cognitive functions, comorbidities, quality of life, and, more in general, the functional outcome [7].

Therefore, besides the symptomatic remission and the prevention of acute relapses, also the prevention and treatment of comorbidities, as well as the improvement in functional outcome and the subjective well-being, are now considered important targets of the care of people with schizophrenia [3, 6, 8, 13–17]. Within this frame, different stakeholders, such as patients, family members, advocates, and scientists, contributed to the development of the recovery concept. Recovery is a multifaceted and a broad umbrella construct [18]. Different conceptualizations have been described, e.g., internal vs. external recovery; clinical vs. social recovery; subjective or personal recovery vs. objective or clinical/functional recovery [3, 9, 13]. Internal factors refer mainly to hope and health, while external factors to human and patient's rights and opportunities for vocational and social integration [9]. Clinical recovery corresponds to symptoms reduction and improvement in functioning, while social recovery corresponds to economic and social independence [9, 19]. Subjective recovery, also named as personal recovery, refers to the subjective experience of recovery, defined by the quality of life, hope, reliance on others, and not feeling overwhelmed by symptoms [20, 21]. This concept has been developed based especially on narratives of individuals who have experienced mental illness and, therefore, has also been named patient-based recovery. Within this conceptualization, recovery has been defined as "a deeply personal, unique process of changing one's attitudes, values, feelings, goals, skills and roles … living a satisfying, hopeful, and contributing life even with limitations caused by the illness … the development of new meaning and purpose in one's life, as one grows beyond the catastrophic effects of mental illness" [22]. Therefore, recovery means a transformation in which the patient accepts what he or she cannot do or be and discovers who he or she can be and what he or she can do. In this sense, recovery is not a return to a "premorbid state," not an end product or a result, but it is a transformative and developmental process, which changes from person to person and also over time in the same individual [9, 18]. Different authors have tried to define important aspects of personal recovery and described different components and characteristics that are fundamental for reaching recovery: hope, reestablishment of identity, finding meaning in life, connectedness, empowerment, self-direction, individualized and person centered, holistic, nonlinear, strengths based, peer support, respect, and responsibility [6, 18, 22–29]. A systematic review conducted by Leamy et al. (2011) [28] has identified four fundamental components of personal recovery: hope, reestablishment of identity, finding meaning in life, connectedness and empowerment. Different assessment instruments have been developed to assess these aspects of subjective recovery; some are based entirely on the perspective of mental health service users while others also on the perspective of clinicians, scientists, family members, and legislators [13, 30–33].

Objective recovery, named by some authors as clinical or functional recovery, refers to remission of symptoms and improvement in functioning, in particular in the ability to function in the community, socially and vocationally. In this meaning, recovery is conceptualized as an outcome influenced by several factors [7]. Liberman et al. (2002) [34] defined recovery as the stage at which a patient is socially and professionally well functioning and he or she is relatively free of psychotic symptoms (BPRS<4, moderate) [34]. Other authors have also included living independently, having friends and scores of >65 on the Global Assessment of Functioning (GAF). Therefore, two aspects are crucial in determining clinical recovery, symptomatic remission and satisfactory real-life functioning.

In this chapter we will describe the major determinants of clinical recovery, i.e., symptomatic remission and improvement in real-life functioning. In particular, we will focus on those factors that have an impact on functional outcome, whose identification has a crucial role in the development of integrated and individualized targeted treatments aimed at achieving recovery. Factors most consistently reported in association with functional outcome are deficit of neurocognition, functional capacity and social cognition, as well as the severity of negative symptoms; however, several other psychopathological, personal and environmental variables have shown a potential role in determining functional outcome [14–17, 35].

The literature on the topic has shown that: (1) determinants of functional outcome in subjects with schizophrenia are multifactorial; (2) their relationship with functional outcome is not always direct; therefore, it is extremely important to clarify multiple direct and indirect pathways between potential predictors and functioning, as well as identify the role of mediating variables; and (3) variables explored as potential predictors of functional outcome and variables chosen as indices of functioning represent complex domains, whose assessment modality plays a fundamental role in the reliability of study findings.

In the following paragraphs, main findings on determinants of functional outcome in subjects with schizophrenia and their direct and indirect relationship with indices of functioning will be described.

2.2 Cross-Sectional Assessment of Determinants of Clinical Recovery

2.2.1 Neurocognitive Deficits

The impairment of cognitive functions has been regarded since the early description of the syndrome [10, 36] as a basic characteristic of schizophrenia. Cognitive deficits have been reported in 75–80% of subjects with schizophrenia who showed a performance on the majority of cognitive tests from 1.5 to 2 standard deviations below normative values [37–41]. Deficits involve different cognitive domains, such as general cognitive abilities (as assessed by IQ), attention, executive functions, speed of processing, secondary memory, working memory, and semantic memory [40, 42–46]. Several findings bring to the assumption that cognitive deficits in schizophrenia are primary and therefore not due to known factors, such as symptoms severity and pharmacological treatments [39, 47, 48]. In fact, an impairment of cognitive functions is observable before the onset of the disorder [49, 50] and often persists after symptom remission [37]. Moreover, cognitive deficits similar to those found in patients with schizophrenia, though less severe, have been found in their unaffected first-degree relatives [41, 51–53], suggesting that they may represent a vulnerability factor for the disorder.

According to the findings of a large body of literature, cognitive deficits are strong predictors of functional outcome in subjects with schizophrenia [14, 35, 42, 54] and have a greater impact on social functioning than positive and negative symptoms [14, 35, 55–57].

Some studies found that deficits of specific cognitive domains influence all or some aspects of functional outcome. According to a meta-analysis [42], specific patterns of associations can be identified: for instance, secondary verbal memory associated with all areas of functioning; immediate verbal memory with psychosocial skill acquisition of basic life skills such as conversation and leisure skills; executive functioning with daily activities; and sustained attention with social problem solving. However, this meta-analysis underlined that effect sizes of the associations tended to be medium, while more robust associations were found when global measures of neurocognition were used. Other domain-specific associations included attention/working memory with work skills; executive functions with interpersonal behavior; and processing speed with all areas of functioning [58]. In other papers, no domain-specific associations were found between neurocognition and functioning [59–63].

One point arising from studies investigating these relationships is that the deficit in neurocognition, although widely recognized as a factor associated to real-life functioning, is not sufficient by itself to predict functional outcome and other factors contribute with a direct or indirect impact to functional outcome or act as mediators of the relationship between neurocognitive deficits and functional outcome [14–17, 35, 42, 54, 64–66]. Social cognition, functional capacity, and negative symptoms are more frequently reported as predictors of functioning or mediators, but many other variables have been taken into account, although less frequently. The definition of these factors and their role in the pathways between potential predictors and functional outcome are reported in the next paragraphs.

2.2.2 Deficits of Functional Capacity

Functional capacity is the ability to perform everyday life activities measured with tests or role plays in laboratory settings [67]. Its association with functional performance in everyday life is inconsistent since the latter can be influenced by several aspects such as motivation and environmental factors [54]. An impairment of functional capacity has been reported in patients with schizophrenia, even in early-onset patients, and is considered a key aspect of the disorder [68, 69].

The majority of studies including functional capacity in pathways between potential predictors and functional outcome found that it acts as a mediator between neurocognitive performance and real-life functioning [35]. Bowie et al. [54] reported that neurocognitive performance has a small direct contribution to real-life performance, while it is in large part associated to functional capacity that, in turn, is significantly associated to all domains of real-life functioning. According to the findings of this study, functional capacity represents the stronger predictor of functional outcome with additional variance explained by the direct effect of negative and depressive symptoms.

A network analysis carried out in a large sample of patients within the Italian Network for Research on Psychoses (INRP) showed that functional capacity and everyday life skills were the most central and interconnected nodes in the network and that the former bridged both neurocognition and social cognition with "Everyday life skills" domain, which, in turn, was connected to other areas of real-life functioning, i.e., "Work skills" and "Interpersonal relationships" [15].

A study examining the relationships of specific neurocognitive domains and two different aspects of functional capacity (everyday living skills and social competence) with distinct aspects of real-life functioning reported a complex pattern of associations: both domains of functional capacity mediated the relationship between neurocognition and two domains of functioning, community activities and work skills, while only social competence predicted the interpersonal functioning domain [58]. In addition, social competence seems to act as mediator between social cognition and everyday functioning, suggesting that the impairment of both neurocognition and social cognition predicts the deficit of functional capacity which, in its turn, predicts impairment in different domains of functional outcome [66].

Discrepant findings have also been reported, such as lack of correlation between neurocognitive indices or functional capacity and self-reported functional outcome [70], or an impact of neurocognitive dysfunction on everyday life functioning without influence of functional capacity [71].

2.2.3 Deficits of Social Cognition

Social cognition is the subject's ability to perceive, interpret, and process social stimuli for adaptive social interactions. It is currently considered a domain relatively independent of neurocognition, although related to it [72–74]. It is a complex construct for which four different domains have been identified by a consensus of experts [75]: emotion processing, social perception, theory of mind (ToM), and attributional bias. Deficits of one or more domains of social cognition have been reported in subjects with schizophrenia, even early in the disease process, as well as in subjects at risk to develop the disorder, and have been found to be stable over time [76–78].

Given its impact on social interactions, social cognition has been considered a candidate as mediator in the relationships between functional outcome and its potential predictors. Several studies found that social cognition is associated to functional outcome even more strongly than neurocognition, acting as mediator between the latter and functional outcome [14–17, 65, 66, 72, 74, 79–83].

Patterns of association between specific domains of social cognition, neurocognition, and functional outcome vary among studies depending on the investigated indices. Some examples include social perception as mediator in the relationship between early visual processing and functional outcome, the association of social cognition only with the domain of interpersonal functioning, the role of ToM as mediator between cognition and social competence that, in turn, showed a direct path of association with self-reported functioning [83, 84].

Some studies also found that different domains of social cognition are mediators in the relationship between neurocognition and social aspects of functional capacity (social competence), which then have a direct impact on social functioning [84–86].

Although heterogeneous, these findings, together with those reported in the previous paragraphs, strongly suggest the need to focus on specific therapeutic targets, such as deficits of social cognition and deficit of functional capacity, in addition to neurocognitive deficits.

2.2.4 Negative Symptoms

Negative symptoms are a core clinical dimension of schizophrenia. They have been described in prodromal phases of schizophrenia, as well as in unaffected first-degree relatives of subjects with the disorder [57, 87]. Negative symptoms represent an unmet need in the care of the disorder, as they are associated to poor response to available treatments and to poor functional outcome [88–91]. In fact, several data suggest that their presence negatively influences functional outcome of patients with schizophrenia [92–94].

Both direct and indirect relationships between negative symptoms and functional outcome have been reported, as well as evidence of their role as mediators in pathways of functional outcome. In a study exploring the impact of several factors on three different areas of functioning, negative symptoms showed a direct relationship with interpersonal skills, independent of other predictors such as neurocognition and functional capacity, while they did not contribute to the prediction of everyday life skills and work skills [54]. In a further paper of the same authors, the direct relationship between negative symptoms and interpersonal skills was confirmed, but also an indirect effect on all the three areas of functioning (interpersonal skills, community activities, and work skills), mediated by a reduction of social competence, was reported [58]. The finding of a direct relationship of negative symptoms with indices of functional outcome suggests that they may have an impact on functioning that is independent of cognition. Both direct and indirect impact (the latter mediated by social competence) of negative symptoms on outcome were confirmed in a study using self-reported functioning as outcome index [84]. In a paper investigating the impact of specific PANSS negative symptoms on functioning in the areas of interpersonal functioning and everyday activities, blunted affect and passive-apathetic social withdrawal were found to predict outcome in the former area, while lack of spontaneity in the latter. These specific negative symptoms resulted stronger predictors than the PANSS negative total score and served as mediators between functional capacity and real-world functioning, suggesting that subjects may have the competence for a good functioning but the presence of those specific negative symptoms limits patient's ability to use such competences in real life [55].

The influence of negative symptoms on functioning was confirmed in a meta-analysis showing that they mediate the relationship between neurocognition and functional outcome [95]. In a more recent paper, negative symptoms, together with general psychopathology and insight, were associated to cognition and predicted functioning acting as mediators in the relationship between cognition and functioning [96]. These findings suggest that cognitive deficits have a negative impact on symptoms and insight that, in turn, exert a negative impact on functioning. Some other studies found a prominent role of the negative construct amotivation in influencing functioning in people with schizophrenia [97, 98].

Taken together, these findings confirm that negative symptoms have an impact on functional outcome. However, the heterogeneity of results does not allow conclusions on either the identification of specific negative symptoms associated to functional outcome or on the definition of pathways of associations with other predictors of functioning. Actually, negative symptoms represent a complex and heterogeneous psychopathological dimension, including different constructs that can be grouped, according to studies based on factor analysis, in two main domains: the expressive domain (including blunted affect and alogia) and the experiential domain (including avolition, asociality, and anhedonia) [93, 94, 99]. The two domains seem to be associated with different neurobiological abnormalities and psychosocial outcome [94, 100, 101]. Moreover, within the construct of anhedonia, two different aspects have been described: consummatory anhedonia (reduced experience of pleasure derived from ongoing enjoyable activities) and anticipatory anhedonia (reduced ability to anticipate future pleasure): the former one seems to be relatively intact in schizophrenia, while the latter one seems to be impaired [102, 103]. It has been hypothesized that patients with schizophrenia with persistent cognitive deficits may be unable to retrieve their memories of previous positive experiences, leading to a difficulty in anticipating pleasurable consequences of actions [35]. Therefore, these two aspects of anhedonia may have different patterns of association with functional outcome. Finally, a valid and reliable assessment of negative symptoms is challenging and, as matter of fact, rating scales used in the above-reported studies for the assessment of negative symptoms have been criticized for the inclusion of items assessing neurocognition and the focus on behavioral aspects, as opposed to internal experience, which may lead to artifactual associations with functional outcome measures [104, 105].

To overcome these limitations, second-generation rating scales, such as the Brief Negative Symptom Scale (BNSS) [104, 106] and the Clinical Assessment Interview for Negative Symptoms [105], should be preferred. The BNSS is a new-generation rating scale for the assessment of negative symptoms that has several advantages with respect to the older ones: it does not include symptoms previously considered as part of the negative dimension but now clearly identified as aspects of other dimensions, such as the cognitive or depressive one [93, 104, 106–108]; it provides a separate assessment of the consummatory and anticipatory anhedonia, a total score as well as a separate score for each of the five negative symptom domains, a separate assessment of behavior and inner experience for items referring to experiential deficits such as avolition, thus enabling a better differentiation from social functioning and other subjective experiences such as decreased interest or energy. According to several studies, the BNSS five negative symptom domains can be grouped in the two main domains: the Expressive domain, including blunted affect and alogia, and the Experiential domain consisting of anhedonia, asociality, and avolition.

Based on this evidence, in all studies of the Italian Network for Research on Psychoses aimed at identifying factors that affect real-life functioning of subjects with schizophrenia and defining their relative contribution, the BNSS was used to assess the negative psychopathological dimension. In those studies, we found a different impact of the two main domains of negative symptoms on functioning: the Experiential domain showed a direct and indirect effect on real-life functioning and was connected to the areas of real-life functioning "Interpersonal relationships" and "Work skills" in the network analysis, while the Expressive domain was only indirectly and weakly related to real-life functioning and, in the network analysis, resulted connected to "Everyday Life Activities" [14, 15].

2.2.5 Other Potential Predictors or Mediators of Clinical Recovery

Besides the negative ones, other symptoms have been investigated as potential predictors of functioning. Depression has been found to be directly associated to some areas of functioning [54, 58]. However, no impact was found in other studies [14, 109]. Several studies found that disorganization is associated with real-life functioning [14, 15, 57, 63, 95, 110]. The presence of severe disorganization has a negative impact on outcome as it interferes with functioning in the acute phase of the illness and with the achievement of symptomatic remission [111–113]. The role of positive symptoms has been explored in a few studies reporting heterogeneous results, including lack of association with functioning [114], a direct effect on Work skills and Everyday life skills [58], or an association with Community activities only [55]. The presence of autism spectrum disorders symptoms has been found associated to poor functional capacity, real-life interpersonal relationships, and participation in community-living activities [115]. Poor premorbid level of functioning has been also found in association with worse functional outcome [116, 117].

Some studies also investigated the role of personal resources: patients with comparable severity of psychopathology present heterogeneous real-life functioning because of differences in coping strategies, recovery style, and resilience [118, 119]. As to the coping strategies, those defined as "emotion-oriented," together with those "avoidance oriented," are associated with a worse real-life functioning [119, 120]. Resilience has been found in association with patterns of patients' engagement with mental health services, which can affect real-life functioning [121].

Among personal resources, physical health status plays an important role in quality of life and functioning of people with schizophrenia. In these subjects, indeed, high medical comorbidity was reported, and attributed to several factors, including lifestyle and treatment with antipsychotics [122, 123]. Deficit in neurocognition and functional capacity may also impair patients' ability to choose and cook food and contribute to the risk of obesity and other metabolic issues in patients with schizophrenia [66].

Several environmental factors have been found in association to real-world functioning, including poor economic status, lack of disability compensation and of support services, and living in poor neighborhoods [35]. All these factors obviously influence real-life functioning and should be included in studies investigating predictors of functional outcome; however, the identification of the most appropriate indices to capture the complexity of these variables may be difficult [14].

A higher level of internalized stigma (i.e., the incorporation of others' prejudices and stereotypes about people with mental illnesses into beliefs about oneself with consequent anticipation of social rejection) [124] has been found in association with several psychosocial variables such as hope, self-esteem, and empowerment [125]. In addition, an indirect association mediated by resilience has been found between internalized stigma and real-life functioning [14]. Therefore, it is likely to influence real-life functioning and should be included in relevant studies.

Other demographic and clinical factors have been reported as predictors of clinical recovery, including female gender, higher educational level, older age at onset, shorter duration of untreated psychosis, and less cannabis use [3].

2.3 Longitudinal Assessment of Determinants of Clinical Recovery

As emerged from previous paragraphs, factors most consistently reported in association with functional outcome are deficit of neurocognition, functional capacity and social cognition, as well as the severity of negative symptoms. However, the majority of studies investigating factors affecting functional outcome had a cross-sectional design, which, unfortunately, prevented inferences about the direction of causality. Only few studies had a longitudinal design investigating pathway towards functional outcome. Findings arising from these studies are summarized below.

2.3.1 Neurocognitive Deficits

Several studies with a longitudinal design found that deficits in cognitive domains were associated with later functional outcome at follow-up time points ranging from 6 months to 10 years (20 years in the case of a retrospective study) [16, 17, 43, 126–128]. Lack of such an association has also been found in some studies [43, 129]. More in detail, the review by Green et al. (2004) [43], which included 18 longitudinal studies, reported that the majority of them ($N = 14$) found associations between baseline impairment of various cognitive indices and later functional outcome with an effect size in the medium to large range. Two studies included in the review did not find any relationships between baseline cognition and outcome, and two more studies reported not clear results (one found associations only for one out of two samples, and the other for one out of two types of community outcome). Among more recent papers not included in the review, one [126] reported that, in a small sample of patients with first-episode schizophrenia, the baseline cognitive domains attention, verbal learning, and verbal working memory were associated with social outcome at follow-up, while attention, verbal working memory, and reasoning/problem solving with role functioning at follow-up. Another paper [127] found that the cognitive domain processing speed predicted self-care, vocational outcome, and social functioning at 6-month follow-up. Baseline global cognition resulted a predictor of 1-year functional outcome, although at a weaker level with respect to avolition in a sample of 114 Chinese patients with first-episode schizophrenia [128]. No associations were found between baseline neurocognition and everyday functioning in a paper conducted in 111 patients with chronic schizophrenia [129].

From the majority of longitudinal studies emerges that cognitive deficits predict later functional outcome; however different patterns of associations have been described in the abovementioned studies, involving different cognitive domains and indices of outcome. This is probably due to methodological problems, including the heterogeneity of instrument used to assess cognitive functions, mainly measured combining tests to evaluate different cognitive domains, and only in one study [126] assessed by means of the MATRICS (Measurement and Treatment Research to Improve Cognition in Schizophrenia) Consensus Cognitive Battery (MCCB) that is regarded as the state-of-the-art neuropsychological battery for research purposes in schizophrenia [130, 131]; the heterogeneity of indices of functional outcome; and the small sample size included in the majority of studies.

These points were addressed in a recent study carried out within the Italian Network for Research on Psychosis aimed to verify whether factors identified as predictors and mediators of real-life functioning at the baseline were confirmed as such in a 4-year longitudinal design [16, 17]: state-of-the-art instruments were adopted to assess psychopathology, neurocognitive functions, social cognition, personal resources, and real-life functioning in 618 patients out of the 921 recruited in the cross-sectional study. The study adopted three main strategies of statistical analysis. Two of them—Structural Equation Model (SEM) and Latent Change Score (LCS) modeling—were used to investigate, respectively, whether variables that showed an impact on real-life functioning in the cross-sectional study confirmed their influence at follow-up and which variables affected changes at follow-up in real-life functioning [17]. Furthermore, also a network analysis with a longitudinal design was conducted to test whether the pattern of relationships among all variables investigated in the cross-sectional study was similar at follow-up and to compare the network structure of patients who were classified as recovered at follow-up versus those who did not recover [16]. The network analysis has the advantage of not requiring the a priori modeling of relationships among variables needed in SEM, but produces spatially ordered networks in which variables are nodes and causal interactions between variables are connections between nodes expressing direction and magnitude of correlations. Strongly related nodes at the center of the graph and weakly related ones at the periphery. Moreover, closeness of nodes, as well as strength and number of their connections, provides estimates of the extent to which variables belong to the same construct and how different constructs are mutually interacting and reinforcing each other [132].

Both SEM and LCS analyses in the longitudinal study consistently confirmed that neurocognition is among factors predicting functional outcome at 4-year follow-up. In particular, according to the SEM, better baseline neurocognition predicted better everyday life and work skills. The LCS model, used as a control analysis, showed that better baseline neurocognitive functioning predicted improved everyday life skills, work skills, social cognition, and functional capacity at follow-up. As regard to the network analysis [16], the network structure in the longitudinal study did not change significantly with respect to the cross-sectional one. In fact, at both time points, neurocognition, together with social cognition, resilience, and real-life functioning, was spatially contiguous and highly interconnected, confirming the central role of these variables in impacting real-life functioning.

2.3.2 Deficits of Functional Capacity and Social Cognition

Very few longitudinal studies investigated the association between functional capacity and/or social cognition with functional outcome [16, 17, 129, 133, 134]. It has been reported that worsening in measures of functional capacity and of social competence predicts worsening of everyday functioning in the domains everyday life and working skills of the real-life functioning after 18 months [129]. In patients with first-episode schizophrenia, social cognition assessed with three different instruments was found to predict work, independent living, and social functioning at 1-year follow-up [133]. The study of McCleery et al. [134] found a cross-sectional association between social cognition and community functioning, while no association was observed between baseline social cognition and community functioning at 5 years follow-up, suggesting the hypothesis that social cognition may have a short-term rather than long-term implications for outcome. In the longitudinal study of the Italian Network for Research on Psychosis [16, 17] SEM analysis showed that better baseline social cognition predicted better work skills and interpersonal relationships at follow-up, and LCS analysis confirmed the association between the same baseline variables and interpersonal relationships. As mentioned above, network analysis showed that social cognition is among variables highly interconnected to real-life functioning and that functional capacity and everyday life skills had a high betweenness and closeness in the network.

Overall, although a few studies are available on this topic, findings of longitudinal studies confirm the contribution of social cognition and functional capacity in predicting later functional outcome.

2.3.3 Negative Symptoms

Longitudinal studies exploring the role of negative symptoms in predicting functional outcome showed positive results [16, 17, 90, 97, 128, 135–138]. Different domains and categories of negative symptoms have been explored in the various papers, given the already mentioned complexity and heterogeneity of this psychopathological construct. The presence of persistent negative symptoms in two different cohorts of patients with first-episode schizophrenia was found to be associated to worse psychosocial functioning after 1 year [135] and after 4 weeks [136]. Studies exploring the Experiential and the Expressive domain found that the former has a higher predictive value than the latter on functional outcome [16, 17, 90, 128, 137]. In line with these findings, two more studies reported the role of amotivation in predicting functional outcome [97, 138]. Some discrepancies emerge on the functional domain predicted by negative symptoms, as in one study [138] amotivation was found to predict poor work but not social functioning, while in another paper [16] more severe avolition predicted worse interpersonal relationships. The use of outdated instruments for the evaluation of negative symptoms is among the main limitations of the above-reported studies, as only two of them [16, 17] used a new-generation rating scale (BNSS) for the assessment of this psychopathological domain. In spite of the above limitations, longitudinal studies confirmed that negative symptoms are among strongest predictors of later functional outcome.

2.4 Conclusions

Findings summarized in this chapter confirm that several variables are involved as predictors or mediators of clinical outcome and that their interactions and pathways towards functional outcome are complex.

Social and nonsocial cognition show a key role as predictors of real-life functioning, suggesting that rehabilitation interventions addressing their impairment should be routinely included in integrated treatments aimed at clinical recovery in patients with schizophrenia. Such interventions should be provided as early as possible given the fact that the above-reported impairments have been described since early stage of illness and even before clinical onset.

Negative symptoms have certainly an impact on clinical outcome, although the complexity of this psychopathological domain leads to some heterogeneity in findings regarding the most involved subdomains and their role as direct/indirect predictors or mediators. The search for effective treatments for negative symptoms should represents a priority for research in schizophrenia.

The reported role of many other factors in influencing clinical outcome, either those related to personal resource—such as resilience or physical health status—or those related to the context, underlines the importance of personalized treatments based on a detailed characterization of each individual patient [139].

References

1. Owen MJ, Sawa A, Mortensen PB. Schizophrenia. Lancet. 2016;388(10039):86–97. https://doi.org/10.1016/S0140-6736(15)01121-6.
2. Jablensky A. The diagnostic concept of schizophrenia: its history, evolution, and future prospects. Dialogues Clin Neurosci. 2010;12(3):271–87.
3. Vita A, Barlati S. Recovery from schizophrenia: is it possible? Curr Opin Psychiatry. 2018;31(3):246–55. https://doi.org/10.1097/YCO.0000000000000407.
4. Jaaskelainen E, Juola P, Hirvonen N, McGrath JJ, Saha S, Isohanni M, et al. A systematic review and meta-analysis of recovery in schizophrenia. Schizophr Bull. 2013;39(6):1296–306. https://doi.org/10.1093/schbul/sbs130.
5. Zipursky RB, Agid O. Recovery, not progressive deterioration, should be the expectation in schizophrenia. World Psychiatry. 2015;14(1):94–6. https://doi.org/10.1002/wps.20194.
6. Frese FJ, Knight EL, Saks E. Recovery from schizophrenia: with views of psychiatrists, psychologists, and others diagnosed with this disorder. Schizophr Bull. 2009;35(2):370–80. https://doi.org/10.1093/schbul/sbn175.
7. Harvey PD, Bellack AS. Toward a terminology for functional recovery in schizophrenia: is functional remission a viable concept? Schizophr Bull. 2009;35(2):300–6. https://doi.org/10.1093/schbul/sbn171.
8. Farkas M. The vision of recovery today: what it is and what it means for services. World Psychiatry. 2007;6(2):68–74.
9. Amering M, Schmolke M. Recovery in mental health. Chichester [England]: Wiley-Blackwell; 2009.
10. Kraepelin E. Dementia praecox and paraphrenia. Edinburgh, UK: E and S Livingstone; 1919.
11. Correll CU, Kishimoto T, Nielsen J, Kane JM. Quantifying clinical relevance in the treatment of schizophrenia. Clin Ther. 2011;33(12):B16–39. https://doi.org/10.1016/j.clinthera.2011.11.016.
12. Andreasen NC, Carpenter WT Jr, Kane JM, Lasser RA, Marder SR, Weinberger DR. Remission in schizophrenia: proposed criteria and rationale for consensus. Am J Psychiatry. 2005;162(3):441–9. https://doi.org/10.1176/appi.ajp.162.3.441.
13. Van Eck RM, Burger TJ, Vellinga A, Schirmbeck F, de Haan L. The relationship between clinical and personal recovery in patients with schizophrenia spectrum disorders: a systematic review and meta-analysis. Schizophr Bull. 2018;44(3):631–42. https://doi.org/10.1093/schbul/sbx088.
14. Galderisi S, Rossi A, Rocca P, Bertolino A, Mucci A, Bucci P, et al. The influence of illness-related variables, personal resources and context-related factors on real-life functioning of people with schizophrenia. World Psychiatry. 2014;13(3):275–87. https://doi.org/10.1002/wps.20167.

15. Galderisi S, Rucci P, Kirkpatrick B, Mucci A, Gibertoni D, Rocca P, et al. Interplay among psychopathologic variables, personal resources, context-related factors, and real-life functioning in individuals with schizophrenia: a network analysis. JAMA Psychiat. 2018;75(4):396–404. https://doi.org/10.1001/jamapsychiatry.2017.4607.
16. Galderisi S, Rucci P, Mucci A, Rossi A, Rocca P, Bertolino A, et al. The interplay among psychopathology, personal resources, context-related factors and real-life functioning in schizophrenia: stability in relationships after 4 years and differences in network structure between recovered and non-recovered patients. World Psychiatry. 2020;19(1):81–91. https://doi.org/10.1002/wps.20700.
17. Mucci A, Galderisi S, Gibertoni D, Rossi A, Rocca P, Bertolino A, et al. Factors associated with real-life functioning in persons with schizophrenia in a 4-year follow-up study of the italian network for research on psychoses. JAMA Psychiat. 2021;78(5):550–9. https://doi.org/10.1001/jamapsychiatry.2020.4614.
18. Slade M, Amering M, Farkas M, Hamilton B, O'Hagan M, Panther G, et al. Uses and abuses of recovery: implementing recovery-oriented practices in mental health systems. World Psychiatry. 2014;13(1):12–20. https://doi.org/10.1002/wps.20084.
19. Shrivastava A, Johnston M, Shah N, Bureau Y. Redefining outcome measures in schizophrenia: integrating social and clinical parameters. Curr Opin Psychiatry. 2010;23(2):120–6. https://doi.org/10.1097/YCO.0b013e328336662e.
20. Silverstein SM, Bellack AS. A scientific agenda for the concept of recovery as it applies to schizophrenia. Clin Psychol Rev. 2008;28(7):1108–24. https://doi.org/10.1016/j.cpr.2008.03.004.
21. Roe D, Mashiach-Eizenberg M, Lysaker PH. The relation between objective and subjective domains of recovery among persons with schizophrenia-related disorders. Schizophr Res. 2011;131(1–3):133–8. https://doi.org/10.1016/j.schres.2011.05.023.
22. Anthony WA. Recovery from mental illness: the guiding vision of the mental health service system in the 1990s. Psychosoc Rehabil J. 1993;16(4):11–23. https://doi.org/10.1037/h0095655.
23. Mead S, Copeland ME. What recovery means to us: consumers' perspectives. Community Ment Health J. 2000;36(3):315–28. https://doi.org/10.1023/a:1001917516869.
24. Deegan P. Recovery as a self-directed process of healing and transformation. Occup Ther Ment Health. 2001;17:5–21. https://doi.org/10.1300/J004v17n03_02.
25. Lysaker PH, Roe D, Buck KD. Recovery and wellness amidst schizophrenia: definitions, evidence, and the implications for clinical practice. J Am Psychiatr Nurses Assoc. 2010;16(1):36–42. https://doi.org/10.1177/1078390309353943.
26. Andresen R, Oades L, Caputi P. The experience of recovery from schizophrenia: towards an empirically validated stage model. Aust N Z J Psychiatry. 2003;37(5):586–94. https://doi.org/10.1046/j.1440-1614.2003.01234.x.
27. Bird V, Leamy M, Tew J, Le Boutillier C, Williams J, Slade M. Fit for purpose? Validation of a conceptual framework for personal recovery with current mental health consumers. Aust N Z J Psychiatry. 2014;48(7):644–53. https://doi.org/10.1177/0004867413520046.
28. Leamy M, Bird V, Le Boutillier C, Williams J, Slade M. Conceptual framework for personal recovery in mental health: systematic review and narrative synthesis. Br J Psychiatry. 2011;199(6):445–52. https://doi.org/10.1192/bjp.bp.110.083733.
29. Slade M. Personal recovery and mental illness: a guide for mental health professionals. Cambridge: Cambridge University Press; 2009.
30. Bellack AS, Drapalski A. Issues and developments on the consumer recovery construct. World Psychiatry. 2012;11(3):156–60. https://doi.org/10.1002/j.2051-5545.2012.tb00117.x.
31. Gordon S, Ellis P. My voice, my life: a measure based on the consumer model of recovery. World Psychiatry. 2013;12(3):277. https://doi.org/10.1002/wps.20055.
32. Rose D, Sweeney A, Leese M, Clement S, Jones IR, Burns T, et al. Developing a user-generated measure of continuity of care: brief report. Acta Psychiatr Scand. 2009;119:320–4. https://doi.org/10.1111/j.1600-0447.2008.01296.x.

2 Determinants of Clinical Recovery in Schizophrenia

33. Callard F. The vicissitudes of the recovery construct; or, the challenge of taking "subjective experience" seriously. World Psychiatry. 2012;11(3):168–9. https://doi.org/10.1002/j.2051-5545.2012.tb00124.x.

34. Liberman RP, Kopelowicz A, Ventura J, Gutkind D. Operational criteria and factors related to recovery from schizophrenia. Int Rev Psychiatry. 2002;14(4):256–72. https://doi.org/10.1080/0954026021000016905.

35. Harvey PD, Strassnig M. Predicting the severity of everyday functional disability in people with schizophrenia: cognitive deficits, functional capacity, symptoms, and health status. World Psychiatry. 2012;11(2):73–9. https://doi.org/10.1016/j.wpsyc.2012.05.004.

36. Bleuler E. Dementia praecox or the group of schizophrenias. Oxford, England: International Universities Press; 1950.

37. Heinrichs RW, Zakzanis KK. Neurocognitive deficit in schizophrenia: a quantitative review of the evidence. Neuropsychology. 1998;12(3):426–45. https://doi.org/10.1037//0894-4105.12.3.426.

38. Keefe RS. Should cognitive impairment be included in the diagnostic criteria for schizophrenia? World Psychiatry. 2008;7(1):22–8. https://doi.org/10.1002/j.2051-5545.2008.tb00142.x.

39. Galderisi S, Davidson M, Kahn RS, Mucci A, Boter H, Gheorghe MD, et al. Correlates of cognitive impairment in first episode schizophrenia: the EUFEST study. Schizophr Res. 2009;115(2–3):104–14. https://doi.org/10.1016/j.schres.2009.09.022.

40. Reichenberg A. The assessment of neuropsychological functioning in schizophrenia. Dialogues Clin Neurosci. 2010;12(3):383–92. https://doi.org/10.31887/DCNS.2010.12.3/areichenberg.

41. Mucci A, Galderisi S, Green MF, Nuechterlein K, Rucci P, Gibertoni D, et al. Familial aggregation of MATRICS Consensus Cognitive Battery scores in a large sample of outpatients with schizophrenia and their unaffected relatives. Psychol Med. 2018;48(8):1359–66. https://doi.org/10.1017/S0033291717002902.

42. Green MF, Kern RS, Braff DL, Mintz J. Neurocognitive deficits and functional outcome in schizophrenia: are we measuring the "right stuff"? Schizophr Bull. 2000;26(1):119–36. https://doi.org/10.1093/oxfordjournals.schbul.a033430.

43. Green MF, Kern RS, Heaton RK. Longitudinal studies of cognition and functional outcome in schizophrenia: implications for MATRICS. Schizophr Res. 2004;72(1):41–51. https://doi.org/10.1016/j.schres.2004.09.009.

44. Galderisi S, Maj M, Mucci A, Cassano GB, Invernizzi G, Rossi A, et al. Historical, psychopathological, neurological, and neuropsychological aspects of deficit schizophrenia: a multicenter study. Am J Psychiatry. 2002;159(6):983–90. https://doi.org/10.1176/appi.ajp.159.6.983.

45. Galderisi S, Maj M, Kirkpatrick B, Piccardi P, Mucci A, Invernizzi G, et al. Catechol-O-methyltransferase Val158Met polymorphism in schizophrenia: associations with cognitive and motor impairment. Neuropsychobiology. 2005;52(2):83–9. https://doi.org/10.1159/000087096.

46. Bora E, Yucel M, Pantelis C. Cognitive impairment in schizophrenia and affective psychoses: implications for DSM-V criteria and beyond. Schizophr Bull. 2010;36(1):36–42. https://doi.org/10.1093/schbul/sbp094.

47. Nuechterlein KH, Dawson ME, Gitlin M, Ventura J, Goldstein MJ, Snyder KS, et al. Developmental processes in schizophrenic disorders: longitudinal studies of vulnerability and stress. Schizophr Bull. 1992;18(3):387–425. https://doi.org/10.1093/schbul/18.3.387.

48. Mohamed S, Rosenheck R, Swartz M, Stroup S, Lieberman JA, Keefe RS. Relationship of cognition and psychopathology to functional impairment in schizophrenia. Am J Psychiatry. 2008;165(8):978–87. https://doi.org/10.1176/appi.ajp.2008.07111713.

49. Kravariti E, Morris RG, Rabe-Hesketh S, Murray RM, Frangou S. Comparative profile analysis of cognitive function in recent-onset and chronic patients with adolescent-onset schizophrenia. Schizophr Res. 2007;94(1–3):240–4. https://doi.org/10.1016/j.schres.2007.05.014.

50. Mesholam-Gately RI, Giuliano AJ, Goff KP, Faraone SV, Seidman LJ. Neurocognition in first-episode schizophrenia: a meta-analytic review. Neuropsychology. 2009;23:315–36. https://doi.org/10.1037/a0014708.

51. Staal WG, Hijman R, Hulshoff Pol HE, Kahn RS. Neuropsychological dysfunctions in siblings discordant for schizophrenia. Psychiatry Res. 2000;95(3):227–35. https://doi.org/10.1016/s0165-1781(00)00172-4.

52. Sponheim SR, Steele VR, McGuire KA. Verbal memory processes in schizophrenia patients and biological relatives of schizophrenia patients: intact implicit memory, impaired explicit recollection. Schizophr Res. 2004;71(2–3):339–48. https://doi.org/10.1016/j.schres.2004.04.008.

53. Sitskoorn MM, Aleman A, Ebisch SJ, Appels MC, Kahn RS. Cognitive deficits in relatives of patients with schizophrenia: a meta-analysis. Schizophr Res. 2004;71(2–3):285–95. https://doi.org/10.1016/j.schres.2004.03.007.

54. Bowie CR, Reichenberg A, Patterson TL, Heaton RK, Harvey PD. Determinants of real-world functional performance in schizophrenia subjects: correlations with cognition, functional capacity, and symptoms. Am J Psychiatry. 2006;163(3):418–25. https://doi.org/10.1176/appi.ajp.163.3.418.

55. Leifker FR, Bowie CR, Harvey PD. Determinants of everyday outcomes in schizophrenia: the influences of cognitive impairment, functional capacity, and symptoms. Schizophr Res. 2009;115(1):82–7. https://doi.org/10.1016/j.schres.2009.09.004.

56. Kurtz MM, Jeffrey SB, Rose J. Elementary neurocognitive function, learning potential and everyday life skills in schizophrenia: what is their relationship? Schizophr Res. 2010;116(2–3):280–8. https://doi.org/10.1016/j.schres.2009.08.011.

57. Galderisi S, Rossi A, Rocca P, Bertolino A, Mucci A, Bucci P, et al. Pathways to functional outcome in subjects with schizophrenia living in the community and their unaffected first-degree relatives. Schizophr Res. 2016;175(1–3):154–60. https://doi.org/10.1016/j.schres.2016.04.043.

58. Bowie CR, Leung WW, Reichenberg A, McClure MM, Patterson TL, Heaton RK, et al. Predicting schizophrenia patients' real-world behavior with specific neuropsychological and functional capacity measures. Biol Psychiatry. 2008;63(5):505–11. https://doi.org/10.1016/j.biopsych.2007.05.022.

59. Dickerson F, Boronow JJ, Ringel N, Parente F. Neurocognitive deficits and social functioning in outpatients with schizophrenia. Schizophr Res. 1996;21(2):75–83. https://doi.org/10.1016/0920-9964(96)00040-0.

60. Dickerson F, Boronow JJ, Ringel N, Parente F. Social functioning and neurocognitive deficits in outpatients with schizophrenia: a 2-year follow-up. Schizophr Res. 1999;37(1):13–20. https://doi.org/10.1016/s0920-9964(98)00134-0.

61. Evans JD, Heaton RK, Paulsen JS, Palmer BW, Patterson T, Jeste DV. The relationship of neuropsychological abilities to specific domains of functional capacity in older schizophrenia patients. Biol Psychiatry. 2003;53(5):422–30. https://doi.org/10.1016/s0006-3223(02)01476-2.

62. Twamley EW, Thomas KR, Burton CZ, Vella L, Jeste DV, Heaton RK, et al. Compensatory cognitive training for people with severe mental illnesses in supported employment: a randomized controlled trial. Schizophr Res. 2019;203:41–8. https://doi.org/10.1016/j.schres.2017.08.005.

63. Norman RM, Malla AK, Cortese L, Cheng S, Diaz K, McIntosh E, et al. Symptoms and cognition as predictors of community functioning: a prospective analysis. Am J Psychiatry. 1999;156(3):400–5. https://doi.org/10.1176/ajp.156.3.400.

64. Green AR, Segal J, Tian J, Oh E, Roth DL, Hilson L, et al. Use of bladder antimuscarinics in older adults with impaired cognition. J Am Geriatr Soc. 2017;65(2):390–4. https://doi.org/10.1111/jgs.14498.

65. Green MF, Horan WP, Lee J. Nonsocial and social cognition in schizophrenia: current evidence and future directions. World Psychiatry. 2019;18(2):146–61. https://doi.org/10.1002/wps.20624.

66. Harvey PD, Strassnig MT. Cognition and disability in schizophrenia: cognition-related skills deficits and decision-making challenges add to morbidity. World Psychiatry. 2019;18(2):165–7. https://doi.org/10.1002/wps.20647.

2 Determinants of Clinical Recovery in Schizophrenia

67. Harvey PD, Velligan DI, Bellack AS. Performance-based measures of functional skills: usefulness in clinical treatment studies. Schizophr Bull. 2007;33(5):1138–48. https://doi.org/10.1093/schbul/sbm040.
68. Harvey PD, Isner EC. Cognition, social cognition, and functional capacity in early-onset schizophrenia. Child Adolesc Psychiatr Clin N Am. 2020;29(1):171–82. https://doi.org/10.1016/j.chc.2019.08.008.
69. Vesterager L, Christensen TO, Olsen BB, Krarup G, Melau M, Forchhammer HB, et al. Cognitive and clinical predictors of functional capacity in patients with first episode schizophrenia. Schizophr Res. 2012;141(2–3):251–6. https://doi.org/10.1016/j.schres.2012.08.023.
70. McKibbin CL, Brekke JS, Sires D, Jeste DV, Patterson TL. Direct assessment of functional abilities: relevance to persons with schizophrenia. Schizophr Res. 2004;72(1):53–67. https://doi.org/10.1016/j.schres.2004.09.011.
71. Heinrichs RW, Ammari N, Miles AA, McDermid VS. Cognitive performance and functional competence as predictors of community independence in schizophrenia. Schizophr Bull. 2010;36(2):381–7. https://doi.org/10.1093/schbul/sbn095.
72. Couture SM, Penn DL, Roberts DL. The functional significance of social cognition in schizophrenia: a review. Schizophr Bull. 2006;32(Suppl 1):S44–63. https://doi.org/10.1093/schbul/sbl029.
73. Green MF, Penn DL, Bentall R, Carpenter WT, Gaebel W, Gur RC, et al. Social cognition in schizophrenia: an NIMH workshop on definitions, assessment, and research opportunities. Schizophr Bull. 2008;34(6):1211–20. https://doi.org/10.1093/schbul/sbm145.
74. Fett AK, Viechtbauer W, Dominguez MD, Penn DL, van Os J, Krabbendam L. The relationship between neurocognition and social cognition with functional outcomes in schizophrenia: a meta-analysis. Neurosci Biobehav Rev. 2011;35(3):573–88. https://doi.org/10.1016/j.neubiorev.2010.07.001.
75. Pinkham AE, Penn DL, Green MF, Buck B, Healey K, Harvey PD. The social cognition psychometric evaluation study: results of the expert survey and RAND panel. Schizophr Bull. 2014;40(4):813–23. https://doi.org/10.1093/schbul/sbt081.
76. Harvey PD, Penn D. Social cognition: the key factor predicting social outcome in people with schizophrenia? Psychiatry (Edgmont). 2010;7(2):41–4.
77. Hoekert M, Kahn RS, Pijnenborg M, Aleman A. Impaired recognition and expression of emotional prosody in schizophrenia: review and meta-analysis. Schizophr Res. 2007;96(1–3):135–45. https://doi.org/10.1016/j.schres.2007.07.023.
78. Langdon R, Flynn M, Connaughton E, Brune M. Impairments of spontaneous and deliberative mentalizing co-occur, yet dissociate, in schizophrenia. Br J Clin Psychol. 2017;56(4):372–87. https://doi.org/10.1111/bjc.12144.
79. Pinkham AE. Social cognition in schizophrenia. J Clin Psychiatry. 2014;75(Suppl 2):14–9. https://doi.org/10.4088/JCP.13065su1.04.
80. Pinkham AE, Penn DL, Green MF, Harvey PD. Social cognition psychometric evaluation: results of the initial psychometric study. Schizophr Bull. 2016;42(2):494–504. https://doi.org/10.1093/schbul/sbv056.
81. Green MF. Impact of cognitive and social cognitive impairment on functional outcomes in patients with schizophrenia. J Clin Psychiatry. 2016;77(Suppl 2):8–11. https://doi.org/10.4088/JCP.14074su1c.02.
82. Javed A, Charles A. The importance of social cognition in improving functional outcomes in schizophrenia. Front Psych. 2018;9:157. https://doi.org/10.3389/fpsyt.2018.00157.
83. Sergi MJ, Rassovsky Y, Nuechterlein KH, Green MF. Social perception as a mediator of the influence of early visual processing on functional status in schizophrenia. Am J Psychiatry. 2006;163(3):448–54. https://doi.org/10.1176/appi.ajp.163.3.448.
84. Couture SM, Granholm EL, Fish SC. A path model investigation of neurocognition, theory of mind, social competence, negative symptoms and real-world functioning in schizophrenia. Schizophr Res. 2011;125(2–3):152–60. https://doi.org/10.1016/j.schres.2010.09.020.
85. Brekke J, Kay DD, Lee KS, Green MF. Biosocial pathways to functional outcome in schizophrenia. Schizophr Res. 2005;80(2–3):213–25. https://doi.org/10.1016/j.schres.2005.07.008.

86. Addington J, Saeedi H, Addington D. Influence of social perception and social knowledge on cognitive and social functioning in early psychosis. Br J Psychiatry. 2006;189:373–8. https://doi.org/10.1192/bjp.bp.105.021022.
87. Fanous A, Gardner C, Walsh D, Kendler KS. Relationship between positive and negative symptoms of schizophrenia and schizotypal symptoms in nonpsychotic relatives. Arch Gen Psychiatry. 2001;58(7):669–73. https://doi.org/10.1001/archpsyc.58.7.669.
88. Leucht S, Corves C, Arbter D, Engel RR, Li C, Davis JM. Second-generation versus first-generation antipsychotic drugs for schizophrenia: a meta-analysis. Lancet. 2009;373(9657):31–41. https://doi.org/10.1016/S0140-6736(08)61764-X.
89. Fusar-Poli P, Papanastasiou E, Stahl D, Rocchetti M, Carpenter W, Shergill S, et al. Treatments of negative symptoms in schizophrenia: meta-analysis of 168 randomized placebo-controlled trials. Schizophr Bull. 2015;41(4):892–9. https://doi.org/10.1093/schbul/sbu170.
90. Galderisi S, Bucci P, Mucci A, Kirkpatrick B, Pini S, Rossi A, et al. Categorical and dimensional approaches to negative symptoms of schizophrenia: focus on long-term stability and functional outcome. Schizophr Res. 2013;147(1):157–62. https://doi.org/10.1016/j.schres.2013.03.020.
91. Foussias G, Agid O, Fervaha G, Remington G. Negative symptoms of schizophrenia: clinical features, relevance to real world functioning and specificity versus other CNS disorders. Eur Neuropsychopharmacol. 2014;24(5):693–709. https://doi.org/10.1016/j.euroneuro.2013.10.017.
92. Kirkpatrick B, Galderisi S. Deficit schizophrenia: an update. World Psychiatry. 2008;7(3):143–7. https://doi.org/10.1002/j.2051-5545.2008.tb00181.x.
93. Marder SR, Galderisi S. The current conceptualization of negative symptoms in schizophrenia. World Psychiatry. 2017;16(1):14–24. https://doi.org/10.1002/wps.20385.
94. Galderisi S, Mucci A, Buchanan RW, Arango C. Negative symptoms of schizophrenia: new developments and unanswered research questions. Lancet Psychiatry. 2018;5(8):664–77. https://doi.org/10.1016/S2215-0366(18)30050-6.
95. Ventura J, Hellemann GS, Thames AD, Koellner V, Nuechterlein KH. Symptoms as mediators of the relationship between neurocognition and functional outcome in schizophrenia: a meta-analysis. Schizophr Res. 2009;113(2–3):189–99. https://doi.org/10.1016/j.schres.2009.03.035.
96. Lee EHM, Hui CLM, Chan KPK, Chan PY, Law EYL, Chong CSY, et al. The role of symptoms and insight in mediating cognition and functioning in first episode psychosis. Schizophr Res. 2019;206:251–6. https://doi.org/10.1016/j.schres.2018.11.009.
97. Foussias G, Mann S, Zakzanis KK, van Reekum R, Agid O, Remington G. Prediction of longitudinal functional outcomes in schizophrenia: the impact of baseline motivational deficits. Schizophr Res. 2011;132(1):24–7. https://doi.org/10.1016/j.schres.2011.06.026.
98. Beck AT, Himelstein R, Bredemeier K, Silverstein SM, Grant P. What accounts for poor functioning in people with schizophrenia: a re-evaluation of the contributions of neurocognitive v. attitudinal and motivational factors. Psychol Med. 2018;48(16):2776–85. https://doi.org/10.1017/S0033291718000442.
99. Galderisi S, Mucci A, Dollfus S, Nordentoft M, Falkai P, Kaiser S, et al. EPA guidance on assessment of negative symptoms in schizophrenia. Eur Psychiatry. 2021;64:1–91. https://doi.org/10.1192/j.eurpsy.2021.11.
100. Stiekema AP, Liemburg EJ, van der Meer L, Castelein S, Stewart R, van Weeghel J, et al. Confirmatory factor analysis and differential relationships of the two subdomains of negative symptoms in chronically ill psychotic patients. PLoS One. 2016;11(2):e0149785. https://doi.org/10.1371/journal.pone.0149785.
101. Kaiser S, Lyne J, Agartz I, Clarke M, Morch-Johnsen L, Faerden A. Individual negative symptoms and domains—relevance for assessment, pathomechanisms and treatment. Schizophr Res. 2017;186:39–45. https://doi.org/10.1016/j.schres.2016.07.013.
102. Gard DE, Kring AM, Gard MG, Horan WP, Green MF. Anhedonia in schizophrenia: distinctions between anticipatory and consummatory pleasure. Schizophr Res. 2007;93(1–3):253–60. https://doi.org/10.1016/j.schres.2007.03.008.

103. Mucci A, Dima D, Soricelli A, Volpe U, Bucci P, Frangou S, et al. Is avolition in schizophrenia associated with a deficit of dorsal caudate activity? A functional magnetic resonance imaging study during reward anticipation and feedback. Psychol Med. 2015;45(8):1765–78. https://doi.org/10.1017/S0033291714002943.
104. Kirkpatrick B, Strauss GP, Nguyen L, Fischer BA, Daniel DG, Cienfuegos A, et al. The brief negative symptom scale: psychometric properties. Schizophr Bull. 2011;37(2):300–5. https://doi.org/10.1093/schbul/sbq059.
105. Kring AM, Gur RE, Blanchard JJ, Horan WP, Reise SP. The Clinical Assessment Interview for Negative Symptoms (CAINS): final development and validation. Am J Psychiatry. 2013;170(2):165–72. https://doi.org/10.1176/appi.ajp.2012.12010109.
106. Mucci A, Galderisi S, Merlotti E, Rossi A, Rocca P, Bucci P, et al. The Brief Negative Symptom Scale (BNSS): independent validation in a large sample of Italian patients with schizophrenia. Eur Psychiatry. 2015;30(5):641–7. https://doi.org/10.1016/j.eurpsy.2015.01.014.
107. Daniel DG. Issues in selection of instruments to measure negative symptoms. Schizophr Res. 2013;150(2–3):343–5. https://doi.org/10.1016/j.schres.2013.07.005.
108. Garcia-Portilla MP, Garcia-Alvarez L, Saiz PA, Al-Halabi S, Bobes-Bascaran MT, Bascaran MT, et al. Psychometric evaluation of the negative syndrome of schizophrenia. Eur Arch Psychiatry Clin Neurosci. 2015;265(7):559–66. https://doi.org/10.1007/s00406-015-0595-z.
109. Strassnig MT, Raykov T, O'Gorman C, Bowie CR, Sabbag S, Durand D, et al. Determinants of different aspects of everyday outcome in schizophrenia: the roles of negative symptoms, cognition, and functional capacity. Schizophr Res. 2015;165(1):76–82. https://doi.org/10.1016/j.schres.2015.03.033.
110. Rocca P, Galderisi S, Rossi A, Bertolino A, Rucci P, Gibertoni D, et al. Disorganization and real-world functioning in schizophrenia: results from the multicenter study of the Italian Network for Research on Psychoses. Schizophr Res. 2018;201:105–12. https://doi.org/10.1016/j.schres.2018.06.003.
111. Reed RA, Harrow M, Herbener ES, Martin EM. Executive function in schizophrenia: is it linked to psychosis and poor life functioning? J Nerv Ment Dis. 2002;190(11):725–32. https://doi.org/10.1097/00005053-200211000-00001.
112. Metsänen M, Wahlberg KE, Hakko H, Saarento O, Tienari P. Thought disorder index: a longitudinal study of severity levels and schizophrenia factors. J Psychiatr Res. 2006;40:258–66. https://doi.org/10.1016/j.jpsychires.2005.03.004.
113. Metsänen M, Ke W, Saarento O, Tarvainen T, Miettunen J, Koistinen P, et al. Early presence of thought disorder as a prospective sign of mental disorder. Psychiatry Res. 2004;125:193–203. https://doi.org/10.1016/j.psychres.2004.01.002.
114. Harvey PD, Howanitz E, Parrella M, White L, Davidson M, Mohs RC, et al. Symptoms, cognitive functioning, and adaptive skills in geriatric patients with lifelong schizophrenia: a comparison across treatment sites. Am J Psychiatry. 1998;155(8):1080–6. https://doi.org/10.1176/ajp.155.8.1080.
115. Vita A, Barlati S, Deste G, Rocca P, Rossi A, Bertolino A, et al. The influence of autistic symptoms on social and non-social cognition and on real-life functioning in people with schizophrenia: evidence from the Italian Network for Research on Psychoses multicenter study. Eur Psychiatry. 2020;63(1):e98. https://doi.org/10.1192/j.eurpsy.2020.99.
116. Treen Calvo D, Gimenez-Donoso S, Setien-Suero E, Toll Privat A, Crespo-Facorro B, Arriola RA. Targeting recovery in first episode psychosis: the importance of neurocognition and premorbid adjustment in a 3-year longitudinal study. Schizophr Res. 2018;195:320–6. https://doi.org/10.1016/j.schres.2017.08.032.
117. Bucci P, Galderisi S, Mucci A, Rossi A, Rocca P, Bertolino A, et al. Premorbid academic and social functioning in patients with schizophrenia and its associations with negative symptoms and cognition. Acta Psychiatr Scand. 2018;138(3):253–66. https://doi.org/10.1111/acps.12938.
118. MacDonald EM, Pica S, McDonald S, Hayes RL, Baglioni AJ. Stress and coping in early psychosis: role of symptoms, self-efficacy, and social support in coping with stress. Br J Psychiatry. 1998;172(S33):122–7. https://doi.org/10.1192/S0007125000297778.

119. Rossi A, Galderisi S, Rocca P, Bertolino A, Mucci A, Rucci P, et al. The relationships of personal resources with symptom severity and psychosocial functioning in persons with schizophrenia: results from the Italian Network for Research on Psychoses study. Eur Arch Psychiatry Clin Neurosci. 2017;267(4):285–94. https://doi.org/10.1007/s00406-016-0710-9.

120. Ritsner MS, Ratner Y. The long-term changes in coping strategies in schizophrenia: temporal coping types. J Nerv Ment Dis. 2006;194(4):261–7. https://doi.org/10.1097/01.nmd.0000207361.81947.52.

121. Tait L, Birchwood M, Trower P. Adapting to the challenge of psychosis: personal resilience and the use of sealing-over (avoidant) coping strategies. Br J Psychiatry. 2004;185:410–5. https://doi.org/10.1192/bjp.185.5.410.

122. Casey DA, Rodriguez M, Northcott C, Vickar G, Shihabuddin L. Schizophrenia: medical illness, mortality, and aging. Int J Psychiatry Med. 2011;41(3):245–51. https://doi.org/10.2190/PM.41.3.c.

123. De Hert M, Correll CU, Bobes J, Cetkovich-Bakmas M, Cohen D, Asai I, et al. Physical illness in patients with severe mental disorders. I. Prevalence, impact of medications and disparities in health care. World Psychiatry. 2011;10(1):52–77. https://doi.org/10.1002/j.2051-5545.2011.tb00014.x.

124. Gerlinger G, Hauser M, De Hert M, Lacluyse K, Wampers M, Correll CU. Personal stigma in schizophrenia spectrum disorders: a systematic review of prevalence rates, correlates, impact and interventions. World Psychiatry. 2013;12(2):155–64. https://doi.org/10.1002/wps.20040.

125. Livingston JD, Boyd JE. Correlates and consequences of internalized stigma for people living with mental illness: a systematic review and meta-analysis. Soc Sci Med. 2010;71:2150–61. https://doi.org/10.1016/j.socscimed.2010.09.030.

126. Fu S, Czajkowski N, Rund BR, Torgalsboen AK. The relationship between level of cognitive impairments and functional outcome trajectories in first-episode schizophrenia. Schizophr Res. 2017;190:144–9. https://doi.org/10.1016/j.schres.2017.03.002.

127. Sanchez P, Ojeda N, Pena J, Elizagarate E, Yoller AB, Gutierrez M, et al. Predictors of longitudinal changes in schizophrenia: the role of processing speed. J Clin Psychiatry. 2009;70(6):888–96. https://doi.org/10.4088/JCP.08m04294.

128. Chang WC, Hui CL, Chan SK, Lee EH, Chen EY. Impact of avolition and cognitive impairment on functional outcome in first-episode schizophrenia-spectrum disorder: a prospective one-year follow-up study. Schizophr Res. 2016;170(2–3):318–21. https://doi.org/10.1016/j.schres.2016.01.004.

129. Reichenberg A, Feo C, Prestia D, Bowie CR, Patterson TL, Harvey PD. The course and correlates of everyday functioning in schizophrenia. Schizophr Res Cogn. 2014;1(1):e47–52. https://doi.org/10.1016/j.scog.2014.03.001.

130. Kern RS, Nuechterlein KH, Green MF, Baade LE, Fenton WS, Gold JM, et al. The MATRICS Consensus Cognitive Battery, part 2: co-norming and standardization. Am J Psychiatry. 2008;165(2):214–20. https://doi.org/10.1176/appi.ajp.2007.07010043.

131. Nuechterlein KH, Green MF, Kern RS, Baade LE, Barch DM, Cohen JD, et al. The MATRICS Consensus Cognitive Battery, part 1: test selection, reliability, and validity. Am J Psychiatry. 2008;165(2):203–13. https://doi.org/10.1176/appi.ajp.2007.07010042.

132. Costantini G, Epskamp S, Borsboom D, Perugini M, Mõttus R, Waldorp L, et al. State of the aRt personality research: a tutorial on network analysis of personality data in R. J Res Pers. 2015;54:13–29. https://doi.org/10.1016/j.jrp.2014.07.003.

133. Horan WP, Green MF, DeGroot M, Fiske A, Hellemann G, Kee K, et al. Social cognition in schizophrenia, Part 2: 12-month stability and prediction of functional outcome in first-episode patients. Schizophr Bull. 2012;38(4):865–72. https://doi.org/10.1093/schbul/sbr001.

134. McCleery A, Lee J, Fiske AP, Ghermezi L, Hayata JN, Hellemann GS, et al. Longitudinal stability of social cognition in schizophrenia: a 5-year follow-up of social perception and emotion processing. Schizophr Res. 2016;176(2–3):467–72. https://doi.org/10.1016/j.schres.2016.07.008.

135. Galderisi S, Mucci A, Bitter I, Libiger J, Bucci P, Fleischhacker WW, et al. Persistent negative symptoms in first episode patients with schizophrenia: results from the European First

Episode Schizophrenia Trial. Eur Neuropsychopharmacol. 2013;23(3):196–204. https://doi.org/10.1016/j.euroneuro.2012.04.019.

136. Bucci P, Mucci A, van Rossum IW, Aiello C, Arango C, Baandrup L, et al. Persistent negative symptoms in recent-onset psychosis: relationship to treatment response and psychosocial functioning. Eur Neuropsychopharmacol. 2020;34:76–86. https://doi.org/10.1016/j.euroneuro.2020.03.010.

137. Ahmed AO, Murphy CF, Latoussakis V, McGovern KE, English J, Bloch A, et al. An examination of neurocognition and symptoms as predictors of post-hospital community tenure in treatment resistant schizophrenia. Psychiatry Res. 2016;236:47–52. https://doi.org/10.1016/j.psychres.2016.01.001.

138. Fulford D, Piskulic D, Addington J, Kane JM, Schooler NR, Mueser KT. Prospective relationships between motivation and functioning in recovery after a first episode of schizophrenia. Schizophr Bull. 2018;44(2):369–77. https://doi.org/10.1093/schbul/sbx096.

139. Maj M, van Os J, De Hert M, Gaebel W, Galderisi S, Green MF, et al. The clinical characterization of the patient with primary psychosis aimed at personalization of management. World Psychiatry. 2021;20(1):4–33. https://doi.org/10.1002/wps.20809.

Personal Recovery in Schizophrenia: A Narrative Review

3

Rodolfo Rossi, Valentina Socci, and Alessandro Rossi

3.1 Introduction

Historically, schizophrenia has been considered a severe mental disorder with an inconstant prognosis [1].

The severity of schizophrenia depends on the interaction between the disorder itself and several variables, including social factors and access to proper treatment delivery. In this view, clinical and functional outcomes are not a predetermined destiny; rather, they depend on a multifactorial trajectory in which stakeholders, including professionals and patients, play a central role.

Beyond the medical and psychopathological domains, social factors have been repeatedly reported and taken into account in the pathogenesis, course, and outcome of schizophrenia [2, 3].

In a meta-analysis of schizophrenia or dementia praecox's outcomes, Hegarthy et al. [4] concluded that … *overall, less than half of patients diagnosed with schizophrenia have shown substantial clinical improvement after follow-up averaging*

R. Rossi
Department of Systems Medicine, University of Rome Tor Vergata, Rome, Italy
e-mail: rudy86.rossi@gmail.com

V. Socci
Department of Biotechnological and Applied Clinical Sciences, University of L'Aquila,
L'Aquila, Italy
e-mail: valentinasocci@gmail.com

A. Rossi (✉)
Department of Biotechnological and Applied Clinical Sciences, University of L'Aquila,
L'Aquila, Italy

Department of Mental Health, ASL1, L'Aquila, Italy
e-mail: alessandro.rossi@univaq.it

© The Author(s), under exclusive license to Springer Nature
Switzerland AG 2022
B. Carpiniello et al. (eds.), *Recovery and Major Mental Disorders*,
Comprehensive Approach to Psychiatry 2,
https://doi.org/10.1007/978-3-030-98301-7_3

nearly as 6 years. Despite considerable gains in improvement rates after mid-century, there has been a decline since the 1970s. These historical changes probably reflect improved treatment, a shift in diagnostic criteria, and selection bias related to changes in health care.

However, literature about the long-term course of schizophrenia is mixed. While most cases seem to have an undulating course, characterized by remissions and recurrences, or a chronic, unremitting course with poor outcome, recent observations suggest that recovery with good outcome in psychoses is a possible achievement.

Remission and recovery in schizophrenia have received increasing attention in the last decades, offering new clinical practice opportunities, health services research, and clinical trials [5–7].

From a psychopathological perspective, symptoms reduction and social functioning improvement have always been regarded as the two most important outcomes in schizophrenia. However, the variations in these domains are not always closely correlated [8, 9]. In recent years a new psychiatric practice is emerging, aiming not merely to achieve symptoms relief and social abilities but also to a broader 'recovery' [10, 11].

Recovery, defined as 'a way of living a satisfying, hopeful, and contributing life even with any limitations caused by illness' [12], has received increasing attention in mental health practice. However, the term 'recovery' has been used in different ways with different meaning [10]. The recovery concept can be broken down into clinical, or objective, and personal, or subjective, domains. Subjective and objective recovery reflect different perspectives in schizophrenia outcome, not necessarily matching with each other, and usually representing the consumer's or the therapist's different points of view [13].

The principal purpose of this narrative review is to provide a comprehensive overview of personal recovery and to highlight the most relevant fields of research and clinical practice perspectives.

3.2 From Remission to Recovery

What has led, during the last 30 years, the transition from a Kraepelinian view of schizophrenia outcomes towards a more optimistic one, based on a remission/recovery perspective?

Maybe more than one reason prompted clinicians and stakeholders to consider alternative views other than that rooted in the Kraepelin-Bleuler-Schneider concepts [14].

Since the Hegarty work, second-generation antipsychotics renewed the interest of professionals and stakeholders in treatment and outcome assessment.

Growing attention into remission in psychiatry and, more recently, schizophrenia [5] as a critical component of recovery dominated the century's early decade. In a naturalistic cohort, about 30% of patients diagnosed with schizophrenia or schizoaffective disorder met the criteria for remission at the study endpoint. However, the remission concept and the remission criteria [5] were rooted in the medical model of treatment response and underlined the need for a systematic quantitative symptoms rating over 6 months. The discussion of the Andreasen criteria is beyond the scope of this chapter. Anyway, the scientific literature reports a favourable acceptance of the criteria mentioned above, even though with some criticism [15].

Parallel to the development and acceptance of the 'remission' construct, the rehabilitation moved from traditional vocational rehabilitation programmes, typically involving low-level activities in sheltered workshops, to supported employment programmes, which support the consumer in finding and maintaining a job in the real-world marketplace [3, 10, 16].

These changes have promoted a general evolution in public opinion, as well as in patterns of service delivery and relationships between providers and consumers. Recovery is a central issue in this paradigm shift. There is increasing recognition that recovery is not only possible but that it may even be common. Consequently, increasing consumer and political pressure aims to ensure that mental health services are recovery-oriented [16].

3.3   How Many Types of Recovery

While all the clinicians agree that recovery is a multidimensional and multidetermined concept, not all of them agree about the construct's content.

Bert-Jan Roosenschoon et al. [17] propose three types of not mutually exclusive but complementary recovery: a clinical or symptomatic recovery, related to the degree of psychiatric symptoms; a functional recovery, also named objective recovery—some authors equate this type of recovery with functional remission or consider it a part of clinical recovery; and a personal recovery that underlines the personal nature of the recovery process, also named subjective recovery.

Subjective or personal resource domains have been shown to mediate the impact of symptoms and cognitive impairment on real-life functioning in subjects with schizophrenia [9, 18, 19], suggesting that the two recovery domains are complementary rather than incompatible [20].

The real-world functioning of people with schizophrenia depends on several variables related to the disorder itself, to the person's resources, and to the person's context [19]. Several studies report that patients with comparable severity of psychopathology may differ in their real-life functioning because of differences in personal resources [21–23].

Resilience, coping abilities, recovery style, the relationship with services and therapists, and stigma are all constructs encompassing several aspects of personal resources. These variables can be considered within the subjective elements of recovery (SER) domains. Nonetheless, few studies investigated these factors from a recovery perspective. Several SERs, such as resilience, self-esteem, coping styles, internalized stigma, and happiness, have been associated with a positive outcome in schizophrenia [24–26].

Research concerning the relationship between objective and subjective elements of recovery reported inconsistent findings. Different studies found a significant correlation of subjective recovery with the severity of symptoms [27–29], a moderate link between symptoms and social function [30], or no direct correlation between symptom severity and self-reported recovery [20].

3.4 The Content of Personal Recovery

As many aspects of personal life and subjectivity can be included in the 'personal recovery' concept, there is a risk to enumerate several positive issues that have been only poorly conceptualized in relation to outcome measure of schizophrenia. Many of them overlap with the quality of life concept and measurements.

Hope, self-esteem, resilience, happiness, self-stigma, adult attachment style, social connectedness, and empowerment [13, 31, 32] have all been related to recovery.

'Personal recovery' stands for '*a deeply personal, unique process of changing one's attitudes, values, feelings, goals, skills and/or roles. It is a way of living a satisfying, hopeful, and contributing life even within the limitations caused by illness. Recovery involves the development of new meaning and purpose in one's life as one grows beyond the catastrophic effects of mental illness*' [12]. In simple terms, personal recovery principles are based on the belief that a meaningful life is possible, despite symptoms' persistence. This positive approach to mental illness is not limited to full symptom resolution; rather, it promotes resilience and control over problems and life, endorsing the idea that people with severe mental illness have vocational, educational, and residential needs beyond symptoms reduction. People suffering from schizophrenia have the right to be treated and to play an active role in therapeutic decisions. They are indeed able to establish independent and healthy lives, even in the presence of symptoms [10, 33].

Recovering from schizophrenia includes four phases: (1) feeling overwhelmed by the disease; (2) struggling with the disease; (3) living with disability; and (4) living beyond the disability [34].

People with schizophrenia reported lower levels of happiness, but there was substantial heterogeneity within the schizophrenia group. Happiness in persons with schizophrenia correlates with higher mental health-related quality of life and several positive psychosocial outcomes, such as lower perceived stress, higher resilience, optimism and personal mastery [31].

Lysaker et al. [35] also mention the quality of the personal narrative of one's own life and challenges as a meaningful aspect of recover *from* schizophrenia. Furthermore, he suggested that personal narratives might be a unique recovery domain relevant to wellness in daily life. Soundy et al. [36], in a systematic review, reported three types of psychosocial factors which promoted and influenced recovery: (1) adjustment, coping and reappraisal, (2) responding to the illness, and (3) social support. The factors which challenged recovery included (1) negative interaction and isolation, (2) internal barriers, and (3) uncertainty and hopelessness.

It is easy to recognize that all these factors are qualitatively 'personal' and may interact with service engagement and orientation.

Other researchers tried to operationalize and measure personal recovery. Even though it could be challenging to operationalize and catch the personal and subjective recovery experiences, several authors attempted to develop different instruments for this purpose [37–39]. It could be that no single measure of 'personal recovery' exists', but more dimensions and tools could be necessary to assess personal experience, contextual factors, and service engagement [13].

3.5 Consumer Models of Recovery

Jose et al. [40] reviewed the consumer perspective of recovery from schizophrenia, identifying five areas: process orientation, self-orientation, family orientation, social interaction, and illness orientation.

Patient or client-based definition of recovery mainly involved factors related to personal well-being and social inclusion. These aspects were distant from the clinical recovery measure. However, the scientific and consumer literature continue to have quite different opinions and views of the meaning (and perhaps practice) of 'recovery'. Bellack [16] summarized these different positions in terms of historical context, perspectives and practice. While the scientific definition arises from a biomedical perspective, the consumers' one evolved from a civil rights perspective, endorsing a sociopolitical meaning towards a change in public attitude about mental illness and services practice. Recovery-oriented services describe mental health treatments and interventions aimed at the recovery model. Likewise, the recovery model and movement deeply informed mental health services stimulating the synthesis of hope, identity, dignity and respect, partnership and communication [39, 41]. Despite the broad consensus about these issues, several limitations, and cross-cultural variation in dissemination and principles applications still exist [42].

3.6 Stigma and Resilience

Internalized stigma, also referred to as self-stigma, is characterized by a subjective perception of devaluation, marginalization, secrecy, shame, and withdrawal [43]. People with a severe mental illness, such as schizophrenia, anticipate social rejection and consider themselves devalued society members [44]. They may internalize negative stereotypes about mental illness and respond by self-stigma [45]. According to the current literature, both stigma and lack of empowerment may lead to depression [46, 47].

Resilience is a construct encompassing several aspects of personal resources. It is usually defined as a dynamic adaptation process to challenging life conditions that could be protective against mental disorders. In patients with schizophrenia, resilience and psychosocial functioning are tightly correlated [24, 48].

Clinical strategies targeting resilience should be further addressed and tested within the recovery approach [25, 49]. Because of the complex interaction between subjective and objective recovery elements [28], strategies to improve resilience could ultimately improve recovery. This approach could be further reshaped into the *'subjective recovery perspective'*, as suggested by Hofer et al. [25].

Several variables related to personal resources such as resilience, self-esteem, coping styles, internalized stigma, and happiness have been associated with a positive outcome in schizophrenia. These variables could explain the different real-life functioning outcomes in persons with comparable psychopathology severity [13]. The relationship of these variables with symptom severity and psychosocial functioning was explored, suggesting that specific treatments aimed to reduce stigma, improve coping strategies and shape recovery styles might be effective in producing considerable clinical and functional improvements [9, 13].

The role of personal resources suggests that some positive features of 'adjustment to psychosis' may reduce the burden of depression, which, in turn, could have a positive impact on the disorder itself.

In addition to personal resources, personal styles to cope with psychosis or to react to a psychotic experience have been described [50]. Integration and sealing over have been identified as two clinically distinct recovery styles from schizophrenia. Mc Glashan et al. [50] suggested that 'sealing over' could represent a dysfunctional attitude towards psychosis while an 'integration Style ' could favour recovery. Low 'sealing over' and higher 'integration' could be conceived as a resilient personal adaptation to psychosis [51].

Within the positive psychological adjustment to psychosis, happiness has been suggested as an achievable goal among people with schizophrenia [31], but the 'wellness within illness' issue [52] deserves further exploration.

3.7 From Values to Recovery

Personal recovery could be pursued through spiritual, ethical, and human rights/social capital approaches if we scientifically characterize its conceptual framework. Kasai and Fukuda stated that users, caregivers, and professionals could contribute to the users' personal recovery and subjective well-being if we scientifically redefine a person's 'value' or 'personalized value' [11]. Values are motivational constructs guiding behaviour, abstract trans-situational goals that reflect what people think and state about themselves and regulate principles in people's lives [53]. In the proposed model, living in the 'real-world' affects values development, which then influences behavioural patterns in life and induces plasticity in the brain circuit [11]. These interactions acquire importance, especially in adolescence. Schizophrenia research is a promising field for the exploration of the value-based approach since developmental psychopathology, psychology and neuroscience in adolescence and functional impairment are core domains of pathological pathways [11].

3 Personal Recovery in Schizophrenia: A Narrative Review

Huguelet and colleagues [54] found that values mediated the association between symptoms and meaning. 'Meaning' is concerned with one's goal in life. Spirituality, self-esteem and close relationship are determinants of meaning. More significantly, the fulfilment of values allows subjects to achieve a sense of purpose. Hence, depression, hopelessness, self-esteem, and the number of relationships influenced values in a heterogeneous clinical sample; the presence and enactment of values were associated with meaning that, in turn, was associated with some symptoms and social characteristics.

Many authors have studied the usefulness of values in influencing actions, predicting attitudes, preferences, goals, and their association with personality traits. Personal values predict mental health indicators in non-clinical samples [55] and stigmatization in clinical samples [56]. Personal values can be directly related to 'negative' behaviours, such as interpersonal violence [53]. It is reasonable to assume that the enactment of these behaviours is related to the motivational structure of a given value for a given person. It can be argued that, for some people, the motivational drive could deviate from a harmonic development [53]. Differences in value orientation have been observed among subjects with severe mental illness compared to a non-clinical sample (Socci et al., 2021 unpublished data). Persons with a severe mental illness were characterized by a higher 'conservation' value compared to the non-clinical sample. The expression of conservation value in individuals with a mental disorder could reflect an orientation towards conformity underlying fundamental affiliative goals. It has been shown that goals related to affiliation and social approval are strongly activated when one's self-esteem is threatened by the prospect or actual occurrence of not fitting in with the group and stigmatization.

These observations open new scenarios relevant to the recovery process. The type and extent of treatment could be adapted to one's own clinical and personal variables. In other words, recovery-oriented practices develop person-centred tailored interventions, promote resilience, personal skills, and hope, facilitate self-determination, and enhance individual strengths, preferences, and aspirations. These practices support people with severe mental illness to pursue their goals and achieve subjective well-being in terms of health and social outcomes.

Emerging literature supports the relevance of addressing values and meaning in the recovery-oriented care of patients with persistent psychiatric disorders [54]. Since recovery is a personal and subjective experience, and values influence the sense of meaning in life by interacting with behaviour and mental indicators, tailored interventions targeting personal values and purpose in life should be fulfilled [13]. Moreover, preliminary findings suggest that tailoring psychological interventions according to values in clinical populations could help reduce risky behaviours [53], which is associated with better psychopathological outcomes and social functioning.

In conclusion, the integration of subjective and clinical models would yield a better assessment and overall understanding of recovery and contribute to design individualized and integrated treatment programmes aimed to help individuals to live a meaningful and satisfying life [13].

3.8 A Pragmatic View About Personal Recovery

The pendulum of research interest into treatment and outcome in schizophrenia swings from scepticism and pessimism to optimism, depending on several factors related to the medical discipline (i.e. medical discoveries, change in diagnostic criteria, new drug development) [57], socio-economic factors (i.e. urbanizations, migration, mental health care system changes, economic crisis, fundings), and personal attitude of the stakeholders (i.e. individuals with the disorders and their caregiver) [58].

We will try to maintain the more pragmatic attitude explaining, supporting, and applying the *current* status of the art in psychiatry in connection to all the other discipline and resources within the so-called mental health arena. The conceptualization of 'positive psychiatry' and 'personal recovery' could inform the development of *optimism-based mental health* [39].

The construct of 'personal recovery' is a double-faced one, with an undoubted positive force moving all mental health citizens towards a more integrative, holistic, positive, optimistic, and right-respective practice.

On the other side, we cannot *reduce* the 'medical component' of this alliance in a *minority role.* We know how much we need medical and neuroscientific innovation to cope with mental disorder's dramatic burden [57]. A brilliant example of this synthesis could be traced in the field of early detection psychosis, where many aspects mentioned above found a proper place with an Optimism Based Practice [59]. We suggest that an 'evidence-based optimism' could better trace how to improve mental health outcomes and practice.

3.9 Conclusions

Schizophrenia recovery has long divided opinion: do it for everyone or for a minority? Is it a political statement or a reasonable hope for patients and their families? That controversies are not as polarized at present is perhaps a sign of increased knowledge. However, as should be clear from this debate, evidence-based literature does not support 'recovery either symptomatic or personal' for everyone (i.e. recovery *from* schizophrenia). However, the process in which people can live a fulfilling and productive life despite disability should be a goal for all patient/user and services (i.e. recovery *in* schizophrenia).

As only about 25% of patients with serious mental illness receive treatment consistent with evidence-based recommendations, recovery-orientated rehabilitation services and person-centred care planning through assessment and formulation are recommended by international agencies (NICE guidelines 2020) [60].

Many debates and uncertainties remain: should we use a rating instrument to assess recovery? How to ameliorate the climate of our department? What type of training, or change in training, do we need [7]?

The different meaning and adjective of the 'term' recovery should not be considered a limitation [41] but a potential for enrichment and improvement with a

3 Personal Recovery in Schizophrenia: A Narrative Review

medically oriented approach better integrated with a person-centred one [58]. However, a new paradigm shift from symptom control to recovery is needed. As current underpowered services are 'broken and demoralized' in most even developed countries [2], mental health policies and practice changes are urgent [61].

References

1. An Der Heiden W, Häfner H. The epidemiology of onset and course of schizophrenia. Eur Arch Psychiatry Clin Neurosci. 2000;250(6):292–303. https://pubmed.ncbi.nlm.nih.gov/11153964/.
2. Owen MJ, Sawa A, Mortensen PB. Schizophrenia. Lancet. 2016;388:86–97. https://pubmed.ncbi.nlm.nih.gov/26777917/.
3. Warner R. Recovery from schizophrenia and the recovery model. Curr Opin Psychiatry. 2009;22:374–80. https://pubmed.ncbi.nlm.nih.gov/19417668/.
4. Hegarty JD, Baldessarini RJ, Tohen M, Waternaux C, Oepen G. One hundred years of schizophrenia: a meta-analysis of the outcome literature. Am J Psychiatry. 1994;151(10):1409–16. https://ajp.psychiatryonline.org/doi/abs/10.1176/ajp.151.10.1409.
5. Andreasen NC, Carpenter WT, Kane JM, Lasser RA, Marder SR, Weinberger DR. Remission in schizophrenia: proposed criteria and rationale for consensus. Am J Psychiatry. 2005;162:441–9. https://pubmed.ncbi.nlm.nih.gov/15741458/.
6. Rossi A, Bagalà A, Del Curatolo V, Scapati F, Bernareggi MM, Giustra MG. Remission in schizophrenia: one-year Italian prospective study of risperidone long-acting injectable (RLAI) in patients with schizophrenia or schizoaffective disorder. Hum Psychopharmacol. 2009;24(7):574–83. https://pubmed.ncbi.nlm.nih.gov/19790173/.
7. Davidson L, Schmutte T, Dinzeo T, Andres-Hyman R. Remission and recovery in schizophrenia: practitioner and patient perspectives. Schizophr Bull. 2008;34:5–8.
8. Gorwood P, Burns T, Juckel G, Rossi A, San L, Hargarter L, et al. Psychiatrists' perceptions of the clinical importance, assessment and management of patient functioning in schizophrenia in Europe, the Middle East and Africa. Ann General Psychiatry. 2013;12(1):8.
9. Rossi A, Galderisi S, Rocca P, Bertolino A, Mucci A, Rucci P, et al. The relationships of personal resources with symptom severity and psychosocial functioning in persons with schizophrenia: results from the Italian Network for Research on Psychoses study. Eur Arch Psychiatry Clin Neurosci. 2017;267(4):285–94. https://pubmed.ncbi.nlm.nih.gov/27381016/.
10. Martinelli A, Ruggeri M. An overview of mental health recovery-oriented practices: potentiality, challenges, prejudices, and misunderstandings. J Psychopathol. 2020;26:147–54.
11. Kasai K, Fukuda M. Science of recovery in schizophrenia research: brain and psychological substrates of personalized value. NPJ Schizophr. 2017;3:14. https://www.ncbi.nlm.nih.gov/pmc/articles/PMC5441539/.
12. Anthony WA. Recovery from mental illness: the guiding vision of the mental health service system in the 1990s. Psychosoc Rehabil J. 1993;16(4):11–23.
13. Rossi A, Amore M, Galderisi S, Rocca P, Bertolino A, Aguglia E, et al. The complex relationship between self-reported 'personal recovery' and clinical recovery in schizophrenia. Schizophr Res. 2018;192:108–12. http://www.ncbi.nlm.nih.gov/pubmed/28495492.
14. Hoenig J. The concept of schizophrenia Kraepelin-Bleuler-Schneider. Br J Psychiatry. 1983;142(6):547–56. https://pubmed.ncbi.nlm.nih.gov/6349735/.
15. Remington G, Kapur S, Andreasen NC. Remission: what's in a name? [4] (multiple letters). Am J Psychiatry. 2005;162:2393–4. https://pubmed.ncbi.nlm.nih.gov/16330612/.
16. Bellack AS. Scientific and consumer models of recovery in schizophrenia: concordance, contrasts, and implications. Schizophr Bull. 2006;32:432–42. https://pubmed.ncbi.nlm.nih.gov/16461575/.
17. Roosenschoon BJ, Kamperman AM, Deen ML, Van Weeghel J, Mulder CL. Determinants of clinical, functional and personal recovery for people with schizophrenia and other severe

mental illnesses: a cross-sectional analysis. PLoS One. 2019;14(9):e0222378. https://pubmed.ncbi.nlm.nih.gov/31532805/.

18. Galderisi S, Rossi A, Rocca P, Bertolino A, Mucci A, Bucci P, et al. Pathways to functional outcome in subjects with schizophrenia living in the community and their unaffected first-degree relatives. Schizophr Res. 2016;175(1–3):154–60. https://pubmed.ncbi.nlm.nih.gov/27209527/.

19. Galderisi S, Rossi A, Rocca P, Bertolino A, Mucci A, Bucci P, et al. The influence of illness-related variables, personal resources and context-related factors on real-life functioning of people with schizophrenia. World Psychiatry. 2014;13(3):275–87. https://pubmed.ncbi.nlm.nih.gov/25273301/.

20. Roe D, Mashiach-Eizenberg M, Lysaker PH. The relation between objective and subjective domains of recovery among persons with schizophrenia-related disorders. Schizophr Res. 2011;131(1–3):133–8. https://pubmed.ncbi.nlm.nih.gov/21669512/.

21. Hultman CM, Wieselgren IM, Öhman A. Relationships between social support, social coping and life events in the relapse of schizophrenic patients. Scand J Psychol. 1997;38(1):3–13. https://pubmed.ncbi.nlm.nih.gov/9104101/.

22. MacDonald EM, Pica S, McDonald S, Hayes RL, Baglioni AJ. Stress and coping in early psychosis. Br J Psychiatry. 1998;172(S33):122–7.

23. Ritsner MS, Ratner Y. The long-term changes in coping strategies in schizophrenia: temporal coping types. J Nerv Ment Dis. 2006;194(4):261–7. https://pubmed.ncbi.nlm.nih.gov/16614547/.

24. Torgalsbøen AK. Sustaining full recovery in schizophrenia after 15 years: does resilience matter? Clin Schizophr Relat Psychoses. 2012;5(4):193–200. https://pubmed.ncbi.nlm.nih.gov/22182456/.

25. Hofer A, Mizuno Y, Frajo-Apor B, Kemmler G, Suzuki T, Pardeller S, et al. Resilience, internalized stigma, self-esteem, and hopelessness among people with schizophrenia: cultural comparison in Austria and Japan. Schizophr Res. 2016;171(1–3):86–91. https://pubmed.ncbi.nlm.nih.gov/26805413/.

26. Xu ZY, Zu S, Xiang YT, Wang N, Guo ZH, Kilbourne AM, et al. Associations of self-esteem, dysfunctional beliefs and coping style with depression in patients with schizophrenia: a preliminary survey. Psychiatry Res. 2013;209(3):340–5. https://pubmed.ncbi.nlm.nih.gov/23537843/.

27. Corrigan PW, Salzer M, Ralph RO, Sangster Y, Keck L. Examining the factor structure of the recovery assessment scale. Schizophr Bull. 2004;30(4):1035–41. https://pubmed.ncbi.nlm.nih.gov/15957202/.

28. Jørgensen R, Zoffmann V, Munk-Jørgensen P, Buck KD, Jensen SOW, Hansson L, et al. Relationships over time of subjective and objective elements of recovery in persons with schizophreni. Psychiatry Res. 2015;228(1):14–9.

29. Resnick SG, Rosenheck RA, Lehman AF. An exploratory analysis of correlates of recovery. Psychiatr Serv. 2004;55(5):540–7. https://pubmed.ncbi.nlm.nih.gov/15128962/.

30. Kukla M, Lysaker PH, Roe D. Strong subjective recovery as a protective factor against the effects of positive symptoms on quality of life outcomes in schizophrenia. Compr Psychiatry. 2014;55(6):1363–8. https://pubmed.ncbi.nlm.nih.gov/24939703/.

31. Palmer BW, Martin AS, Depp CA, Glorioso DK, Jeste DV. Wellness within illness: happiness in schizophrenia. Schizophr Res. 2014;159(1):151–6.

32. Van Eck RM, Burger TJ, Vellinga A, Schirmbeck F, De Haan L. The relationship between clinical and personal recovery in patients with schizophrenia spectrum disorders: a systematic review and meta-analysis. Schizophr Bull. 2018;44(3):631–42. https://pubmed.ncbi.nlm.nih.gov/29036720/.

33. Martinelli A, Ruggeri M. The impact on psychiatric rehabilitation of personal recovery-oriented approach. J Psychopathol. 2020;2020(3):189–95. https://doi.org/10.36148/2284-0249-355.

34. Spaniol L, Wewiorski NJ, Gagne C, Anthony WA. The process of recovery from schizophrenia. Int Rev Psychiatry. 2002;14(4):327–36. https://www.tandfonline.com/doi/abs/10.1080/0954026021000016978.

35. Lysaker PH, Ringer J, Maxwell C, McGuire A, Lecomte T. Personal narratives and recovery from schizophrenia. Schizophr Res. 2010;121(1–3):271–6.

36. Soundy A, Stubbs B, Roskell C, Williams SE, Fox A, Vancampfort D. Identifying the facilitators and processes which influence recovery in individuals with schizophrenia: a systematic review and thematic synthesis. J Ment Health. 2015;24:103–10. https://pubmed.ncbi.nlm.nih.gov/25643043/.
37. Shanks V, Williams J, Leamy M, Bird VJ, Le Boutillier C, Slade M. Measures of personal recovery: a systematic review. Psychiatr Serv. 2013;64(10):974–80. https://pubmed.ncbi.nlm.nih.gov/23820592/.
38. Cavelti M, Kvrgic S, Beck EM, Kossowsky J, Vauth R. Assessing recovery from schizophrenia as an individual process. A review of self-report instruments. Eur Psychiatry. 2012;27:19–32. https://pubmed.ncbi.nlm.nih.gov/22130177/.
39. Bejerholm U, Roe D. Personal recovery within positive psychiatry. Nord J Psychiatry. 2018;72:420–30.
40. Jose D, Ramachandra LK, Gandhi S, Desai G, Nagarajaiah. Consumer perspectives on the concept of recovery in schizophrenia: a systematic review. Asian J Psychiatr. 2015;14:13–8.
41. Slade M, Amering M, Oades L. Recovery: an international perspective. Epidemiol Psichiatr Soc. 2008;17:128–37. https://pubmed.ncbi.nlm.nih.gov/18589629/.
42. van Weeghel J, van Zelst C, Boertien D, Hasson-Ohayon I. Conceptualizations, assessments, and implications of personal recovery in mental illness: a scoping review of systematic reviews and meta-analyses. Psychiatr Rehabil J. 2019;42(2):169–81. https://pubmed.ncbi.nlm.nih.gov/30843721/.
43. Boyd JE, Adler EP, Otilingam PG, Peters T. Internalized Stigma of Mental Illness (ISMI) scale: a multinational review. Compr Psychiatry. 2014;55:221–31.
44. Corrigan PW, Watson AC, Barr L. The self-stigma of mental illness: implications for self-esteem and self-efficacy Center for Psychiatric Rehabilitation at Evanston Northwestern Healthcare. J Soc Clin Psychol. 2006;25(9):875–84.
45. Mittal D, Sullivan G, Chekuri L, Allee E, Corrigan PW. Empirical studies of self-stigma reduction strategies: a critical review of the literature. Psychiatr Serv. 2012;63(10):974–81. https://pubmed.ncbi.nlm.nih.gov/22855130/.
46. Lysaker PH, Vohs J, Hillis JD, Kukla M, Popolo R, Salvatore G, et al. Poor insight into schizophrenia: contributing factors, consequences and emerging treatment approaches. Expert Rev Neurother. 2013;13:785–93. https://pubmed.ncbi.nlm.nih.gov/23898850/.
47. Sibitz I, Amering M, Unger A, Seyringer ME, Bachmann A, Schrank B, et al. The impact of the social network, stigma and empowerment on the quality of life in patients with schizophrenia. Eur Psychiatry. 2011;26(1):28–33. https://pubmed.ncbi.nlm.nih.gov/21036554/.
48. Kim KR, Song YY, Park JY, Lee EH, Lee M, Lee SY, et al. The relationship between psychosocial functioning and resilience and negative symptoms in individuals at ultra-high risk for psychosis. Aust N Z J Psychiatry. 2013;47(8):762–71. http://journals.sagepub.com/doi/10.1177/0004867413488218.
49. Yoshida K, Suzuki T, Imasaka Y, Kubo K, Mizuno Y, Saruta J, et al. Resilience in schizophrenia: a comparative study between a remote island and an urban area in Japan. Schizophr Res. 2016;171(1–3):92–6. https://keio.pure.elsevier.com/en/publications/resilience-in-schizophrenia-a-comparative-study-between-a-remote-.
50. McGlashan TH. Recovery style from mental illness and long-term outcome. J Nerv Ment Dis. 1987;175(11):681–5. https://pubmed.ncbi.nlm.nih.gov/3681279/.
51. Tait L, Birchwood M, Trower P. Adapting to the challenge of psychosis: personal resilience and the use of sealing-over (avoidant) coping strategies. Br J Psychiatry. 2004;185:410–5. https://pubmed.ncbi.nlm.nih.gov/15516550/.
52. Saks Elyn R. Opinion. Successful and schizophrenic. The New York Times; 2021. https://www.nytimes.com/2013/01/27/opinion/sunday/schizophrenic-not-stupid.html.
53. Rossi A, Talevi D, Collazzoni A, Parnanzone S, Stratta P, Rossi R. From basic human values to interpersonal violence: a mental illness sample. J Aggress Maltreatment Trauma. 2020;29(3):259–71.

54. Huguelet P, Guillaume S, Vidal S, Mohr S, Courtet P, Villain L, et al. Values as determinant of meaning among patients with psychiatric disorders in the perspective of recovery. Sci Rep. 2016;6:27617.
55. Maercker A, Chi Zhang X, Gao Z, Kochetkov Y, Lu S, Sang Z, et al. Personal value orientations as mediated predictors of mental health: a three-culture study of Chinese, Russian, and German university students. Int J Clin Heal Psychol. 2015;15(1):8–17.
56. Norman RMG, Sorrentino R, Windell D, Manchanda R. Are personal values of importance in the stigmatization of people with mental illness? Can J Psychiatr. 2008;53(12):848–56. https://pubmed.ncbi.nlm.nih.gov/19087483/.
57. Insel TR. Rethinking schizophrenia. Nature. 2010;468:187–93. http://www.mentalhealthcommission.gov/.
58. Lloyd K, White J. Democratizing clinical research. Nature. 2011;474:277–8. https://www.nature.com/articles/474277a.
59. Riecher-Rössler A, McGorry PD. Early detection and intervention in psychosis. In: Riecher-Rössler A, McGorry PD, editors. Key issues in mental health. S. Karger AG; 2016. p. 179–89. (Key Issues in Mental Health; vol. 181). https://www.karger.com/Book/Home/270141.
60. Recommendations I Rehabilitation for adults with complex psychosis I Guidance I NICE. 2021. https://www.nice.org.uk/guidance/ng181/chapter/Recommendations.
61. Mohr P, Galderisi S, Boyer P, Wasserman D, Arteel P, Ieven A, et al. Value of schizophrenia treatment I: the patient journey. Eur Psychiatry. 2018;53:107–15. https://pubmed.ncbi.nlm.nih.gov/30036773/.

Personal Recovery Within Forensic Settings

4

Andrew Shepherd 🔟

4.1 Introduction

In this chapter I provide an overview argument in relation to the concept of personal recovery as it is enacted and may be understood within forensic institutional settings—for example, prisons, secure hospitals and probation settings. This is drawn from the perspective of a psychiatrist working in England—with experience particularly in the North West of England. An initial limitation becomes immediately apparent in that this is a sole author chapter—a position that may be seen as anathema to the concept of personal recovery which, by its very nature, represents a process of co-construction. This chapter is therefore partial in its perspective—and there is an inherent power assumption that comes with that situation that is particularly painful and sensitively enacted within forensic settings and practice. This limitation is remarked upon not to dismiss the content of this chapter—but to draw the reader's attention to this partial perspective. This point is returned to at various stages of the argument set out below.

With this in mind the chapter begins with a brief overview of the concept of personal recovery—focusing on the core ideas of personal identity and identity work which will be considered in light of the particular nature of forensic environments and mental health practice within these institutional settings. This leads to a discussion on the nature of forensic recovery before then addressing some particular points of consideration and finally some suggestions for future work and direction of travel. Contextualising remarks are provided throughout for readers unfamiliar with forensic mental health practice in England and Wales.

A. Shepherd (✉)
Health and Justice, Greater Manchester Mental Health NHS Foundation Trust, Prestwich, UK
e-mail: andrew.shepherd@gmmh.nhs.uk

© The Author(s), under exclusive license to Springer Nature Switzerland AG 2022
B. Carpiniello et al. (eds.), *Recovery and Major Mental Disorders*, Comprehensive Approach to Psychiatry 2,
https://doi.org/10.1007/978-3-030-98301-7_4

4.2 Personal Recovery

The conceptualisation of *personal recovery* represents a profoundly political act—building on a legacy of disability activism and the emergent field of mad studies [1]. Two key moves are captured in the claim of personal recovery: Firstly, the introduction of the concept of "the personal" nature of recovery ties this into a legacy of feminist research and argument [2]. Secondly, the word recovery itself is radical—rejecting a historical legacy of mental illness and disorder being seen as untreatable—and, perhaps worse, unmanageable [3]. Moving on from its radical beginning the idea of personal recovery, as a goal for mental health service provision, is perhaps best summarised by one of the most widely cited definitions:

> Recovery is described as a deeply personal, unique process of changing one's attitudes, values, feelings, goals, skills, and/or roles. It is a way of living a satisfying, hopeful, and contributing life even with limitations caused by illness. Recovery involves the development of new meaning and purpose in one's life as one grows beyond the catastrophic effects of mental illness. (Anthony, 1993, p. 527 [4])

This definition has been criticised (for example, in relation to its novelty as a claim [5]) but has been largely accepted and seen as a transformative introduction to the field. Seeking to operationalise the concept into a workable structure a significant piece of research was undertaken by Slade and colleagues [6]—leading to the development of a transtheoretical framework of change in relation to personal recovery [7]. This is often referred to as the CHIMES framework:

- Connectedness
- Hope
- **Identity**
- Meaning
- Empowerment
- Spirituality

For the purpose of the argument in this chapter I would suggest that "identity" can be seen as the core component of this framework—from which each of the other components flows as a facet or emphasis. In this sense then recovery can be understood as a form of *"identity work"*—a process of making sense of personal experience in the face of adversity [8].

4.3 Forensic Settings and Practice

Within England and Wales, through the Royal College of Psychiatry (the organisation responsible for the post-graduate training and certification of psychiatrists—www.rcpsych.ac.uk), forensic psychiatry is defined as: *"…work at the interface between the law and psychiatry, managing patients with mental disorders who have*

4 Personal Recovery Within Forensic Settings

been or have the potential to be, violent." [https://www.rcpsych.ac.uk/become-a-psychiatrist/choose-psychiatry/what-is-psychiatry/types-of-psychiatrist/forensic].

Most forensic psychiatrists will therefore practice in secure hospitals—previously known as special hospitals—these units provide multidisciplinary mental healthcare within a locked setting. Prison psychiatry represents an emerging field of practice and development focusing on the mental health of prisoners. In England and Wales movement between forensic institutions and disposal from court to hospital are handled under a particular section of the Mental Health Act (1983, revised 2007)—known as Part III. A further significant potential role for psychiatrists lies, as above, at the interface with the law—including roles where psychiatrists may be summoned as expert witnesses in relation to ongoing legal proceedings: While beyond the scope of this paper discussion of this role is significant in relation to the concept of recovery calling as it does into focus definitions of power and the role of the mental health professional in relation to a person's experience.

Prisons represent sites of significant mental suffering—with epidemiological studies estimating high levels of mental disorder globally [9]. Rates of deliberate self-harm and suicidal behaviour are also significant [10] and such behaviours are easy to misunderstand or dismiss [11].

Prisons, in a sense, represent a form of community setting in forensic psychiatry—they are chosen here as an illustrative example of a secure environment. A deconstruction of a prison environment would likely highlight the following features: The perimeter wall, gates and doors impeding passage, cells, keys providing access.

The perimeter wall serves a particular function—not simply as a means of containment—but also as the defining boundary for an example of a total institution [12]. Total institutions serve as cultural containers—with the emergence of institutional practice, that is a series of shared practices reaching towards a common goal. In the case of prisons in England and Wales these goals are defined by Her Majesty's Prison and Probation Service (https://www.gov.uk/government/organisations/her-majestys-prison-and-probation-service) as:

- Restriction [preventing escape or free movement]
- Retribution [enacting punishment on behalf of the State]
- Rehabilitation [providing education to allow reintegration into society]
- Restoration [facilitating acts of restorative justice, for example, community service, where appropriate]

Although a controversial point, in England and Wales it is the *loss of time* through incarceration that acts as retribution—not the act of incarceration itself. Beyond containment the perimeter wall serves a wider function—drawing the attention of the general population to the prison, while obscuring the suffering and experience of prisoners within [13].

Inside the prison progress is impeded by the presence of locked doors—keys therefore become a symbol of power and authority within the institution.

4.4 Forensic Recovery

With this context let us now return to the concept of recovery—and particularly recovery in forensic settings. The immediate problems of the concept can be seen through returning to the CHIMES framework:

- Connectedness: By virtue of acts of violence, or potential for violence, people are excluded from their home communities, often with considerable geographical distance. How can connectedness be considered with this restriction and when should this connection be restored?
- Hope: Prisons and other secure settings are often experienced as profoundly hopeless environments.
- Identity: A person introduced into a forensic setting experiences a profound act of personal stigmatisation being marked as a *"forensic patient"* or *"offender"*.
- Meaning: Within prisons and secure settings meaning becomes contested—as discussed in more detail below.
- Empowerment: Secure institutions disempower patients or other residents, for example, through the introduction of locks and gates to impede progress—simultaneously empowering professionals in relation to others.

A systematic review and meta-synthesis, focusing on qualitative research into the process of personal recovery in forensic mental health settings identified three core themes [14]: The need for a sense of safety and security, dynamics of hope during the course of a sentence or hospital admission, and the need for integration with social networks.

Building on the central concept of identity work, outlined above, is perhaps helpful in further illustrating the challenging situation that offenders and forensic psychiatric patients experience. In a sense, offenders going through a court hearing and eventual conviction experienced an enforced identity shift—with the conclusion of a guilty verdict. Without wishing to apologise for criminal acts this represents a form of stigma likely to accompany the individual even after the completion of a prison sentence [15]. Introducing a concept of mental disorder, or substance use, layers on this stigmatised experience—resulting in an experience of double or even triple stigma [16].

Rightly or wrongly therefore the forensic patient's identity if forced—and any act of recovery will have to contend with this. Recovery narratives and experiences in this context may be understood as acts of resistance [17]. Narratives can be understood as a means of expressing personal identity—both to ourselves and to others. Redemption narratives have been shown to have a particular resonance when the act of rehabilitation and *"making good"* in relation to criminal activity are considered [18]. Narrative understanding ties in with the concept of meaning making, and identity work, as outlined in the CHIMES framework and can serve as a helpful means of understanding the experience of offenders who experience mental disorder. Such narratives are, sadly, too often punctuated by acts of trauma and experiences of alienation: There is a pressure therefore to avoid further alienation through the act of incarceration within forensic settings—this is returned to in the concluding section of this essay.

4.5 Particular Issues

Moving beyond this general conceptualisation of recovery in forensic settings we turn now to some of the particular issues that characterise the distress and disorder experienced by individuals within this space, and the challenges facing practitioners.

4.5.1 Ethics

For the past nearly 40 years [19] much of the ethical curriculum in medical education has been dominated by the work of Beauchamp and Childress [20]: Although their approach has been criticised—for example, in relation to the risk of its becoming common ethical understanding as opposed to being drawn from common understanding [21]—the work remains a bulwark for many. Forensic mental health practice raises some key issues in relation to these principles however (for further discussion see Adshead, 2000 [22])—and some of these are highlighted here with a focus on any overlap with the concept of personal recovery.

- Beneficence and Non-maleficence: Acting with the good of the patient in mind seems an uncontroversial aim in medical practice, and this is often held in balance with the need to minimise harm in the pursuit of benefit. In forensic practice there is an essential truth however that any therapeutic interaction essentially introduces a third party—in the form of the wronged state—which complicates the process substantially. How then is the balance of treatment maintained? When an individual, in the context of a mental health crisis, displays aggressive behaviour what is the role of the clinician in managing this? To whom does their responsibility lie? Is there a risk that treatment becomes a means of containing an individual simply within a toxic environment—where mediation of that environment can seem like an impossible endeavour?
- Respect for autonomy: All individuals exist as autonomous agents and respect for that essential dignity and right is essential in all areas of medical practice. Within the CHIMES framework this is captured in the concept of empowerment. How far does this right extend however? An individual suffering from a mental disorder with a relapsing remitting nature may disagree with the benefit of continuous medication and may question the evidence for longitudinal treatment [23]. How can their right to choice in this respect be balanced against a need for public protection however if—in the context once more of a mental health crisis—they have previously acted in a violent manner towards others?

- Justice: In England and Wales the principle of *"equivalence"* is proposed as a means of understanding distribution of resources with respect to prison healthcare [24]. A challenge rises here in terms of interpretation however—does this mean equivalence of resource and treatment availability or equivalence of outcome? If the latter then, given the significant position of disadvantage from which prison populations are drawn, a far larger investment will be required.

4.5.2 Complexity, Co-morbidity and Personality Disruption

Complexity is the norm within forensic healthcare—with individuals often showing signs of distress and need across several different domains of need [25]: For example, an individual may show signs of severe mental illness, such as acute psychosis, exacerbated by personality disorder with dissocial and impulsive traits, and substance misuse. Each of these factors may pose a complication with respect to the understanding an individual's recovery experience and support needs—for example, in relation to personality disorder systematic review has shown that many of the underpinning concepts of personal recovery become problematic [26, 27].

4.5.3 Offending Behaviour

Essential to the nature of experience in forensic mental healthcare is the fact that most patients will have carried out some form of criminal act. This in and of itself can pose a problem for the individual and for any mental health practitioners working to support them—raising challenging interpersonal and intrapersonal psychodynamics [28].

4.6 Future Work and Directions

In this chapter I have attempted to set out the particular issues that arise in relation to the concept of personal recovery in forensic settings. I have argued that placing the concept of identity, and identity work, as central to this process is a helpful means of working to understand individual experience. In this lies the truth that additional work is required to capture the particular experience of individuals within forensic settings—raising them up from beyond the position of subjects to agents in their own rights.

Considering the individual's identity—beyond the experience of mental disorder—also demands particular attention to lived experience, taking account of specific experiences and cultural influences. For example, the experiences of women who offend are radically different from their male counterparts in terms of social response [29] and in terms of their experience within therapy or contact with mental healthcare providers [30, 31].

Recovery narratives are essentially social in their nature—relying as much on audience as performer in terms of credibility [32]—as such forensic recovery focused work must take account of the multiple agencies that are essentially involved in the individual's narrative: For example, courts, parole, probation and wider community and potentially media interest. Building on the idea of connection as essential in recovery it is also important to consider ways in which the individual may wish to forge or re-forge links with their family and social networks. This sense of disconnection, always present for the incarcerated individual, has become more apparent with the atomisation of experience attendant following the emergence of a global viral pandemic [33].

In closing, I set out a proposal for a three-stage process for working in a recovery focussed fashion with individuals in forensic settings:

1. Safety in security: In keeping with Maslow [34] a sense of safety is essential to any therapeutic endeavour and can be provided within forensic environments.
2. Containment and expression: Appropriate witnessing of trauma and containment of this experience is essential in allowing the individual to process trauma in their past.
3. Synthesis and re-direction: Moving beyond their current trapped state allows individuals to develop a new sense of purpose—a positive sense of self, or positive narcissistic construct, in comparison with older internal representations.
4. Individuation and flourishing: Ultimately, as the concept of personal recovery suggests—the act is a personal one and personal narrative accounts and understanding represent a potential means of expressing this growing individuation and sense of eudaimonia [35].

References

1. Howell A, Voronka J. Introduction: the politics of resilience and recovery in mental health care. Stud Soc Justice. 2012;6:1–7.
2. Hanisch C. The personal is political. 2006.
3. Mechanic D. Illness and social disability: some problems in analysis. Sociol Perspect. 1959;2:37–41.
4. Anthony W. Recovery from mental illness: the guiding vision of the mental health service system in the 1990s. Psychosocial Rehabilitation Journal. 1993;16:11–23.
5. Davidson L, O'Connell MJ, Tondora J, Lawless M, Evans AC. Recovery in serious mental illness: a new wine or just a new bottle? Prof Psychology Res Pract. 2005;36:480–7.
6. Slade M, Willia J, Bi V, Leamy M, Boutillier CL. Recovery grows up. J Ment Health. 2012;21:99–103.
7. Leamy M, Bird V, Boutillier CL, Williams J, Slade M. Conceptual framework for personal recovery in mental health: systematic review and narrative synthesis. Brit J Psychiat. 2011;199:445–52.
8. Longden E. Making sense of voices: a personal story of recovery. Psychos. 2010;2:255–9.
9. Fazel S, Baillargeon J. The health of prisoners. Lancet. 2011;377:956–65.
10. Young MH, Justice JV, Erdberg P. Risk of harm: inmates who harm themselves while in prison psychiatric treatment. J Forensic Sci. 2006;51:156–62.

11. Dear GE, Thomson DM, Hills AM. Self-harm in prison. Crim Justice Behav. 2000;27:160–75.
12. Goffman E. Asylums: essays on the social situation of mental patients and other inmates. Doubleday; 1961.
13. Foucault M. Discipline and punish. Gallimard; 1975.
14. Shepherd A, Doyle M, Sanders C, Shaw J. Personal recovery within forensic settings—systematic review and meta-synthesis of qualitative methods studies. Crim Behav Ment Health. 2016;26:59–75.
15. Moore KE, Stuewig JB, Tangney JP. The effect of stigma on criminal offenders' functioning: a longitudinal mediational model. Deviant Behav. 2015;37:196–218.
16. Hartwell S. Triple stigma: persons with mental illness and substance abuse problems in the criminal justice system. Crim Justice Policy Rev. 2004;15:84–99.
17. Nielsen E. Counternarratives of breast cancer and chronic illness: performing disruption, patienthood and narrative repair. Perform Res. 2014;19:97–106.
18. Maruna S. Making good: how ex-convicts reform and rebuild their lives. American Psychological Association. 2001.
19. Rauprich O, Vollmann J. 30 years principles of biomedical ethics: introduction to a symposium on the 6th edition of Tom L Beauchamp and James F Childress' seminal work. J Med Ethics. 2011;37:454.
20. Beauchamp TL, Childress LF. Principles of biomedical ethics. Oxford University Press; 2009.
21. Lee MJH. The problem of 'thick in status, thin in content' in Beauchamp and Childress' principlism. J Med Ethics. 2010;36:525.
22. Adshead G. Care or custody? Ethical dilemmas in forensic psychiatry. J Med Ethics. 2000;26:302.
23. Wunderink L, Nieboer RM, Wiersma D, Sytema S, Nienhuis FJ. Recovery in remitted first-episode psychosis at 7 years of follow-up of an early dose reduction/discontinuation or maintenance treatment strategy: long-term follow-up of a 2-year randomized clinical trial. JAMA Psychiat. 2013;70:913–20.
24. Birmingham L, Wilson S, Adshead G. Prison medicine: ethics and equivalence. Brit J Psychiat. 2006;188:4–6.
25. Forrester A, Till A, Simpson A, Shaw J. Mental illness and the provision of mental health services in prisons. Brit Med Bull. 2018;127:101–9.
26. Shepherd A, Sanders C, Shaw J. Seeking to understand lived experiences of personal recovery in personality disorder in community and forensic settings—a qualitative methods investigation. BMC Psychiatry. 2017;17:282.
27. Shepherd A, Sanders C, Doyle M, Shaw J. Personal recovery in personality disorder: systematic review and meta-synthesis of qualitative methods studies. Int J Soc Psychiatr. 2016;62:41–50.
28. Adshead G. Psychiatric staff as attachment figures. Brit J Psychiat. 1998;172:64–9.
29. Cho S, Crenshaw KW, McCall L. Toward a field of intersectionality studies: theory, applications, and praxis. Signs J Women Cult Soc. 2013;38:785–810.
30. Shaw C, Proctor G. I. Women at the margins: a critique of the diagnosis of borderline personality disorder. Fem Psychol. 2005;15:483–90.
31. Welldon EV. Dancing with death. Br J Psychother. 2009;25:149–82.
32. Hillman A. 'Why must I wait?' The performance of legitimacy in a hospital emergency department. Sociol Health Ill. 2014;36:485–99.
33. Hewson T, Shepherd A, Hard J, Shaw J. Effects of the COVID-19 pandemic on the mental health of prisoners. Lancet Psychiatry. 2020;7:568–70.
34. Maslow AH. A theory of human motivation. Psychol Rev. 1943;50:370–96.
35. Bauer JJ, McAdams DP, Pals JL. Narrative identity and eudaimonic well-being. J Happiness Stud. 2008;9:81–104.

Stigma and Attitude Towards Personal Recovery from Mental Illness Among Italian Mental Health Professionals

5

Rita Roncone ⓘ, Laura Giusti ⓘ, Valeria Bianchini ⓘ, Anna Salza ⓘ, and Massimo Casacchia ⓘ

5.1 Introduction

In the area of mental health, "recovery" is characterized by two distinct connotations used to refer to an individual personal "process" and an outcome, particularly following the widespread adoption of "recovery" as a target treatment for people affected by mental illness.

Personal recovery has been defined as "a way of living a satisfying, hopeful, and contributing life even in the presence of limitations caused by illness" [1]. In contrast to *clinical or social recovery*, comprising a reduction or absence of symptoms and a significant improvement in occupational and social functioning, *personal recovery* is a process that individuals go through to live a satisfying life and achieve life goals [2], a process of helping people to live a life "beyond illness"—i.e., to recover a meaningful life, with or without symptoms is the traditional meaning applied to "personal" recovery [3].

Indeed, the recent definition of "personal recovery" [4], *"Recovery is defined by the person themself and not other people's definition of what recovery means,"*

R. Roncone (✉)
Department of Life, Health and Environmental Sciences, University of L'Aquila, L'Aquila, Italy

Hospital S. Salvatore, University Unit Rehabilitation Treatment, Early Interventions in Mental Health, L'Aquila, Italy
e-mail: rita.roncone@univaq.it

L. Giusti · V. Bianchini · A. Salza · M. Casacchia
Department of Life, Health and Environmental Sciences, University of L'Aquila, L'Aquila, Italy
e-mail: laura.giusti@univaq.it; valeria.bianchini@univaq.it; anna.salza@univaq.it; massimo.casacchia@univaq.it

© The Author(s), under exclusive license to Springer Nature
Switzerland AG 2022
B. Carpiniello et al. (eds.), *Recovery and Major Mental Disorders*,
Comprehensive Approach to Psychiatry 2,
https://doi.org/10.1007/978-3-030-98301-7_5

seems to make it more difficult to scientifically investigate this important construct that has garnered considerable attention over the last two decades. Based on a recent systematic review and meta-analysis of factors associated with personal recovery in people with a psychotic disorder, meaning in life, empowerment, and hope seem to be the main dimensions on which to focus [5].

In Italy, the term "recovery," borrowed from the English language, is present in the everyday language of mental health professionals, and is highly popular in mental health services focused on becoming recovery-oriented. Numerous parallelisms can be identified between the relatively "new," "recovery-orientated" approach and the Italian community psychiatry established by Law 180. Over the last 40 years, following the abolishment of mental hospitals, Italy has seen a progressive consolidation of a community-based system of mental healthcare [6]; indeed, continuity of care provided in the context of the subject's life domain and multi-professional care represent the main approach in the psychiatric care of severe mental disorders in a psychosocial rehabilitation setting [7].

Despite the relevant interregional variability, development of the Individual Treatment Plan (ITP), based on the user's personal goals rather than those imposed by professionals, represents an important step not only from a clinical perspective, but also at a social and functional level in terms of quality of life, care needs, and user satisfaction for the treatments received, in what could be defined as "the recovery process."

Although not particularly frequent in Italy, qualitative research, innovative experiences of peer support, accounts from a "first-person" and "evidence-based hope" perspective have contributed to the understanding of the paradigm of recovery in severe mental illness [8–10].

In an Italian context, further impetus to the recovery process was provided by multicentric research involving several Mental Health Services that confirmed the validity of the Italian version of the Recovery Assessment Scale (RAS) [11], an instrument developed to detect recovery among users [12]. This Italian Study on Recovery demonstrated the ability of RAS to identify users matching the "in recovery" operational criteria and offered an outcome measure on which to base a recovery-oriented transformation [12, 13].

Our work will examine the "state of the art" of barriers and orientation relating to the recovery principles of mental health professionals in an Italian context. In particular, a lack of theoretical clarity over the practical provision of support recovery hampers the implementation of policies aimed at addressing this ambitious goal.

5.2 Attitudes and Stigma Displayed by Mental Health Professionals Towards the Mentally Ill: Selected Studies Conducted in Italian Facilities

Stigmas relating to mental illness seem to be widely endorsed by the general public [14], with those affected being challenged by the stereotypes and prejudice resulting from misconceptions of mental disorders.

Negative attitudes, such as discrimination, frustration, and lack of respect, at times displayed even by health professionals, may lead to poor health outcomes in those targeted [15, 16], thus representing a major barrier to consumer and carer participation and overall improvement of health [17].

An inverse relationship has been found between recovery orientation and stigmatizing attitudes, in the sense that recovery-oriented individuals may display less negative attitudes with regard to people affected by mental disorders [18]. Stigma represents a major barrier in preventing patients affected by mental disorders from seeking help or achieving personal recovery [19]. Stigmatizing attitudes may also be detected among mental health professionals, thus exerting negative effects on the quality of healthcare [20]. Several interesting Italian studies investigating the attitudes and stigma displayed by mental health professionals towards the mentally ill will be briefly described.

Attitudes displayed by psychiatric nurses and mental health professionals towards patients affected by mental disorders present in a series of different care settings in an Italian healthcare facility were investigated by Cremonini et al. [21]. The authors of the study used the Italian version [22] of the Community Attitudes Mentally Ill inventory (CAMI-I) [23] to investigate authoritarian attitudes, benevolence, and social restrictiveness, and revealed how healthcare professionals displayed fluctuating levels of sensitivity and positive attitudes towards mental illness. Varying attitudes were found to exist between psychiatric care units: healthcare professionals employed on the psychiatric ward displayed less positive attitudes, whereas staff working in the mental health daycare center held more positive views on mental illness. The authors hypothesized that their findings may have been influenced by resource organization, staff-user interaction, care provider stress levels, and the high complexity of users on an acute psychiatric ward [21].

Another European study used the Community Attitudes Mentally Ill inventory (CAMI-I) to compare attitudes towards mental illness and investigate potential differences based on type of professional category, setting and country across a large sample of professionals (1525) working in a wide range of mental health facilities run by a non-profit mental health organization (Sisters Hospitallers) in Spain, Portugal, and Italy [24]. The study included compilation of the Attribution Questionnaire (AQ-27) [25], validated in Italian by Pingani [26]. The AQ-27 provides a vignette about a man with schizophrenia and comprises 27 items that evaluate respective assertions related to the hypothetical case. The AQ-27 evaluates nine factors: (1) personal responsibility; (2) anger; (3) pity; (4) help (provision of assistance to people with mental illness); (5) dangerousness; (6) fear; (7) avoidance; (8) segregation; and (9) coercion. Psychologists and social therapists displayed the most positive attitudes, while nursing assistants the most negative. Community staff displayed more positive attitudes than hospital-based professionals [24]. Comparison of the three countries at AQ-27 revealed how Spanish professionals had the highest inference of attribution of responsibility for the illness and more coercive approaches, but felt more pity and less fear than the other two groups. On the other hand, Italian professionals were at the lowest end of the dimensions of pity and help, and ranked highest in avoidant behaviors. Anger, perceived dangerousness, and segregation did not significantly differ throughout the three countries. On the CAMI scale, Spanish professionals showed more positive attitudes towards benevolence and communitarian ideology, the Italians were the least supportive of community treatment and most supportive of social restriction, while the Portuguese ranked highest in authoritarianism.

Given the primary role of community care within the Italian mental health services, these findings are surprising and confirm the data reported by Chambers et al. [27] from a study conducted on a sample of nurses from five European countries. At the CMHI subscale, Portuguese nurses were found to be significantly more positive about community care than Italian nurses [27].

An association between stigma and personality was observed in an Italian study of mental health professionals working across six Community Mental Health Services (CMHS) in North-East Italy [28]. The personality trait of openness to new experiences was seen to determine lower levels of stigma. People scoring higher on openness may be more prone to developing positive contact experiences and proving more willing to try to understand the feelings of individuals affected by mental disorders. They seem to be more prone to a positive and recovery-oriented attitude, which in turn has been associated with lower levels of stigma [29]. The study highlighted how higher levels of burnout were associated with more negative views of patients, in particular those displaying lower emotional stability [28]. A previous study had addressed a possible connection between personality traits, burnout dimensions, and stigmatizing attitudes in mental health professionals [30]. Perception of poor workplace safety was found to produce a significant negative effect on the burnout dimension of personal efficacy, and, indirectly, negative attitudes towards users. The presence of institutional responses at CMHS to risk situations (namely, protocols for the management of aggressive or violent behaviors) was associated with a higher level of personal efficacy. Emotional Stability and Openness to new experiences were inversely correlated with burnout dimensions and avoidant attitudes, respectively [30].

5.3 Assessment of Staff Knowledge and Attitudes Towards Recovery Principles

For the purpose of operationalizing recovery and assessing the extent of understanding and implementation of the recovery concept, a series of measures were developed to evaluate the knowledge of mental health professionals and their attitudes towards recovery. Studies conducted using both qualitative and quantitative measurement methods have been reported in the literature. We describe below the widely used quantitative scales, deemed to be evidence-based by a very recently published review [31].

5.3.1 Quantitative Methods

A frequently used tool among the quantitative methods is represented by the **Recovery Knowledge Inventory (RKI)**, a questionnaire developed in the United States addressed to evaluating more recovery-oriented health services [32]. The original 36-item scale was reduced to 20 items. The RKI consists of 20 items on a 5-point Likert scale and assesses four different domains of understanding on recovery in mental health: (1) *"Roles and responsibilities in recovery"* (seven items; range score 7–35), relating to risk-taking, decision-making, and the various roles and responsibilities of people in recovery and behavioral health providers, respectively (e.g., people with mental illness should not be burdened with the responsibilities of everyday life); (2) *"Non-linearity of the recovery process"* (six items; range score 6–30), regarding the role of illness and symptom management and the non-linear nature of recovery (e.g., recovery is characterized by a person making gradual steps forward with no major steps back); (3) *"Roles of self-definition and peers in recovery"* (five items; range score 5–25), focusing on the activities undertaken by an affected individual to define an identity for him/herself and a life that goes beyond that of "mental patient," including the valuable roles that peers can play in this process (e.g., the pursuit of hobbies and leisure activities is important for recovery); and (4) *"Expectations regarding recovery"* (two items; range score 2–10), relating to expectations (e.g., not everyone is capable of actively participating in the recovery process). Fifteen out of 20 items are reverse-coded. The maximum score for the 20 items is 100 (range 20–100). Higher scores represent a greater orientation to the concept of recovery (cutoff scores are not reported in the literature).

The **Recovery Attitude Questionnaire (RAQ-7)** is a self-administered instrument developed in the United States by the Recovery Initiative Research Team, consisting of a group of mental health users, mental health professionals, and graduate students and researchers from Hamilton County (Ohio) intended to measure the attitudes displayed towards mental health recovery by a range of stakeholders, including consumers, health professionals, family members, or significant others, and community members [33].

The questionnaire contributes towards assessing feelings relating to recovery and monitoring adherence to the principles of recovery by mental health services. The original 21-item scale was reduced to 7 items, and the addition of a further two items to measure "somewhat unconventional attitudes about mental illness and its treatment but which are important to the idea of recovery." The questionnaire identifies two factors: (1) *"Recovery is possible and needs faith"* (e.g., recovery is possible even if the symptoms of mental illness persist; recovery from mental illness is possible no matter what you think may be the cause; (2) *Recovery is difficult and differs from person to person* (e.g., Stigma associated with mental illness may slow down the recovery process; people differ as to how they recover from a mental illness). The RAQ includes a brief introduction based on the concept of recovery defined by William Anthony [1]. Each item is measured on a 5-point scale ranging from 1, strongly disagree, to 5, strongly agree. Concurrent validity was also found in that consumer respondents who identified themselves as being in recovery, and who were in recovery for longer periods, displayed the most favorable attitudes to recovery [33]. Higher total scores indicate a more positive attitude to the concept of recovery.

The **Recovery approach staff questionnaire** [34] is a structured self-report measure developed by the Southwark Recovery Approach Implementation Group, which included an ex-service user, specifically created for application in forensic services, although the content was guided by published work on the recovery approach [35, 36], where the focus is on teaching and training service users. It consists of 50 closed questions investigating the individual's knowledge and understanding of the principles of the recovery approach and social inclusion. Apart from item 2 ("*I have attended a training course on the recovery approach to care*," which was rated either as "true" or "false" and was the key predictor in the research), the remaining 49 items were rated on a three-point scale: true (3), not sure (2), and false (1). The scoring was reversed for items requiring a negative endorsement: false (3), not sure (2), and true (1). The maximum score for the 49 questions was 147 (range 49–147).

The **Staff attitudes to Recovery Scale (STARS)** is a self-rating instrument consisting of 19 items, developed by Crowe et al. [37] to evaluate staff attitudes and hopefulness related to the goal striving and recovery possibilities for the mental health consumers with whom they work. Principles and constructs that influenced item construction included the interrelatedness of hope, goal setting, and recovery. Three of the STARS items address general hopefulness (e.g., "*All of these clients are capable of positive change*"). Eight items were adapted from the Adult Dispositional Hope Scale [38] (e.g., "*There are lots of ways around any problem*" became "*There are lots of ways to deal with any problems that these clients have*"). Each item was rated on a 5-point scale ranging from 1, strongly disagree, to 5, strongly agree. Scores range from 19 to 95, with higher scores reflecting more positive and hopeful attitudes.

The collaborative **Recovery Knowledge scale**, developed by Crowe et al. [37], consists of 13 multiple-choice items related to knowledge of the key principles and intervention characteristics representing components of the collaborative recovery model that provides an integrative framework combining (a) evidence-based practice; (b) manageable and modularized competencies relevant to case management and psychosocial rehabilitation contexts; and (c) recognition of the subjective experiences of consumers [39]. Sample questions follow: "*Research evidence demonstrates that well-being is related to: a) achieving as many goals as possible, b) achieving autonomous goals, c) not having goals, or d) having only one goal*" and "*Resistance is: a) a treatment opportunity, b) always an obstacle, c) the client's fault, d) proof the client is not motivated, or e) evidence that treatment is failing.*" Each item answered correctly was scored as 1, incorrect items were scored as 0. Possible scores range from 0 to 13, with higher scores indicating better knowledge.

The **Wellness Recovery Action Plan (WRAP) questionnaire** is a self-assessment tool administered to consumers and mental health professionals to evaluate their attitudes towards and knowledge of recovery after attending a WRAP workshop in New Zealand [40]. The tool represents a 5-point Likert-type rating scale (1 = strongly disagree, 5 = strongly agree) consisting of 16 items (e.g., *"I believe that for some recovery is not possible"; "People who experience mental illness should have the opportunity to choose what treatment they will receive"; "I understand what is meant by peer support"; "It is important that non-consumers know about mental health recovery concepts"; "People who experience mental illness should decide whether or not family members and significant others are to be consulted regarding their treatment and recovery process"*).

The two items that vary to allow a negative acceptation are *"I believe that for some recovery is not possible"* and *"The opinions of health professionals should be given more weight than a person receiving treatment,"* both of which were reversed items.

5.4 Measures of Recovery Orientation in Mental Health Services

In addition to investigating the recovery orientation of mental health professionals, numerous measures have been developed to assess the recovery orientation of mental health services. In their systematic review of measures relating to the recovery orientation of mental health services, Williams et al. [41] selected papers in a conceptual framework of recovery comprising five recovery processes: connectedness; hope and optimism; identity; meaning and purpose; and empowerment (CHIME). Comparisons between the measures were hampered by the use of a series of different models of recovery and by the lack of uniformity on the level of organization at which services were assessed [41].

Among the six instruments considered in their review, we selected the **Recovery Self-Assessment (RSA)** [42], which includes 4 different versions for persons in recovery, significant others, service providers, and service directors. The 36-item RSA was developed to "go beyond rhetoric into the routine" in an attempt to assess changes in practice. The scale was intended to reflect objective practices associated with the conceptual domains of recovery: indicators, such as the involvement of service users in management meetings and staff education, activities geared towards expanding social networks and social roles, degree of service user choice and self-determination, and staff attitudes and philosophy towards recovery. Factor analysis revealed five factors: *Life Goals, Involvement, Diversity of Treatment Options, Choice*, and *Individually-Tailored Services.*

Mental health professionals, persons in recovery, and family members generally agreed that their agencies were providing services consistent with recovery orientation, although "providers" assigned significantly lower ratings to three of the five factors, e.g., Life Goals, Involvement, and Individually-Tailored Services. The authors highlighted their efforts to operationalize the principles of recovery into objective practices, offering an effective tool to contribute towards strengthening collaborative evaluation-stakeholder feedback loops [42].

5.5 Italian Study of the Knowledge of and Attitudes Displayed Towards Personal Recovery from Mental Illness by Mental Health Operators

Within the context of Italian psychiatry, the values and recovery-oriented practices of which stemmed largely from the Law of 1978, the authors were keen to verify how closely mental health professionals adhered to the model proposed by the RKI, an internationally recognized tool for use in the assessment of "recovery." The aims of our study were (1) to examine the knowledge of and attitudes displayed towards the concept of personal recovery by Italian mental health professionals and students enrolled in the graduate studies course in psychiatric rehabilitation [43] through administration of a questionnaire survey based on the Recovery Knowledge Inventory (RKI) [44], and (2) to examine the differences among mental health professionals and students in understanding recovery domains [45].

An extensive sample of 436 Italian mental health operators, including 349 professionals from Italian Services and 87 students from Italian Universities, recruited during mental health and psychiatric rehabilitation meetings and conferences, were included in the study [44]. The abovementioned survey also included a specific schedule comprising questions relating to the respondent's professional role, gender, age, level of experience (years), work setting, and questions regarding previous exposure to recovery information and training.

Three groups of mental health operators were evaluated: the first group represented 23% of the total sample and consisted of 100 psychiatrists (50% women; mean age = 49.3, SD = 11.8); the second group of 249 mental health professionals represented 57% of the total sample (nurses, social workers, psychologists, psychiatric rehabilitation technicians, and others, 82% women; mean age = 42.5, SD = 12), and the third group consisting of 87 students of psychiatric rehabilitation techniques (79% women; mean age = 24.6, SD = 5.6) represented 20% of the total sample. The position of Psychiatric Rehabilitation Technician (PRT) refers to an Italian mental-health academic and professional specifically trained in conducting psychosocial interventions, which was created in the wake of the Law 180 [43]. Approximately 57% of participants were working as part of community mental health teams, while 20% were working on acute psychiatric inpatient wards. The majority of participants had received no formal training in personal recovery principles, with those who had previously been exposed to this concept having gained their knowledge by means of informal methods rather than structured programs.

Recovery orientation was reported as "low recovery orientation" and "high recovery orientation." No statistically significant differences in the level of overall orientation towards personal recovery were found among the three groups, as measured by RKI total score. Over the 40 years since the introduction of Law 180 in 1978, which abolished psychiatric hospitals and sought to integrate psychiatric care within the social context of the community, Italian psychiatrists, mental health operators, and students of mental health have come to reflect a recovery-oriented biopsychosocial perspective in their attitudes and their work. Professionals appeared to agree on the principles of user identity, treatment involvement based on their goals, and the validity of support received from individuals affected by mental disorders. However, the same professionals seemed to encounter difficulty in accepting users' well-being "beyond" treatment adherence, and "non-linearity" of the individual "journey" undertaken to achieve personal recovery, viewing psychopathological stability as a key factor.

With regard to *gender-related differences*, women seemed to be more favorable towards accepting the decision-making of consumers and risk-taking in planning their lives (*"Roles and responsibilities in recovery"*) compared to men. In our sample, more than two-thirds of the professionals investigated were women, with the highest percentage of male respondents being represented by psychiatrists. Compared to the other two groups, the older groups of psychiatrists with greater work experience comprised a higher percentage of men. The scarce propensity among male psychiatrists included in the study to acknowledge the issue of "therapeutic risk" for their users may be linked to the potential of professional liability in the medical profession, a highly relevant issue in modern-day Italy. Indeed, recent sentences issued by the Italian courts for crimes such as manslaughter have reiterated the culpability of psychiatrists in view of their obligations of custody and constant monitoring of users in their various care settings, thus prompting a more cautious attitude among mental health professionals [46–48].

Differences between less experienced (respondents with fewer than 15 years' experience in the field of mental health) and *more experienced professionals* were detected with regard to *"expectations of recovery."* Less-experienced staff and graduate students enrolled in psychiatric rehabilitation courses displayed more positive attitudes and knowledge compared to the more experienced respondents with regard to expectations of recovery. Compared to their more experienced colleagues, younger mental health operators and students were characterized by a higher degree of cognitive openness and flexibility, in contrast therefore with the low consumer expectations expressed by the older professionals, which could potentially result in delayed recovery and encourage learned helplessness (Roberts & Wolfson, 2004).

5.6 Conclusions

The absence of institutional responses to situations of risk (namely, protocols for the management of aggressive or violent users) and the professional liability impinging on psychiatrists are heavily linked, the former resulting in negative attitudes towards users, and the latter placing limitations on acknowledging users' rights "to take the risk" they choose, a "milestone" principle in the personal recovery paradigm.

An improved understanding of the concept underlying the personal recovery paradigm would provide an incentive for all mental health professionals to decrease stigmatization and improve their attitudes towards individuals with mental disorders in daily clinical practice. This, in turn, would contribute towards fostering a recovery-oriented reorganization of mental health services.

Although numerous mental health services would tend to assert their "recovery-oriented" status, it is uncommon in everyday clinical practice to witness a focus on the empowerment, identity, meaning, and resilience of facility users [49]. The journey to recovery among the users of mental health services would benefit greatly from an enhanced awareness of hope, empowerment, and meaning in life [5] supported by the relevant mental health professionals. The latter may indeed require time to gain familiarity with the model of personal recovery, but may hopefully already display an effective community-based psychiatry, recovery-oriented biopsychosocial perspective in their attitudes and work.

The principles of recovery, self-determination, and other evidence-based practices for individuals affected by psychiatric disorders should be integrated into professional training courses and medical, social, and behavioral sciences curricula [50], with the aim of disseminating and adding further impetus to the "recovery model" underlying the existing practices envisaged by the Italian Department of Mental Health, with the key goal of fostering inclusion and citizenship of the mentally ill and duly acknowledging their rights to live satisfying lives.

References

1. Anthony WA. Recovery from mental illness: the guiding vision of the mental health system in the 1990s. Innov Res. 1993;2:17–24.
2. Lemos-Giraldez S, Garcia-Alvarez L, Paino M, Fonseca-Pedrero E, Vallina-Fernandez O, Vallejo-Seco G, et al. Measuring stages of recovery from psychosis. Compr Psychiatry. 2015;56:51–8.
3. Slade M. Personal recovery and mental illness: a guide for mental health professionals. Cambridge, UK: Cambridge University Press; 2009.
4. Patel V, Saxena S, Lund C, Thornicroft G, Baingana F, Bolton P, et al. The Lancet Commission on global mental health and sustainable development. Lancet. 2018;392(10157):1553–98.
5. Leendertse JCP, Wierdsma AI, van den Berg D, Ruissen AM, Slade M, Castelein S, et al. Personal recovery in people with a psychotic disorder: a systematic review and meta-analysis of associated factors. Front Psych. 2021;12:622628.
6. Barbui C, Papola D, Saraceno B. Forty years without mental hospitals in Italy. Int J Ment Health Syst. 2018;12:43.
7. Vita A, Corrivetti G, Mannu J, Semisa D, Vigano C. Psychosocial rehabilitation in Italy Today. Int J Ment Health. 2016;45(1):15–23.
8. Basso L, Boggian I, Carozza P, Lamonaca D, Svettini A. Recovery in Italy: an update. Int J Ment Health. 2016;45(1):71–88.
9. Tibaldi G, Govers L. Evidence-based hope. A common perspective proposal. Psichiatria di Comunità. 2009;VIII(3):117–27.
10. Davidson L, Borg M, Marin I, Topor A, Mezzina R, Sells D. Processes of recovery in serious mental illness: findings from a multinational study. Am J Psychiatr Rehabil. 2005;8(3):177–201.
11. Corrigan P, Salzer M, Ralph RO, Sangster Y, Keck L. Examining the factor structure of the recovery assessment scale. Schizophr Bull. 2004;30(4):1035–41.
12. Boggian I, Lamonaca D, Ghisi M, Bottesi G, Svettini A, Basso L, et al. "The Italian study on recovery 2" phase 1: psychometric properties of the Recovery Assessment Scale (RAS), Italian validation of the recovery assessment scale. Front Psych. 2019;10:1000.
13. Boggian I, Lamonaca D, Svettini A, Ghisi M, Gruppo SIR. Studio Italiano sul Recovery—SIR. Fase 1: applicazione italiana della Recovery Assessment Scale. Psichiatria di Comunità. 2011;X(1):38–48.
14. Corrigan PW, Watson AC. Understanding the impact of stigma on people with mental illness. World Psychiatry. 2002;1(1):16–20.

15. Klages D, Usher K, Jackson D. 'Canaries in the mine'. Parents of adult children with schizophrenia: an integrative review of the literature. Int J Ment Health Nurs. 2017;26(1):5–19.
16. Goodwin V, Happell B. Consumer and carer participation in mental health care: the carer's perspective: part 1—the importance of respect and collaboration. Issues Ment Health Nurs. 2007;28(6):607–23.
17. World Health Organization. Recovery and the right to health. WHO QualityRights Core training: mental health and social services. Course guide. Geneva: World Health Organization; 2019.
18. Stacy MA, Rosenheck R. The association of recovery orientation and stigmatizing beliefs. J Ment Health. 2019;28(3):276–81.
19. Henderson C, Noblett J, Parke H, Clement S, Caffrey A, Gale-Grant O, et al. Mental health-related stigma in health care and mental health-care settings. Lancet Psychiat. 2014;1(6):467–82.
20. Lauber C, Anthony M, Ajdacic-Gross V, Rossler W. What about psychiatrists' attitude to mentally ill people? Eur Psychiatry. 2004;19(7):423–7.
21. Cremonini V, Pagnucci N, Giacometti F, Rubbi I. Health care professionals attitudes towards mental illness: observational study performed at a public health facility in Northern Italy. Arch Psychiatr Nurs. 2018;32(1):24–30.
22. Buizza C, Pioli R, Ponteri M, Vittorielli M, Corradi A, Minicuci N, et al. Community attitudes towards mental illness and socio-demographic characteristics: an Italian study. Epidemiol Psichiat Soc. 2005;14(3):154–62.
23. Taylor SM, Dear MJ. Scaling community attitudes toward the mentally ill. Schizophr Bull. 1981;7(2):225–40.
24. Del Olmo-Romero F, Gonzalez-Blanco M, Sarro S, Gracio J, Martin-Carrasco M, Martinez-Cabezon AC, et al. Mental health professionals' attitudes towards mental illness: professional and cultural factors in the INTER NOS study. Eur Arch Psychiatry Clin Neurosci. 2019;269(3):325–39.
25. Corrigan P, Markowitz FE, Watson A, Rowan D, Kubiak MA. An attribution model of public discrimination towards persons with mental illness. J Health Soc Behav. 2003;44(2):162–79.
26. Pingani L, Forghieri M, Ferrari S, Ben-Zeev D, Artoni P, Mazzi F, et al. Stigma and discrimination toward mental illness: translation and validation of the Italian version of the Attribution Questionnaire-27 (AQ-27-I). Soc Psychiatry Psychiatr Epidemiol. 2012;47(6):993–9.
27. Chambers M, Guise V, Valimaki M, Botelho MAR, Scott A, Staniuliene V, et al. Nurses' attitudes to mental illness: a comparison of a sample of nurses from five European countries. Int J Nurs Stud. 2010;47(3):350–62.
28. Solmi M, Granziol U, Danieli A, Frasson A, Meneghetti L, Ferranti R, et al. Predictors of stigma in a sample of mental health professionals: network and moderator analysis on gender, years of experience, personality traits, and levels of burnout. Eur Psychiatry. 2020;63(1):e4.
29. Barczyk AN. Relationship between the public's belief in recovery, level of mental illness stigma, and previous contact. Community Ment Health J. 2015;51(1):38–47.
30. Zaninotto L, Rossi G, Daniel A, Frasson A, Meneghetti L, Zordan M, et al. Exploring the relationships among personality traits, burnout dimensions and stigma in a sample of mental health professionals. Psychiatry Res. 2018;264:327–33.
31. Gyamfi N, Bhullar N, Islam MS, Usher K. Knowledge and attitudes of mental health professionals and students regarding recovery: a systematic review. Int J Ment Health Nurs. 2020;29(3):322–47.
32. Davidson L, O'Connell MJ, Tondora J, Lawless M, Evans AC. Recovery in serious mental illness: a new wine or just a new bottle? Prof Psychol-Res Pr. 2005;36(5):480–7.
33. Borkin JR, Steffen JJ, Ensfield LB, Krzton K, Wishnick H, Wilder K, et al. Recovery attitudes questionnaire: development and evaluation. Psychiatr Rehabil J. 2000;24(2):95–102.
34. Gudjonsson GH, Webster G, Green T. The recovery approach to care in psychiatric services: staff attitudes before and after training. Psychiatrist. 2018;34(8):326–9.
35. Rapper J, Perkins R. Social inclusion and recovery: an approach for mental health practice. 1st ed. Bailliere-Tindall; 2003.
36. England NIfMHi. NIMHE guiding statement on recovery. 2005.

37. Crowe TP, Deane FP, Oades LG, Caputi P, Morland KG. Effectiveness of a collaborative recovery training program in Australia in promoting positive views about recovery. Psychiatr Serv. 2006;57(10):1497–500.
38. Snyder CR, Harris C, Anderson JR, Holleran SA, Irving LM, Sigmon ST, et al. The will and the ways: development and validation of an individual-differences measure of hope. J Pers Soc Psychol. 1991;60(4):570–85.
39. Oades L, Deane F, Crowe T, Lambert WG, Kavanagh D, Lloyd C. Collaborative recovery: an integrative model for working with individuals who experience chronic and recurring mental illness. Australas Psychiatry. 2005;13(3):279–84.
40. Doughty C, Tse S, Duncan N, McIntyre L. The Wellness Recovery Action Plan (WRAP): workshop evaluation. Australas Psychiatry. 2008;16(6):450–6.
41. Williams J, Leamy M, Bird V, Harding C, Larsen J, Le Boutillier C, et al. Measures of the recovery orientation of mental health services: systematic review. Soc Psychiatry Psychiatr Epidemiol. 2012;47(11):1827–35.
42. O'Connell M, Tondora J, Croog G, Evans A, Davidson L. From rhetoric to routine: assessing perceptions of recovery-oriented practices in a state mental health and addiction system. Psychiatr Rehabil J. 2005;28(4):378–86.
43. Roncone R, Ussorio D, Salza A, Casacchia M. Psychiatric rehabilitation in Italy: Cinderella no more—the contribution of psychiatric rehabilitation technicians. Int J Ment Health. 2016;45(1):24–31.
44. Bedregal LE, O'Connell M, Davidson L. The recovery knowledge inventory: assessment of mental health staff knowledge and attitudes about recovery. Psychiatr Rehabil J. 2006;30(2):96–103.
45. Giusti L, Ussorio D, Salza A, Malavolta M, Aggio A, Bianchini V, et al. Italian investigation on mental health workers' attitudes regarding personal recovery from mental illness. Community Ment Health J. 2019;55(4):680–5.
46. Terranova C, Rocca G. Homicide committed by psychiatric patients: psychiatrists' liability in Italian law cases. Med Sci Law. 2016;56(1):58–64.
47. Terranova C, Sartore D. Suicide and psychiatrist's liability in Italian law cases. J Forensic Sci. 2013;58(2):523–6.
48. Montanari Vergallo G, Zaami S, Di Luca NM, Bersani G, Rinaldi R. Italian law n. 24/2017 on physicians' criminal liability: a reform that does not solve the problems of the psychiatric practice. Riv Psichiatr. 2017;52(6):213–9.
49. Maj M, van Os J, De Hert M, Gaebel W, Galderisi S, Green MF, et al. The clinical characterization of the patient with primary psychosis aimed at personalization of management. World Psychiatry. 2021;20(1):4–33.
50. Razzano LA, Jonikas JA, Goelitz MA, Hamilton MM, Marvin R, Jones-Martinez N, et al. The recovery education in the academy program: transforming academic curricula with the principles of recovery and self-determination. Psychiatr Rehabil J. 2010;34(2):130–6.

Psychosocial Recovery-Oriented Interventions in Schizophrenia

6

Stefano Barlati, Valentina Regina, Giacomo Deste, Alessandro Galluzzo, Cesare Turrina, Paolo Valsecchi, and Antonio Vita

6.1 Background

The deinstitutionalization occurred in the second half of the twentieth century in Europe and high-income countries modified the Mental Health Care System (MHCS) and how schizophrenia is understood and treated [1]. Priority has been given to outpatient care and community-based services due to the reduction of psychiatric beds. Not all countries have managed to develop adequate community mental health programmes. Many of them continued to invest in traditional services and only a minority of patients received appropriate outpatients' treatment and evidence-based, person-centred psychiatric rehabilitation interventions [1]. At that time two models have challenged the Kraepelian assumption that schizophrenia is a biological and unchangeable disease: the "Recovery Model" and the "Stress-Vulnerability Model" [2]. According to the latter theory, schizophrenia is determined by genetics and environmental insults. This suggests that the illness trajectory could be

---

S. Barlati · C. Turrina · P. Valsecchi
Department of Mental Health and Addiction Services, ASST Spedali Civili of Brescia, Brescia, Italy

Department of Clinical and Experimental Sciences, University of Brescia, Brescia, Italy
e-mail: stefano.barlati@unibs.it; cesare.turrina@unibs.it; paolo.valsecchi@unibs.it

V. Regina · A. Vita (✉)
Department of Clinical and Experimental Sciences, University of Brescia, Brescia, Italy
e-mail: regina.vale92@gmail.com; antonio.vita@unibs.it

G. Deste · A. Galluzzo
Department of Mental Health and Addiction Services, ASST Spedali Civili of Brescia, Brescia, Italy
e-mail: giacomodeste@mac.com; alessandrogalluzzo@gmail.com

© The Author(s), under exclusive license to Springer Nature
Switzerland AG 2022
B. Carpiniello et al. (eds.), *Recovery and Major Mental Disorders*,
Comprehensive Approach to Psychiatry 2,
https://doi.org/10.1007/978-3-030-98301-7_6

modified and relapses and hospitalization could be prevented by lowering biological vulnerability or reducing stress [2]. Psychiatric rehabilitative interventions have been developed on this principle. The purpose of these interventions is helping individuals suffering from severe and persistent mental disorders to develop the intellectual, emotional and social skills and the conditions necessary to live, learn and work in the community with the minimum amount of professional support [3]. Recovery from mental illness is no more only the absence of symptoms, but also a return to normal functioning and the attainment of a meaningful and valued life for patients [3]. Psychosocial functioning is therefore defined as patients' ability to fulfil their role in society as members of a family or as professional workers [4]. Functional outcome is undoubtedly impaired in severe mental ill patients [5]. A lot of studies investigated the factors that affect functional outcomes in psychiatric consumers. Neurocognition is one of the first factors described, along with functional capacity and social cognition [6]. Symptoms have been associated with functional outcomes, with negative symptoms appearing to interfere more than positive ones [7]. Quality of life (QoL), occupation, family, leisure time, other elements of daily living, finances, physical and mental health are the variables on which to intervene [4]. In this scenario, psychosocial interventions—working on all these variables— in add on drugs and psychotherapy, find an important role in improving functioning in patients with schizophrenia [5]. Psychosocial interventions aim to potentiate the effect of pharmacological treatment and are focused on specific areas of personal functioning, in order to improve the clinical outcome and contribute to reduce the number of relapses and hospitalizations [8].

6.1.1 Evidence-Based Psychosocial Practices

Evidence-based psychosocial practices (EBPs) refer to interventions demonstrated to be effective at improving the outcome of schizophrenia, based on multiple randomized controlled trials (RCTs) with at least two of them conducted by different research groups [9]. EBPs need the standardization of interventions and require taking into account the most relevant symptoms of the disorder and/or its psychosocial functioning as outcome measures [2, 10]. In 1992, the Agency for Health Care Policy and Research and the National Institute of Mental Health funded the Schizophrenia Patient Outcome Research Team (PORT) to spread recommendations for the treatment of schizophrenia based on scientific evidence [11]. In 2004, this team published a consensus list of EBPs that includes 14 pharmacological treatments and six psychosocial interventions [12]. The latter enclose psychoeducation (PE), family interventions, supported employment (SE), social skills training (SST), cognitive behaviourally oriented psychotherapy for psychosis (CBTp) and cognitive remediation (CR). In recent years, the number of psychosocial rehabilitation interventions of proven efficacy has increased [13, 14]. Illness self-management (ISM) and assertive community treatment (ACT) were added to the evidence-based practices [15]. Other interventions—such as healthy lifestyle interventions, treatments for co-occurring substance use disorder, social cognitive and metacognitive

6 Psychosocial Recovery-Oriented Interventions in Schizophrenia

Table 6.1 Evidence-based psychiatric rehabilitation interventions to achieve recovery in schizophrenia

Evidence-based interventions	Main outcomes
Psychoeducation/family interventions	Relapses reduction, social functioning improvement, increase in treatment adherence, illness knowledge, family coping and decrease in family burden
Cognitive behavioural therapy for psychosis	Positive and negative symptoms reduction; mood and social functioning improvement
Social skills training	Negative symptoms reduction, social skills and social functioning improvement
Vocational rehabilitation/supported employment	Improvement in employment rates, hours worked and QoL
Cognitive remediation, including social cognitive and metacognitive training	Cognitive, social cognitive, metacognitive and psychosocial functioning improvement. Reduction in negative symptoms.
Healthy lifestyle interventions, including physical aerobic exercise	Positive and negative symptoms reduction; mood, cognition, QoL and social functioning improvement
Assertive community treatment	Decrease in length hospitalization and homelessness rates
Illness self-management training	Skills improvement to cope with the illness, relapses reduction and social functioning improvement
Integrated early intervention for psychosis	Positive and negative symptoms reduction, treatment adherence, QoL and social functioning improvement
Integrated intervention for comorbidity with SUD	Decrease in substance use and detention, improvement in social functioning

QoL quality of life, *SUD* substance use disorder

training—led to promising findings [2]. Table 6.1 summarizes the current evidence-based psychosocial interventions and their potential benefits in schizophrenia patients.

6.1.2 Psychoeducation and Family Interventions

PE is defined as a "systematic, structured didactic information about the illness and its treatment, and includes integrating emotional aspects in order to enable patients or family to cope with the illness" [16]. The goals of this intervention are to increase the understanding of the disorder in order to prevent relapses and hospitalization, to teach strategies of coping and problem solving and to create a collaborative relationship between health professionals and patients, family members or caregivers [5]. Family interventions shared similarities with PE, providing information to relatives. The burden of schizophrenia is often extended to the relatives and many times they know a little about the illness [17, 18]. Family stress often manifests as expressed emotion, criticism and overinvolvement. Research demonstrates that when levels of emotions are reduced, so are psychosis relapses [17, 18]. Family interventions aim to integrate patient's family members into treatment and rehabilitation, improving their ability to support and their knowledge about the illness [19].

They also have a positive impact on service engagement, resilience and stigma [5, 20]. Several approaches to family PE have been developed and validated by RCTs: they are all long-term interventions, lasting for a minimum of 9 months, but also shorter-term family interventions have been developed [21]. More than 50 RCTs have demonstrated the effectiveness of family PE on reducing relapses and hospitalizations [22]. A recent meta-analysis by Ashcroft et al. (2018) states that caregiver-directed interventions are associated with reductions in hospitalization, relapse and treatment non-adherence [23]. In another study by Ivezić et al. (2017), PE in patients with schizophrenia decreased the level of self-stigma and improved the empowerment [24]. No clinically significant improvement in global functioning was found [25]. The guidelines by National Institute of Health and Care Excellence (NICE) report robust evidence on the efficacy of family intervention and PE [26]. The NICE recommend family intervention and good-quality information for people with complex psychosis. The Scottish Intercollegiate Guidelines Network (SIGN) and the Royal Australian &New Zealand College of Psychiatrists (RANZCP) recommend them too [27, 28]. The American Psychiatric Guidelines (APA) consider PE useful only in the context of family intervention [29].

6.1.3 Cognitive Behavioural Therapy for Psychosis

CBTp was first reported in 1952 by Beck [30]. It is a talking therapy that aims to reduce psychotic symptoms and enhance strategies to reduce delusional beliefs with associated distress and interference [31]. CBTp is also used to reduce negative symptoms, anxiety and depression [31]. It can be provided either in individual or group format and the sessions are conducted weekly or biweekly over a period of 9 months. In this intervention it is important to create a treatment alliance and the patient plays an active role in the therapy [32]. The main techniques used are SST and cognitive therapy (CT). In addition, the lack of social skills in patients with schizophrenia reduces their autonomy and may led to social withdrawal; through the acquisition of new interaction modalities, individuals learn to communicate their emotions and requests [33]. The approach of teaching skills includes goal setting, role modelling, behavioural rehearsal, positive reinforcement, corrective feedback, problem solving techniques and home assignments [2]. Jumping to conclusions and lower belief flexibility are largely described in psychosis [34]. CT aims to modify dysfunctional beliefs by helping people to understand the link between perception and reaction and by exploring new coping-strategies [35]. In this way, CT can reduce functional impairment associated with symptoms. Many studies have shown that CBTp improves social functioning, reduces positive and negative symptoms and decreases mood disturbances compared with control groups [2, 36]. Other studies have not shown significant effects on outcomes such as hospitalizations, suicidality and insight [37]. Current meta-analyses have found small effects on the core symptoms of schizophrenia [38]. However, it has been suggested that the effects of CBTp in areas other than psychotic symptoms are at least as important. A recent meta-analysis by Laws et al. (2018) investigated CBTp effectiveness in functioning, distress and QoL in individuals diagnosed with schizophrenia and related disorders, founding a small therapeutic effect on functioning and on distress, but no evidence in improving QoL [39]. NICE recommends CBTp for people with schizophrenia whose illness has not responded adequately to pharmacological treatment. The guideline development group noted that there was evidence to suggest that CBTp is effective at reducing symptoms and would likely be cost-effective [26]. CBTp is recommended in the first episode of psychosis (FEP), as well as among patients with chronic symptoms or in symptomatic remission [26]. Also, SIGN, APA and RANZCP report the effectiveness of CBTp on symptoms and functioning in schizophrenia [27–29].

6.1.4 Social Skills Training

Psychosocial functioning in patients with schizophrenia is impaired by the lack of social skills, which often predates illness and persists over long term [40]. SST works on the three components necessary for social competence: receiving skills (social perception), processing skills (social cognition) and sending skills (behavioural responding or expression) [41]. SST can have different setting, duration and content, but all programmes use similar approaches to teaching skills. They include goal setting, role modelling, behavioural rehearsal, positive reinforcement, corrective feedback, problem-solving techniques, home assignment to practice skills and promote generalization [2]. SST usually takes place in groups led by two therapists and this provides opportunity for self-help and peer-support [33]. Skills group sessions may focus on basic conversation and communication skills and expressiveness, job finding, symptoms management, medical adherence, assertiveness, and problem solving with peers [42]. More than 23 RCTs and several reviews have been published about SST, most of them supporting positive outcomes in skills acquisition, assertiveness, social functioning and negative symptoms [43, 44]. The effects of SST on other areas of psychopathology such as psychotic symptoms, relapse rates and cognitive function are not consistent [44, 45]. It has been suggested that deficits in cognition may hinder the effectiveness of SST [45]. Silverstein et al. (2008) found that patients with schizophrenia attending SST and attention shaping (AS) were significantly more attentive and acquired more skills than individuals who receive SST alone [46]. This study supports the potential benefit of a multidisciplinary and integrated approach that includes SST and CR, but further researches are needed. On one hand PORT [37], SIGN [27] and APA [29] agree to strongly recommend SST as an integrated psychosocial intervention in schizophrenia, remarking that it should be combined with other treatments (e.g. family intervention); on the other hand, NICE guidelines report no recommendation for routine delivery of SST, considering this intervention not effective, neither in short nor in long term [26].

6.1.5 Vocational Rehabilitation: Supported Employment and Prevocational Training

Less than 15% of people with schizophrenia are employed even temporally, although surveys indicate that about 60% of them are capable of employment and 70% say they would like to be working [47]. Furthermore, work is associated with a lot of benefits for patients, such as improved economic standing, modest improvement in self-esteem, sense of purpose, and reduction in symptoms [48]. Several factors make it difficult for patients with schizophrenia to find and maintain suitable employment; intrinsic factors include neurocognitive deficits, lack of social skills, vulnerability to stress, episodic nature of illness and idiosyncratic beliefs and behaviours. Stigma, lack of access to SE and government disability programmes that discourage employment are extrinsic unfavourable factors [49]. The vocational rehabilitation interventions include prevocational training and SE. The first one aims to teach the requisite skills for succeeding in the competitive workplace. This approach has been generally found to be unsuccessful in helping patients to join competitive employment, but it was beneficial for occupation [50]. NICE supports vocational rehabilitation as an effective intervention in order to obtain a competitive employment after a short period (less than 1 month) of preparation, even though evidence about earnings and being able to maintain job is inconclusive [51, 52]. SE was developed as an alternative model to help patients find a competitive job. Major advantages of this programme are helping patients make person-centred choices based on their preferences, abilities and strengths, and acquire skills to maintain a competitive employment [53]. The most validated model of SE is the Individual Placement and Support (IPS) model, for which the only eligibility criterion is that people want competitive works [2, 54]. A recent meta-analysis by Frederick et al. (2019) found that IPS treatment is more effective than treatment as usual, although subjects still work below full time and may still suffer from their underlying disorder [55]. However, there is some evidence demonstrating that the cost-benefit of SE/IPS is not necessarily better than usual treatment [55].

6.1.6 Cognitive Remediation

Impaired cognitive functioning is a core aspect experienced by around 75% of people with schizophrenia [56]. Cognitive deficits are strongly and consistently related to poor real-world outcomes including residential independence, self-care and social and occupational engagement [6]. Antipsychotic drugs have a small effect, if any, on cognitive symptoms [57]. Consequently, behavioural approaches, such as CR therapies, have been developed to cope with this aspect. CR has been recently defined as "a behavioural training-based intervention that aims to improve cognitive processes (attention, memory, executive function, social cognition or metacognition) with the goal of durability and generalization" [58]. Other goals of CR are improving everyday functioning and reducing disability [58]. The most common methods include drill-and-practice of cognitive exercises, which can be computer-based or handwritten, strategy coaching in order to improve performances on cognitive exercises and teaching cognitive compensatory strategies to reduce the effects of impaired cognitive functioning in everyday life [59]. The evolution of CR has resulted in treatment programmes that use a variety of specific techniques but share common core principles. Generally, programmes consist of two to three sessions per week [60]. A group of experts in CR (2019) identified the core features for an effective CR therapy and made recommendations for its design, conduct, reporting, and implementation [61]. The experts underline the importance of a trained therapist who takes an active role in facilitating discussions, addressing negative beliefs about the participant's cognitive or functional abilities, and promoting activities to motivate behavioural changes in daily life [58]. The expert working group agreed that it is also important for participants to engage in multiple repetitions of an exercise to sustain the activation of the associated neural networks and to practice multiple strategies [61]. It is also important to give a feedback to the participant during the training session. Another goal of CR programme includes procedures to facilitate an enhanced use of problem-solving strategies [61]. Moreover, clinicians should work with patients to set cognitive goals that have clear links to community functioning and are suitable to the patients' cognitive profile [61].

Two comprehensive meta-analysis on CR have been published, both reporting a significant effect of CR on improving cognitive and psychosocial functioning and smaller but significant effects on reducing symptoms [60, 62]. Moreover, in a recent review De Tore et al. (2019) show how participants with greater cognitive impairment benefit differentially more from CR than usual services compared to less cognitively impaired participants [63]. CR programmes appear to be more successful if they are embedded in comprehensive rehabilitation programmes where the skills training or CR exercises are used in combination with psychosocial groups or work rehabilitation programmes [62]. Studies in which benefits of CR added to a rehabilitation programme were compared to the psychiatric rehabilitation (PR) alone result in significantly stronger effect on psychosocial functioning in the first one [2]. In a recent meta-analysis, Van Duin and colleagues have shown that adding cognitive training to PR can improve vocational and social functioning in patients with schizophrenia more than a stand-alone PR intervention [64]. For example, CR was added to SE [65], SST [5], and psychosocial intervention for the early period of the disorder [64–67]. CR may potentiate the effect of PR by simplifying the ability to learn new skills [2]. Finally, since cognitive deficits occur before the onset of psychosis [67] and are significantly associated with poor premorbid adjustment and functional outcome in ultrahigh-risk individuals and in the prodromal phase of schizophrenia [68], there is a clear rationale for further researches into CR in these populations. Given the theoretical and clinical interest of the possible role of treatments for preventing the subsequent conversion to psychosis in subjects with "at-risk mental states" [69], it would be particularly relevant to assess whether non-pharmacological interventions, such as CR, may have a preventive effect [70]. APA guidelines, together with SIGN and RANZCP, suggest that patients with schizophrenia should receive CR [27–29]. NICE guidelines conclude that there is limited evidence about long-lasting benefits of CR if not combined to standard interventions [26]. PORT guidelines do not recommend CR [37].

6.1.7 Social Cognitive Training

Social cognition (SC) refers to the cognitive process involved in perception, interpretation, and social information processing [71]. The inability of individuals with schizophrenia to recognize the emotional states of other people have a strong relationship with functional outcomes [72]. Additionally, social cognitive domains appear to be linked to community functioning, with evidence for an association between functioning, social and emotion perception [73], and theory of mind (ToM) [74]. Social cognition training programmes are based on individual sessions aimed at improving a specific cognitive skill (proof of concept model), multiple sessions focused on a specific SC process (targeted treatments) or programmes that focus on multiple social cognitive processes (i.e. social cognition training programme) [75]. SC training can be performed either alone or in combination with CR or SST (such as in Integrated Psychological Treatment, IPT) [76]. In a RCT study, Lindenmayer and colleagues (2018) showed that supplementing CR with computerized SC training produced greater benefits in neurocognition, including visual learning, memory, executive functions, and SC compared to cognitive training alone [77]. An increasingly group of studies support the efficacy of SC training [2]. A RCT study by Horan and colleagues (2011) indicates that a targeted social cognitive intervention led to improvements in SC among outpatients with psychosis [78]. A meta-analysis by Kurtz and Richardson (2021) found medium-large effect on emotion recognition, ToM, community and institutional functioning [79].

6.1.8 Metacognitive Training

Metacognition refers to the range of mental activities that allow people to be aware of their own thoughts, feelings, and intentions, and those of other people, and ultimately formulate connections between these events into larger complex representations of themselves and the others [80]. Recent evidence suggests that social dysfunction and negative symptoms in schizophrenia depend, among other things, on problems in metacognition [80]. Metacognitive interventions might have the potential to help individuals in better understanding thoughts and feelings they and others are having, allowing them to have an appropriate behaviour and social opportunities [81]. An example of metacognitive intervention programme is the Metacognition-Oriented Social Skills Training (MOSST) and takes place in a group therapy setting led by two metacognition-oriented psychotherapists with backgrounds in conducting psychoeducational groups and that are versed in standard SST [82]. In this intervention metacognitive skill building has been incorporated into SST [81]. In a pilot study, Ottavi and colleagues (2014) proposed MOSST to a group of patients with schizophrenia and noted improvements in evoking adaptive social behaviours during role playing; generalizability to the real world of the skills acquired; and a generally positive impact on QoL following the ability to be mindful of and communicate mental states [81]. In a recent RCT by Inchausti et al. (2018), MOSST appears to have short- and long-term beneficial effects on social functioning and symptoms [82]. Another example of metacognitive intervention is the Metacognitive Training (MCT) developed by Steffen Moritz and Todd Woodward [83]. It is based on the theoretical principles of CBT and focuses on the cognitive biases of schizophrenia [83]. MCT aims to raise patients' insight and self-awareness of cognitive distortions, with the goal of attenuating the positive symptoms of psychosis, particularly paranoid ideation [84]. Several meta-analyses on its effectiveness have been published over the years. The two most recent ones show that the training exerts a small to medium effect on symptoms when compared to other interventions [85, 86].

6.1.9 Healthy Lifestyle Interventions and Physical Exercise

People with schizophrenia die 15–20 years earlier than general population [87]. This premature mortality is the result of a number of factors including poor diet, lack of exercise, high rates of smoking, underdiagnosis of physical illness, decreased access to health care, medication side effects, stigmatization, and increased risk of cardiovascular diseases [88]. It is normal for an individual to gain up to 5 or 6 kg in weight within 2 months by the starting of antipsychotic medications and this increases the risk of obesity, diabetes mellitus or heart diseases [88]. Smoking is a cardiovascular risk factor and it is very common between people with schizophrenia (reaching 65% of patients, compared to 33% in the general population) [89]. Moreover, health care professionals sometimes pay too little attention to treating physical illness in patients with mental illness [90]. Therefore, an increased attention has been paid to healthy lifestyle interventions in people with schizophrenia in order to reduce cardiovascular diseases and mortality in these patients. Studies on the level of fitness of these patients underline the importance of supporting people with severe mental illness (SMI) in maintaining an active lifestyle [91]. Several pilot studies of healthy lifestyle programmes have shown promising results [92–94]. In particular, a lot of studies have investigated the effect of physical exercise on patients with schizophrenia [95]. Recent meta-analyses have shown that physical activity, and particularly structured exercise, can improve positive symptoms, negative symptoms, and social functioning [96]. Sabe and colleagues (2020) found beneficial effects on symptoms especially for aerobic exercise [95]. Furthermore, by increasing cardiorespiratory fitness, exercise can reduce physical health problems related to schizophrenia and its pharmacotherapy, such as obesity and diabetes [87]. Researches have demonstrated that physical activity is associated with a better cognitive performance, greater grey and white matter volumes, and higher levels of neurotrophic factors, which induce neuroplasticity [97–99]. In a well-done meta-analysis, Firth et al. (2017) found that aerobic exercise is widely effective on different cognitive domains, such as working memory, attention/vigilance, and social cognition [100]. In particular, meta-regression analyses indicated that greater amounts of exercise are related to larger improvements in global cognition and interventions supervised by physical activity professionals are more effective [100]. Maurus et al. (2019) suggested that physical activity should be delivered in groups, three sessions of 45–60 min per week, over 12 weeks [101]. NICE guidelines recommend physical activity for people with schizophrenia [26] and SIGN guidelines recommend exercise with a level B of evidence [27].

6.1.10 Assertive Community Treatment

ACT was developed to deal with the rise in relapse and rehospitalization that followed the deinstitutionalization [2]. This approach involves a multidisciplinary team (including a psychiatrist, nurses, and specialists in areas such as substance use disorders or vocational rehabilitation) working in the community [2]. The Program for ACT (PACT) is characterized by a high frequency of patient contact, 24/7 staff availability, and a patient-to-staff ratio of 8–12 patients per worker [11]. The services offered include medication management, practical support (i.e. securing housing, paying bills), and rehabilitation [2]. All these services require substantial health care resources, which not all countries have. Most studies were conducted in the USA and focused on patients at high risk of rehospitalization or homelessness. They have shown that ACT is effective at reducing hospitalization and homelessness, at stabilizing housing in the community and at improving symptoms [102]. ACT can reduce the number of hospital days by 23% and hospitalization by 60–80%, making this intervention cost-effective [103]. Researches have also demonstrated the effectiveness at decreasing costs and at improving QoL [104]. Other studies indicate that PACT has a limited impact on social functioning and employment; one of the reasons is that PACT did not target these areas [2], but in recent times standards of ACT have been upgraded [105]. APA and SIGN guidelines strongly recommend this approach for patients with poor adherence to treatment and residual psychotic symptoms [27, 29]. NICE focuses on the use of this intervention in the minority ethnic groups [26].

6.1.11 Illness Self-Management Training

According to the recovery model, ISM emphasizes the active role of patients in their own treatments [2]. Individuals receive information about schizophrenia and its treatment in order to make informed decisions about their care. They learn how to recognize early sign of relapse and coping strategies [106]. Mueser and colleagues (2002) conducted a systematic review of 40 RCTs in order to develop a programme to teach skills [107]. Authors found four strategies: (1) providing PE about mental illness and its treatment, (2) behavioural tailoring to facilitate adherence by incorporating taking medication into daily routine, (3) developing a relapse prevention plan, and (4) teaching coping strategies for persistent symptoms [107]. The Illness Management and Recovery (IMR) was developed by Gingerich and Mueser with the purpose of integrating the four strategies described above into a single package [108]. Information and skills are taught using a combination of educational, motivational, and cognitive-behavioural techniques. 40–50 individualized or group sessions are needed to complete the programme over 5–10 months [108]. In 2019, Lean and colleagues conducted a systematic review of RCTs related to self-management interventions and found that they conferred benefits in terms of reducing symptoms and length of admission, and improving functioning and QoL both at the end of treatment and at follow-up [109]. Overall, the effect size was small to medium. Self-management has been shown to have a significant effect compared with control on subjective measures of recovery such as hope and empowerment at follow-up, and self-rated recovery and self-efficacy at both time points [109]. Specific programmes like the Wellness Recovery Action Plan (WRAP) and IMR are recommended by the RANZCP guidelines [28]. NICE guidelines identify the importance of PE, medication and symptoms management, self-monitoring of predictors of relapse and skills to improve QoL [26]. Manualized, face-to-face interventions by service users are recommended by NICE [26].

6.1.12 Integrated Interventions

The combination of psychopharmacological treatments and psychosocial interventions is necessary to improve functional outcome in patients with schizophrenia [110]. Integrative programmes (i.e. antipsychotic treatment in combination with CBTp, SST, CR, etc.), adapted for specific phases of the illness, seem to be the best approach to improve clinical and psychosocial difficulties and augment the efficacy of single programmes in the treatment of psychosis [110]. Integrated treatment in FEP reduces the risk of relapses and discontinuation and improves insight, QoL, and functional outcome [111]. At the same time, integrated treatment is also effective at reducing hallucinations and negative symptoms in patients with persistent symptoms [112]. PE seems to have a positive impact on medication adherence [113], while CR integrated to antipsychotic drugs improves functional and cognitive outcomes [114]. Moreover, treatment programmes combining CR and SST for patients with schizophrenia have shown promising results [46]. A recent RCT, investigating a treatment protocol composed of computer-assisted cognitive remediation (CACR) and SST, has shown positive effects on working memory and QoL in schizophrenia patients [115]. In 2020, a pilot study by Nibbio and colleagues has shown that an integrated evidence-based treatment programme, consisting of stable pharmacological therapy, CACR, and SST, has good feasibility and effectiveness in schizophrenia [116]. A RCT examining a CBTp intervention, enhanced with CR, has shown a significant improvement in work performance and in neurocognition [117]. Recent practice guidelines have recommended a combination of treatment modalities, to meet the complex health needs of people with schizophrenia. In this perspective, the use of multifaceted illness management programmes—different combinations of physical, psychological, and social interventions—seems to be effective to achieve recovery in this population [118].

6.1.13 Integrated Early Intervention for Psychosis

Poor social functioning usually starts at the onset or in the prodromal phase of schizophrenia, but in many cases it is already present in subjects at clinical high risk for psychosis (CHR) [119]. The greatest psychosocial and clinical declines seem to occur in the first 5 years after the onset of schizophrenia [120]. Although impairment in social functioning seems to be a predictor of transition to psychosis [121], only few studies have developed interventions targeting social functioning in people with FEP or CHR [122–124]. In addiction to drugs, there are two common psychosocial approaches to treat FEP: single element interventions (i.e. CBTp, PE) and multi-element interventions (i.e. community outreach, individual or family therapy, case management) [2]. A systematic review of RCTs of single element interventions has indicated that family psychoeducation was superior to standard care in reducing rehospitalization and relapses, while CBTp has been shown to be effective at reducing symptoms and improving QoL, but not relapses and hospitalization [125]. Also, multi-element interventions are more effective than standard care at improving outcomes at 1–2 years of follow-up [125, 126], even though the enhancement may not be sustainable in the long term [127]. Programmes for FEP were not widely developed in the USA until 2015, when the National Institute of Mental Health has developed a new project focused on the development and evaluation of first-episode treatment called NAVIGATE [128]. NAVIGATE is a multi-element programme with particular attention to psychosocial components, such as family education therapy, individual resilience training (IRT), SE, and individualized medication treatment [128]. Evidence suggest the need of more extended and effective interventions, but it seems that early intervention programmes in psychosis, which focus in enhancing personal strengths and utilize integrative psychosocial therapy, improve social functioning and promote recovery [122]. Psychosocial interventions seem to be effective also for individuals at-risk for psychosis or in the prodromal phase [129]. Recent findings suggest the effectiveness of family-focused therapy (FFT), in particular for individuals at the highest levels of clinical risk for psychosis [130, 131].

6.1.14 Integrated Interventions for Co-occurring Substance Use Disorder

Substance abuse is common in people with schizophrenia: 50% have a substance use disorder (SUD) lifetime, compared with about 15% of the general population [132]. SUD is associated with a higher number of hospitalizations, relapses, homelessness, medical problems, impaired social functioning, and death [133]. Therefore, treating SUD in patients with schizophrenia is of great importance. Ideally, the best way to treat this problem is applying an integrated model: the same clinician or a team of clinicians who treat both the psychiatric area and the substance abuse disorders [134]. In this way, it can be reduced dropouts, lack of follow-up, and miscommunication between services [2]. Integrated programmes are characterized by a combination of pharmacological treatments, motivational enhancement, cognitive behaviour strategy, and minimization of stress, in order to facilitate substance use reduction and abstinence [2]. Residential treatment programmes have demonstrated beneficial effects [135]. Brunette and Mueser (2006) have supported how integrated treatment of mental health and SUD was more effective than treating each disorder separately [136].

6.2 Critical Issues and Future Challenges

Despite the growing scientific literature on the efficacy of psychosocial interventions in improving functioning and in achieving recovery in schizophrenia, the most serious problem is their application in real-world practice [15]. There is a science-to-service gap, which is between the practices knowledge effective and what is available and provided in mental health services [137]. Moreover, there are still some doubts and uncertainties regarding the feasibility in daily clinical practice of mental health services [15]. For many years, high-income European countries continued to invest in old and expensive not evidence-based, not recovery-oriented and not person-centred care services, such as acute care, hospitalization and residency [1]. This results in only few patients with SMI receiving suitable EB psychosocial rehabilitation treatments [138]. In addition, different beliefs coexist between professionals and between patients and professionals, which prevent the realization of a harmonic project [139]. In the USA the situation is not so different: the quality of rehabilitative services seems to be behind the other high-income countries and most of funds are addressed to hospitals, residential treatments and psychotropic drugs [140]. The biggest challenge in modern psychiatry is improving efficient skills at the organizational level, able to allocate the resources according to a clear understanding of the real needs of a mental health service [1]. In this contest, it is important to invest in different dissemination strategies (training events, written materials, practical guidelines) and reinforcement strategies to increase skills between professionals [141]. Current psychosocial rehabilitation practices are highly variable in terms of methodology and contents, with relevant differences from one country to another, and also within the same country, according to the specific orientation and tradition characterizing each mental health service [15]. Adopting a recovery-oriented approach by mental health services means to involve patients, family members and professionals in a common effort, integrating EB psychosocial rehabilitative interventions in an anti-stigma context, in order to obtain not only symptoms remission, but also the increase of life skills and the improvement of psychosocial functioning in people with SMI [142]. Only improving attitudes and actions of all the stakeholders, with the aim to achieve empowerment, self-responsibility, hope and user satisfaction, a mental health service can be defined as "recovery-oriented" [143]. There is the need to design specific pathways with the aim to overcome personal, social, organizational and political barriers that deny evidence-based practices for patients [15]. Finally, it is also crucial to increase knowledge on psychosocial interventions to be able to promote a patient-centred, evidence-based and recovery-oriented psychosocial rehabilitation [15].

References

1. Rössler W, Drake RE. Psychiatric rehabilitation in Europe. Epidemiol Psychiatr Sci. 2017;26(3):1–7. https://doi.org/10.1017/S2045796016000858.
2. Mueser KT, Deavers F, Penn DL, Cassisi JE. Psychosocial treatments for schizophrenia. Annu Rev Clin Psychol. 2013;9:465–97. https://doi.org/10.1146/annurev-clinpsy-050212-185620.
3. Vita A, Corrivetti G, Mannu J, Semisa D, Vigano C. Psychosocial rehabilitation in Italy today. Int J Ment Health. 2016;45:15–23. https://doi.org/10.1080/00207411.2015.1119375.
4. Vita A, Barlati S. Recovery from schizophrenia: is it possible? Curr Opin Psychiatry. 2018;31(3):246–55. https://doi.org/10.1097/YCO.0000000000000407.
5. Morin L, Franck N. Rehabilitation interventions to promote recovery from schizophrenia: a systematic review. Front Psych. 2017;8:100. https://doi.org/10.3389/fpsyt.2017.00100.
6. Harvey PD, Strassnig M. Predicting the severity of everyday functional disability in people with schizophrenia: cognitive deficits, functional capacity, symptoms, and health status. World Psychiatry. 2012;11(2):73–9. https://doi.org/10.1016/j.wpsyc.2012.05.004.
7. Ventura J, Hellemann GS, Thames AD, Koellner V, Nuechterlein KH. Symptoms as mediators of the relationship between neurocognition and functional outcome in schizophrenia: a meta-analysis. Schizophr Res. 2009;113(2–3):189–99. https://doi.org/10.1016/j.schres.2009.03.035.
8. Ventriglio A, Ricci F, Magnifico G, Chumakov E, Torales J, Watson C, Castaldelli-Maia JM, Petito A, Bellomo A. Psychosocial interventions in schizophrenia: focus on guidelines. Int J Soc Psychiatry. 2020;66(8):735–47. https://doi.org/10.1177/0020764020934827.
9. Drake RE, Rosenberg SD, Teague GB, Bartels SJ, Torrey WC. Fundamental principles of evidence-based medicine applied to mental health care. Psychiatr Clin North Am 2003;26(4):811–20, vii. doi: https://doi.org/10.1016/s0193-953x(03)00063-7.
10. Drake RE, Goldman HH, Leff HS, Lehman AF, Dixon L, Mueser KT, Torrey WC. Implementing evidence-based practices in routine mental health service settings. Psychiatr Serv. 2001;52(2):179–82. https://doi.org/10.1176/appi.ps.52.2.179.
11. Shean GD. Evidence-based psychosocial practices and recovery from schizophrenia. Psychiatry. 2009;72(4):307–20. https://doi.org/10.1521/psyc.2009.72.4.307.
12. Lehman AF, Kreyenbuhl J, Buchanan RW, Dickerson FB, Dixon LB, Goldberg R, Green-Paden LD, et al. The Schizophrenia Patient Outcomes Research Team (PORT): updated treatment recommendations 2003. Schizophr Bull. 2004;30(2):193–217. https://doi.org/10.1093/oxfordjournals.schbul.a007071.
13. Kern RS, Glynn SM, Horan WP, Marder SR. Psychosocial treatments to promote functional recovery in schizophrenia. Schizophr Bull. 2009;35(2):347–61. https://doi.org/10.1093/schbul/sbn177.
14. Fleischhacker WW, Arango C, Arteel P, Barnes TR, Carpenter W, Duckworth K, Galderisi S, Halpern L, Knapp M, Marder SR, Moller M, Sartorius N, Woodruff P. Schizophrenia—time to commit to policy change. Schizophr Bull. 2014;40(Suppl 3):S165–94. https://doi.org/10.1093/schbul/sbu006.

15. Vita A, Barlati S. The implementation of evidence-based psychiatric rehabilitation: challenges and opportunities for mental health services. Front Psych. 2019;10:147. https://doi.org/10.3389/fpsyt.2019.00147.
16. Rummel-Kluge C, Kissling W. Psychoeducation in schizophrenia: new developments and approaches in the field. Curr Opin Psychiatry. 2008;21(2):168–72. https://doi.org/10.1097/YCO.0b013e3282f4e574.
17. Atadokht A, Hajloo N, Karimi M, Narimani M. The role of family expressed emotion and perceived social support in predicting addiction relapse. Int J High Risk Behav Addict. 2015;4(1):e21250. https://doi.org/10.5812/ijhrba.21250.
18. Koutra K, Triliva S, Roumeliotaki T, Basta M, Simos P, Lionis C, Vgontzas AN. Impaired family functioning in psychosis and its relevance to relapse: a two-year follow-up study. Compr Psychiatry. 2015;62:1–12. https://doi.org/10.1016/j.comppsych.2015.06.006.
19. Lyman DR, Braude L, George P, Dougherty RH, Daniels AS, Ghose SS, Delphin-Rittmon ME. Consumer and family psychoeducation: assessing the evidence. Psychiatr Serv. 2014;65(4):416–28. https://doi.org/10.1176/appi.ps.201300266.
20. Cohen AN, Glynn SM, Murray-Swank AB, Barrio C, Fischer EP, McCutcheon SJ, Perlick DA, Rotondi AJ, Sayers SL, Sherman MD, Dixon LB. The family forum: directions for the implementation of family psychoeducation for severe mental illness. Psychiatr Serv. 2008;59(1):40–8. https://doi.org/10.1176/ps.2008.59.1.40.
21. Pharoah F, Mari J, Rathbone J, Wong W. Family intervention for schizophrenia. Cochrane Database Syst Rev. 2010;(12):CD000088. https://doi.org/10.1002/14651858.CD000088.pub2.
22. Morgan AJ, Reavley NJ, Ross A, Too LS, Jorm AF. Interventions to reduce stigma towards people with severe mental illness: systematic review and meta-analysis. J Psychiatr Res. 2018;103:120–33. https://doi.org/10.1016/j.jpsychires.2018.05.017.
23. Ashcroft K, Kim E, Elefant E, Benson C, Carter JA. Meta-analysis of caregiver-directed psychosocial interventions for schizophrenia. Community Ment Health J. 2018;54(7):983–91. https://doi.org/10.1007/s10597-018-0289-x.
24. Ivezić SŠ, Sesar MA, Mužinić L. Effects of a group psychoeducation program on self-stigma, empowerment and perceived discrimination of persons with schizophrenia. Psychiatr Danub. 2017;29(1):66–73.
25. Xia J, Merinder LB, Belgamwar MR. Psychoeducation for schizophrenia. Cochrane Database Syst Rev. 2011;2011(6):CD002831. https://doi.org/10.1002/14651858.CD002831.pub2.
26. National Institute for Health and Care Excellence. Rehabilitation for adults with complex psychosis. London, UK; 2020.
27. SIGN guideline, Management of Schizophrenia. 2013.
28. Galletly C, Castle D, Dark F, et al. Royal Australian and New Zealand College of Psychiatrists clinical practice guidelines for the management of schizophrenia and related disorders. Aust N Z J Psychiatry. 2016;50(5):410–72.
29. Keepers GA, Fochtmann LJ, Anzia JM, Benjamin S, Lyness JM, Mojtabai R, Servis M, et al. The American Psychiatric Association Practice guideline for the treatment of patients with schizophrenia. Am J Psychiatry. 2020;177(9):868–72. https://doi.org/10.1176/appi.ajp.2020.177901.
30. Beck AT. Successful outpatient psychotherapy of a chronic schizophrenic with a delusion based on borrowed guilt. Psychiatry. 1952;15(3):305–12. https://doi.org/10.1080/00332747.1952.11022883.
31. Morrison AP, Renton JC, Dunn H, Williams S, Bentall RP. Cognitive therapy for psychosis: a case formulation approach. Brighton: Psychology Press Ltd; 2003.
32. Turkington D, Kingdon D, Weiden PJ. Cognitive behavior therapy for schizophrenia. Am J Psychiatry. 2006;163(3):365–73. https://doi.org/10.1176/appi.ajp.163.3.365.
33. Kopelowicz A, Liberman RP, Zarate R. Recent advances in social skills training for schizophrenia. Schizophr Bull. 2006;32(Suppl 1):S12–23. https://doi.org/10.1093/schbul/sbl023.

34. Beck AT, Rector NA. Cognitive approaches to schizophrenia: theory and therapy. Annu Rev Clin Psychol. 2005;1:577–606. https://doi.org/10.1146/annurev.clinpsy.1.102803.144205.
35. Mander H, Kingdon D. The evolution of cognitive-behavioral therapy for psychosis. Psychol Res Behav Manag. 2015;8:63–9. https://doi.org/10.2147/PRBM.S52267.
36. Wykes T, Steel C, Everitt B, Tarrier N. Cognitive behavior therapy for schizophrenia: effect sizes, clinical models, and methodological rigor. Schizophr Bull. 2008;34(3):523–37. https://doi.org/10.1093/schbul/sbm114.
37. Dixon LB, Dickerson F, Bellack AS, Bennett M, Dickinson D, Goldberg RW, Lehman A, et al. Schizophrenia Patient Outcomes Research Team (PORT). The 2009 schizophrenia PORT psychosocial treatment recommendations and summary statements. Schizophr Bull. 2010;36(1):48–70. https://doi.org/10.1093/schbul/sbp115.
38. Jauhar S, McKenna PJ, Radua J, Fung E, Salvador R, Laws KR. Cognitive-behavioural therapy for the symptoms of schizophrenia: systematic review and meta-analysis with examination of potential bias. Br J Psychiatry. 2014;204(1):20–9. https://doi.org/10.1192/bjp.bp.112.116285.
39. Laws KR, Darlington N, Kondel TK, McKenna PJ, Jauhar S. Cognitive behavioural therapy for schizophrenia—outcomes for functioning, distress and quality of life: a meta-analysis. BMC Psychol. 2018;6(1):32. https://doi.org/10.1186/s40359-018-0243-2.
40. Bellack AS, Mueser KT. Psychosocial treatment for schizophrenia. Schizophr Bull. 1993;19(2):317–36. https://doi.org/10.1093/schbul/19.2.317.
41. Rector NA, Beck AT. Cognitive therapy for schizophrenia: from conceptualization to intervention. Can J Psychiatr. 2002;47(1):39–48.
42. Pilling S, Bebbington P, Kuipers E, Garety P, Geddes J, Martindale B, Orbach G, et al. Psychological treatments in schizophrenia: II. Meta-analyses of randomized controlled trials of social skills training and cognitive remediation. Psychol Med. 2002;32(5):783–91. https://doi.org/10.1017/s0033291702005640.
43. Mueser KT, Penn DL. Meta-analysis examining the effects of social skills training on schizophrenia. Psychol Med. 2004;34(7):1365–7. https://doi.org/10.1017/s0033291704213848.
44. Pfammatter M, Junghan UM, Brenner HD. Efficacy of psychological therapy in schizophrenia: conclusions from meta-analyses. Schizophr Bull. 2006;32(Suppl 1):S64–80. https://doi.org/10.1093/schbul/sbl030.
45. Kurtz MM, Mueser KT. A meta-analysis of controlled research on social skills training for schizophrenia. J Consult Clin Psychol. 2008;76(3):491–504. https://doi.org/10.1037/0022-006X.76.3.491.
46. Silverstein SM, Spaulding WD, Menditto AA, Savitz A, Liberman RP, Berten S, Starobin H. Attention shaping: a reward-based learning method to enhance skills training outcomes in schizophrenia. Schizophr Bull. 2009;35(1):222–32. https://doi.org/10.1093/schbul/sbm150.
47. Turner DT, McGlanaghy E, Cuijpers P, van der Gaag M, Karyotaki E, MacBeth A. A meta-analysis of social skills training and related interventions for psychosis. Schizophr Bull. 2018;44(3):475–91. https://doi.org/10.1093/schbul/sbx146.
48. Leff J, Warner R. Social inclusion of people with mental illness. Cambridge University Press; 2006.
49. Mueser KT, Becker DR, Torrey WC, Xie H, Bond GR, Drake RE, Dain BJ. Work and nonvocational domains of functioning in persons with severe mental illness: a longitudinal analysis. J Nerv Ment Dis. 1997;185(7):419–26. https://doi.org/10.1097/00005053-199707000-00001.
50. Gold PB, Waghorn G. Supported employment for people with severe mental illness. Lancet. 2007;370(9593):1108–9. https://doi.org/10.1016/S0140-6736(07)61491-3.
51. Bond GB. Vocational rehabilitation, Handbook of psychiatric rehabilitation; 1992. p. 244–25.
52. Hoffmann H, Jäckel D, Glauser S, Kupper Z. A randomised controlled trial of the efficacy of supported employment. Acta Psychiatr Scand. 2012;125(2):157–67. https://doi.org/10.1111/j.1600-0447.2011.01780.
53. Lehman AF, Goldberg R, Dixon LB, McNary S, Postrado L, Hackman A, McDonnell K. Improving employment outcomes for persons with severe mental illnesses. Arch Gen Psychiatry. 2002;59(2):165–72. https://doi.org/10.1001/archpsyc.59.2.165.

54. Becker DR, Drake RE. A working life for people with severe mental illness. Oxford University Press; 2003.
55. Frederick DE, VanderWeele TJ. Supported employment: meta-analysis and review of randomized controlled trials of individual placement and support. PLoS One. 2019;14(2):e0212208. https://doi.org/10.1371/journal.pone.0212208.
56. Heinrichs RW, Miles AA, Ammari N, Muharib E. Cognition as a central illness feature in schizophrenia. In: Harvey PD, editor. Cognitive impairment in schizophrenia: characteristics, assessment and treatment. Cambridge University Press; 2013. p. 1–23. https://doi.org/10.1017/CBO9781139003872.002.
57. Keefe RS, Bilder RM, Davis SM, Harvey PD, Palmer BW, Gold JM, Meltzer HY, et al. Neurocognitive effects of antipsychotic medications in patients with chronic schizophrenia in the CATIE Trial. Arch Gen Psychiatry. 2007;64(6):633–47. https://doi.org/10.1001/archpsyc.64.6.633.
58. Kambeitz-Ilankovic L, Betz LT, Dominke C, Haas SS, Subramaniam K, Fisher M, Vinogradov S, Koutsouleris N, Kambeitz J. Multi-outcome meta-analysis (MOMA) of cognitive remediation in schizophrenia: revisiting the relevance of human coaching and elucidating interplay between multiple outcomes. Neurosci Biobehav Rev. 2019;107:828–45. https://doi.org/10.1016/j.neubiorev.2019.09.031.
59. McGurk SR, Mueser KT, Covell NH, Cicerone KD, Drake RE, Silverstein SM, Medialia A, et al. Mental health system funding of cognitive enhancement interventions for schizophrenia: summary and update of the New York Office of Mental Health expert panel and stakeholder meeting. Psychiatr Rehabil J. 2013;36(3):133–45. https://doi.org/10.1037/prj0000020.
60. Wykes T, Huddy V, Cellard C, McGurk SR, Czobor P. A meta-analysis of cognitive remediation for schizophrenia: methodology and effect sizes. Am J Psychiatry. 2011;168(5):472–85. https://doi.org/10.1176/appi.ajp.2010.10060855.
61. Bowie CR, Bell MD, Fiszdon JM, Johannesen JK, Lindenmayer JP, McGurk SR, Medalia AA, et al. Cognitive remediation for schizophrenia: an expert working group white paper on core techniques. Schizophr Res. 2020;215:49–53. https://doi.org/10.1016/j.schres.2019.10.047.
62. McGurk SR, Twamley EW, Sitzer DI, McHugo GJ, Mueser KT. A meta-analysis of cognitive remediation in schizophrenia. Am J Psychiatry. 2007;164(12):1791–802. https://doi.org/10.1176/appi.ajp.2007.07060906.
63. DeTore NR, Mueser KT, Byrd JA, McGurk SR. Cognitive functioning as a predictor of response to comprehensive cognitive remediation. J Psychiatr Res. 2019;113:117–24. https://doi.org/10.1016/j.jpsychires.2019.03.012.
64. Van Duin D, de Winter L, Oud M, Kroon H, Veling W, van Weeghel J. The effect of rehabilitation combined with cognitive remediation on functioning in persons with severe mental illness: systematic review and meta-analysis. Psychol Med. 2019;49(9):1414–25. https://doi.org/10.1017/S003329171800418X.
65. McGurk SR, Mueser KT, Pascaris A. Cognitive training and supported employment for persons with severe mental illness: one-year results from a randomized controlled trial. Schizophr Bull. 2005;31(4):898–909. https://doi.org/10.1093/schbul/sbi037.
66. Hogarty GE, Flesher S, Ulrich R, Carter M, Greenwald D, Pogue-Geile M, Kechavan M, et al. Cognitive enhancement therapy for schizophrenia: effects of a 2-year randomized trial on cognition and behavior. Arch Gen Psychiatry. 2004;61(9):866–76. https://doi.org/10.1001/archpsyc.61.9.866.
67. Pukrop R, Schultze-Lutter F, Ruhrmann S, Brockhaus-Dumke A, Tendolkar I, Bechdolf A, Matuschek E, et al. Neurocognitive functioning in subjects at risk for a first episode of psychosis compared with first- and multiple-episode schizophrenia. J Clin Exp Neuropsychol. 2006;28(8):1388–407. https://doi.org/10.1080/13803390500434425.
68. Lin A, Wood SJ, Nelson B, Brewer WJ, Spiliotacopoulos D, Bruxner A, Broussard C, et al. Neurocognitive predictors of functional outcome two to 13 years after identification as ultra-high risk for psychosis. Schizophr Res. 2011;132(1):1–7. https://doi.org/10.1016/j.schres.2011.06.014.

69. Ruhrmann S, Schultze-Lutter F, Klosterkötter J. Intervention in the at-risk state to prevent transition to psychosis. Curr Opin Psychiatry. 2009;22(2):177–83. https://doi.org/10.1097/YCO.0b013e328324b687.
70. Barlati S, Deste G, De Peri L, Ariu C, Vita A. Cognitive remediation in schizophrenia: current status and future perspectives. Schizophr Res Treatment. 2013;2013:156084. https://doi.org/10.1155/2013/156084.
71. Pinkham AE, Hopfinger JB, Pelphrey KA, Piven J, Penn DL. Neural bases for impaired social cognition in schizophrenia and autism spectrum disorders. Schizophr Res. 2008;99(1–3):164–75. https://doi.org/10.1016/j.schres.2007.10.024.
72. Pinkham AE, Penn DL. Neurocognitive and social cognitive predictors of interpersonal skill in schizophrenia. Psychiatry Res. 2006;143(2–3):167–78. https://doi.org/10.1016/j.psychres.2005.09.005.
73. Couture SM, Penn DL, Roberts DL. The functional significance of social cognition in schizophrenia: a review. Schizophr Bull. 2006;32(Suppl 1):S44–63. https://doi.org/10.1093/schbul/sbl029.
74. Fett AK, Viechtbauer W, Dominguez MD, Penn DL, van Os J, Krabbendam L. The relationship between neurocognition and social cognition with functional outcomes in schizophrenia: a meta-analysis. Neurosci Biobehav Rev. 2011;35(3):573–88. https://doi.org/10.1016/j.neubiorev.2010.07.001.
75. Fiszdon JM. Introduction to social cognitive treatment approaches for schizophrenia. In: Roberts DL, Penn DL, editors. Social cognition in schizophrenia: from evidence to treatment. Oxford University Press; 2013. p. 285–310. https://doi.org/10.1093/med:psych/9780199777587.003.0012.
76. Roder V, Mueller DR, Schmidt SJ. Effectiveness of integrated psychological therapy (IPT) for schizophrenia patients: a research update. Schizophr Bull. 2011;37(Suppl 2):S71–9. https://doi.org/10.1093/schbul/sbr072.
77. Lindenmayer JP, Khan A, McGurk SR, Kulsa MKC, Ljuri I, Ozog V, Fregenti S, et al. Does social cognition training augment response to computer-assisted cognitive remediation for schizophrenia? Schizophr Res. 2018;201:180–6. https://doi.org/10.1016/j.schres.2018.06.012.
78. Horan WP, Kern RS, Tripp C, Hellemann G, Wynn JK, Bell M, Marder SR, et al. Efficacy and specificity of social cognitive skills training for outpatients with psychotic disorders. J Psychiatr Res. 2011;45(8):1113–22. https://doi.org/10.1016/j.jpsychires.2011.01.015.
79. Kurtz MM, Richardson CL. Social cognitive training for schizophrenia: a meta-analytic investigation of controlled research. Schizophr Bull. 2012;38(5):1092–104. https://doi.org/10.1093/schbul/sbr036.
80. Lysaker PH, Shea AM, Buck KD, Dimaggio G, Nicolò G, Procacci M, Salvatore G, Rand KL. Metacognition as a mediator of the effects of impairments in neurocognition on social function in schizophrenia spectrum disorders. Acta Psychiatr Scand. 2010;122(5):405–13. https://doi.org/10.1111/j.1600-0447.2010.01554.x.
81. Ottavi P, D'Alia D, Lysaker P, Kent J, Popolo R, Salvatore G, Dimaggio G. Metacognition-oriented social skills training for individuals with long-term schizophrenia: methodology and clinical illustration. Clin Psychol Psychother. 2014;21(5):465–73. https://doi.org/10.1002/cpp.1850.
82. Inchausti F, García-Poveda NV, Ballesteros-Prados A, Ortuño-Sierra J, Sánchez-Reales S, Prado-Abril J, Aldaz-Armendáriz JA, Mole J, Dimaggio G, Ottavi P, Fonseca-Pedrero E. The effects of metacognition-oriented social skills training on psychosocial outcome in schizophrenia-spectrum disorders: a randomized controlled trial. Schizophr Bull. 2018;44(6):1235–44. https://doi.org/10.1093/schbul/sbx168.
83. Moritz S, Woodward TS. Metacognitive training in schizophrenia: from basic research to knowledge translation and intervention. Curr Opin Psychiatry. 2007;20(6):619–25. https://doi.org/10.1097/YCO.0b013e3282f0b8ed.

84. Moritz S, Andreou C, Schneider BC, Wittekind CE, Menon M, Balzan RP, Woodward TS. Sowing the seeds of doubt: a narrative review on metacognitive training in schizophrenia. Clin Psychol Rev. 2014;34(4):358–66. https://doi.org/10.1016/j.cpr.2014.04.004.
85. Liu YC, Tang CC, Hung TT, Tsai PC, Lin MF. The efficacy of metacognitive training for delusions in patients with schizophrenia: a meta-analysis of randomized controlled trials informs evidence-based practice. Worldviews Evid-Based Nurs. 2018;15(2):130–9. https://doi.org/10.1111/wvn.12282.
86. Philipp R, Kriston L, Lanio J, Kühne F, Härter M, Moritz S, Meister R. Effectiveness of meta-cognitive interventions for mental disorders in adults—a systematic review and meta-analysis (METACOG). Clin Psychol Psychother. 2019;26(2):227–40. https://doi.org/10.1002/cpp.2345.
87. Laursen TM. Life expectancy among persons with schizophrenia or bipolar affective disorder. Schizophr Res. 2011;131(1–3):101–4. https://doi.org/10.1016/j.schres.2011.06.008.
88. Leucht S, Burkard T, Henderson J, Maj M, Sartorius N. Physical illness and schizophrenia: a review of the literature. Acta Psychiatr Scand. 2007;116(5):317–33. https://doi.org/10.1111/j.1600-0447.2007.01095.x.
89. The Schizophrenia Commission. The abandoned illness: a report from the Schizophrenia Commission. London: Rethink Mental Illness; 2012.
90. Thornicroft G. Physical health disparities and mental illness: the scandal of premature mortality. Br J Psychiatry. 2011;199(6):441–2. https://doi.org/10.1192/bjp.bp.111.092718.
91. Vancampfort D, Rosenbaum S, Schuch F, Ward PB, Richards J, Mugisha J, Probst M, et al. Cardiorespiratory fitness in severe mental illness: a systematic review and meta-analysis. Sports Med. 2017;47(2):343–52. https://doi.org/10.1007/s40279-016-0574-1.
92. Hutchison SL, Terhorst L, Murtaugh S, Gross S, Kogan JN, Shaffer SL. Effectiveness of a staff promoted wellness program to improve health in residents of a mental health long-term care facility. Issues Ment Health Nurs. 2016;37(4):257–64. https://doi.org/10.3109/01612840.2015.1126774.
93. Gill KJ, Zechner M, Zambo Anderson E, Swarbrick M, Murphy A. Wellness for life: a pilot of an interprofessional intervention to address metabolic syndrome in adults with serious mental illnesses. Psychiatr Rehabil J. 2016;39(2):147–53. https://doi.org/10.1037/prj0000172.
94. Looijmans A, Jörg F, Bruggeman R, Schoevers RA, Corpeleijn E. Multimodal lifestyle intervention using a web-based tool to improve cardiometabolic health in patients with serious mental illness: results of a cluster randomized controlled trial (LION). BMC Psychiatry. 2019;19(1):339. https://doi.org/10.1186/s12888-019-2310-5.
95. Sabe M, Kaiser S, Sentissi O. Physical exercise for negative symptoms of schizophrenia: systematic review of randomized controlled trials and meta-analysis. Gen Hosp Psychiatry. 2020;62:13–20. https://doi.org/10.1016/j.genhosppsych.2019.11.002.
96. Firth J, Cotter J, Elliott R, French P, Yung AR. A systematic review and meta-analysis of exercise interventions in schizophrenia patients. Psychol Med. 2015;45(7):1343–61. https://doi.org/10.1017/S0033291714003110.
97. Leutwyler H, Hubbard EM, Jeste DV, Miller B, Vinogradov S. Associations of schizophrenia symptoms and neurocognition with physical activity in older adults with schizophrenia. Biol Res Nurs. 2014;16(1):23–30. https://doi.org/10.1177/1099800413500845.
98. McEwen SC, Hardy A, Ellingson BM, Jarrahi B, Sandhu N, Subotnik KL, Ventura J, et al. Prefrontal and hippocampal brain volume deficits: role of low physical activity on brain plasticity in first-episode schizophrenia patients. J Int Neuropsychol Soc. 2015;21(10):868–79. https://doi.org/10.1017/S1355617715000983.
99. Kimhy D, Vakhrusheva J, Bartels MN, Armstrong HF, Ballon JS, Khan S, Chang RW, et al. Aerobic fitness and body mass index in individuals with schizophrenia: implications for neurocognition and daily functioning. Psychiatry Res. 2014;220(3):784–91. https://doi.org/10.1016/j.psychres.2014.08.052.

100. Firth J, Stubbs B, Rosenbaum S, Vancampfort D, Malchow B, Schuch F, Elliott R, et al. Aerobic exercise improves cognitive functioning in people with schizophrenia: a systematic review and meta-analysis. Schizophr Bull. 2017;43(3):546–56. https://doi.org/10.1093/schbul/sbw115.
101. Maurus I, Röh A, Falkai P, Malchow B, Schmitt A, Hasan A. Nonpharmacological treatment of dyscognition in schizophrenia: effects of aerobic exercise. Dialogues Clin Neurosci. 2019;21(3):261–9. https://doi.org/10.31887/DCNS.2019.21.3/aschmitt.
102. Bond GR, Drake RE, Mueser KT, et al. Assertive community treatment for people with severe mental illness. Dis-Manage-Health-Outcomes. 2001;9:141–59. https://doi.org/10.2165/00115677-200109030-00003.
103. Latimer EA. Economic impacts of assertive community treatment: a review of the literature. Can J Psychiatr. 1999;44(5):443–54. https://doi.org/10.1177/070674379904400504.
104. Latimer E. Economic considerations associated with assertive community treatment and supported employment for people with severe mental illness. J Psychiatry Neurosci. 2005;30(5):355–9.
105. Monroe-DeVita M, Teague GB, Moser LL. The TMACT: a new tool for measuring fidelity to assertive community treatment. J Am Psychiatr Nurses Assoc. 2011;17(1):17–29. https://doi.org/10.1177/1078390310394658.
106. Tarrier N, Wittkowski A, Kinney C, McCarthy E, Morris J, Humphreys L. Durability of the effects of cognitive-behavioural therapy in the treatment of chronic schizophrenia: 12-month follow-up. Br J Psychiatry. 1999;174:500–4. https://doi.org/10.1192/bjp.174.6.500.
107. Mueser KT, Corrigan PW, Hilton DW, Tanzman B, Schaub A, Gingerich S, Essock SM, et al. Illness management and recovery: a review of the research. Psychiatr Serv. 2002;53(10):1272–84. https://doi.org/10.1176/appi.ps.53.10.1272.
108. Gingerich S, Mueser KT. Illness management and recovery: personalized skills and strategies for those with mental illness. Centre City, MN: Hazelden; 2011.
109. Lean M, Fornells-Ambrojo M, Milton A, Lloyd-Evans B, Harrison-Stewart B, Yesufu-Udechuku A, Kendall T, et al. Self-management interventions for people with severe mental illness: systematic review and meta-analysis. Br J Psychiatry. 2019;214(5):260–8. https://doi.org/10.1192/bjp.2019.54
110. Valencia M, Fresan A, Juárez F, Escamilla R, Saracco R. The beneficial effects of combining pharmacological and psychosocial treatment on remission and functional outcome in outpatients with schizophrenia. J Psychiatr Res. 2013;47(12):1886–92. https://doi.org/10.1016/j.jpsychires.2013.09.006.
111. Guo X, Zhai J, Liu Z, Fang M, Wang B, Wang C, Hu B, et al. Effect of antipsychotic medication alone vs combined with psychosocial intervention on outcomes of early-stage schizophrenia: a randomized, 1-year study. Arch Gen Psychiatry. 2010;67(9):895–904. https://doi.org/10.1001/archgenpsychiatry.2010.105.
112. Menezes NM, Arenovich T, Zipursky RB. A systematic review of longitudinal outcome studies of first-episode psychosis. Psychol Med. 2006;36(10):1349–62. https://doi.org/10.1017/S0033291706007951.
113. Linden M, Pyrkosch L, Hundemer HP. Frequency and effects of psychosocial interventions additional to olanzapine treatment in routine care of schizophrenic patients. Soc Psychiatry Psychiatr Epidemiol. 2008;43(5):373–9. https://doi.org/10.1007/s00127-008-0318-0.
114. Sato S, Iwata K, Furukawa S, Matsuda Y, Hatsuse N, Ikebuchi E. The effects of the combination of cognitive training and supported employment on improving clinical and working outcomes for people with schizophrenia in Japan. Clin Pract Epidemiol Ment Health. 2014;10:18–27. https://doi.org/10.2174/1745017901410010018.
115. Kurtz MM, Mueser KT, Thime WR, Corbera S, Wexler BE. Social skills training and computer-assisted cognitive remediation in schizophrenia. Schizophr Res. 2015;162(1–3):35–41. https://doi.org/10.1016/j.schres.2015.01.020.
116. Nibbio G, Barlati S, Cacciani P, Corsini P, Mosca A, Ceraso A, Deste G, et al. Evidence-based integrated intervention in patients with schizophrenia: a pilot study of feasibility and effectiveness in a real-world rehabilitation setting. Int J Environ Res Public Health. 2020;17(10):3352. https://doi.org/10.3390/ijerph17103352.

6 Psychosocial Recovery-Oriented Interventions in Schizophrenia 97

117. Kukla M, Bell MD, Lysaker PH. A randomized controlled trial examining a cognitive behavioral therapy intervention enhanced with cognitive remediation to improve work and neurocognition outcomes among persons with schizophrenia spectrum disorders. Schizophr Res. 2018;197:400–6. https://doi.org/10.1016/j.schres.2018.01.012.

118. Chien WT, Yip AL. Current approaches to treatments for schizophrenia spectrum disorders, part I: an overview and medical treatments. Neuropsychiatr Dis Treat. 2013;9:1311–32. https://doi.org/10.2147/NDT.S37485.

119. Addington J, Penn D, Woods SW, Addington D, Perkins DO. Social functioning in individuals at clinical high risk for psychosis. Schizophr Res. 2008;99(1–3):119–24. https://doi.org/10.1016/j.schres.2007.10.001.

120. Lieberman JA, Perkins D, Belger A, Chakos M, Jarskog F, Boteva K, Gilmore J. The early stages of schizophrenia: speculations on pathogenesis, pathophysiology, and therapeutic approaches. Biol Psychiatry. 2001;50(11):884–97. https://doi.org/10.1016/s0006-3223(01)01303-8. Erratum in: Biol Psychiatry 2002 Feb 15;51(4):346.

121. Fusar-Poli P, Byrne M, Valmaggia L, Day F, Tabraham P, Johns L, McGuire P, et al. Social dysfunction predicts two years clinical outcome in people at ultra high risk for psychosis. J Psychiatr Res. 2010;44(5):294–301. https://doi.org/10.1016/j.jpsychires.2009.08.016.

122. Santesteban-Echarri O, Rice S, González-Blanch C, Alvarez-Jimenez M. Chapter 18: Promoting psychosocial functioning and recovery in schizophrenia spectrum and other psychotic disorders. In: Johanna C, editor. A clinical introduction to psychosis: foundations for clinical psychologists and neuropsychologist; 2019. https://doi.org/10.1016/B978-0-12-815012-2.00018-3.

123. Robinson DG, Woerner MG, McMeniman M, Mendelowitz A, Bilder RM. Symptomatic and functional recovery from a first episode of schizophrenia or schizoaffective disorder. Am J Psychiatry. 2004;161(3):473–9. https://doi.org/10.1176/appi.ajp.161.3.473.

124. Jaracz K, Górna K, Kiejda J, Grabowska-Fudala B, Jaracz J, Suwalska A, Rybakowski JK. Psychosocial functioning in relation to symptomatic remission: a longitudinal study of first episode schizophrenia. Eur Psychiatry. 2015;30(8):907–13. https://doi.org/10.1016/j.eurpsy.2015.08.001.

125. Bird V, Premkumar P, Kendall T, Whittington C, Mitchell J, Kuipers E. Early intervention services, cognitive-behavioural therapy and family intervention in early psychosis: systematic review. Br J Psychiatry. 2010;197(5):350–6. https://doi.org/10.1192/bjp.bp.109.074526.

126. Grawe RW, Falloon IR, Widen JH, Skogvoll E. Two years of continued early treatment for recent-onset schizophrenia: a randomised controlled study. Acta Psychiatr Scand. 2006;114(5):328–36. https://doi.org/10.1111/j.1600-0447.2006.00799.x.

127. Bosanac P, Patton GC, Castle DJ. Early intervention in psychotic disorders: faith before facts? Psychol Med. 2010;40(3):353–8. https://doi.org/10.1017/s0033291709990341.

128. Mueser KT, Penn DL, Addington J, Brunette MF, Gingerich S, Glynn SM, Lynde DW, et al. The NAVIGATE program for first-episode psychosis: rationale, overview, and description of psychosocial components. Psychiatr Serv. 2015;66(7):680–90. https://doi.org/10.1176/appi.ps.201400413.

129. Bechdolf A, Wagner M, Ruhrmann S, Harrigan S, Putzfeld V, Pukrop R, Brockhaus-Dumke A, et al. Preventing progression to first-episode psychosis in early initial prodromal states. Br J Psychiatry. 2012;200(1):22–9. https://doi.org/10.1192/bjp.bp.109.066357.

130. Miklowitz DJ, O'Brien MP, Schlosser DA, Addington J, Candan KA, Marshall C, Domingues I, Walsh BC, Zinberg JL, De Silva SD, Friedman-Yakoobian M, Cannon TD. Family-focused treatment for adolescents and young adults at high risk for psychosis: results of a randomized trial. J Am Acad Child Adolesc Psychiatry. 2014;53(8):848–58. https://doi.org/10.1016/j.jaac.2014.04.020.

131. Worthington MA, Miklowitz DJ, O'Brien M, Addington J, Bearden CE, Cadenhead KS, Cornblatt BA, et al. Selection for psychosocial treatment for youth at clinical high risk for psychosis based on the North American Prodrome Longitudinal Study individualized risk calculator. Early Interv Psychiatry. 2021;15(1):96–103. https://doi.org/10.1111/eip.12914.

132. Kessler RC, Crum RM, Warner LA, Nelson CB, Schulenberg J, Anthony JC. Lifetime co-occurrence of DSM-III-R alcohol abuse and dependence with other psychiatric disorders in the National Comorbidity Survey. Arch Gen Psychiatry. 1997;54(4):313–21. https://doi.org/10.1001/archpsyc.1997.01830160031005.

133. Schmidt LM, Hesse M, Lykke J. The impact of substance use disorders on the course of schizophrenia—a 15-year follow-up study: dual diagnosis over 15 years. Schizophr Res. 2011;130(1–3):228–33. https://doi.org/10.1016/j.schres.2011.04.011.

134. Barrowclough C, Haddock G, Wykes T, Beardmore R, Conrod P, Craig T, Davies L, et al. Integrated motivational interviewing and cognitive behavioural therapy for people with psychosis and comorbid substance misuse: randomised controlled trial. BMJ. 2010;341:c6325. https://doi.org/10.1136/bmj.c6325.

135. Brunette MF, Mueser KT, Drake RE. A review of research on residential programs for people with severe mental illness and co-occurring substance use disorders. Drug Alcohol Rev. 2004;23(4):471–81. https://doi.org/10.1080/09595230412331324590.

136. Brunette MF, Mueser KT. Psychosocial interventions for the long-term management of patients with severe mental illness and co-occurring substance use disorder. J Clin Psychiatry. 2006;67(Suppl 7):10–7.

137. Drake RE, Essock SM. The science-to-service gap in real-world schizophrenia treatment: the 95% problem. Schizophr Bull. 2009;35(4):677–8. https://doi.org/10.1093/schbul/sbp047.

138. Liberman RP. Recovery from schizophrenia: form follows functioning. World Psychiatry. 2012;11(3):161–2. https://doi.org/10.1002/j.2051-5545.2012.tb00118.x.

139. Deegan PE. The importance of personal medicine: a qualitative study of resilience in people with psychiatric disabilities. Scand J Public Health Suppl. 2005;66:29–35. https://doi.org/10.1080/14034950510033345.

140. Bond GR, Drake RE. New directions for psychiatric rehabilitation in the USA. Epidemiol Psychiatr Sci. 2017;26(3):223–7. https://doi.org/10.1017/S2045796016000834.

141. Williamson A, Makkar SR, McGrath C, Redman S. How can the use of evidence in mental health policy be increased? A systematic review. Psychiatr Serv. 2015;66(8):783–97. https://doi.org/10.1176/appi.ps.201400329.

142. Farkas M, Gagne C, Anthony W, Chamberlin J. Implementing recovery oriented evidence based programs: identifying the critical dimensions. Community Ment Health J. 2005;41(2):141–58. https://doi.org/10.1007/s10597-005-2649-6.

143. Winsper C, Crawford-Docherty A, Weich S, Fenton SJ, Singh SP. How do recovery-oriented interventions contribute to personal mental health recovery? A systematic review and logic model. Clin Psychol Rev. 2020;76:101815. https://doi.org/10.1016/j.cpr.2020.101815.

Recovery from Psychosis: Emerging Definitions, Research and Select Clinical Application

7

Paul H. Lysaker, Courtney N. Wiesepape, Jay A. Hamm, and Bethany L. Leonhardt

7.1 Introduction

Contrary to what had been accepted as fact for decades, research has confirmed that psychosis is, by definition, not a process of continuous decline ending in chronic dysfunction and disability. Instead, people can recover in meaningful and measurable ways from psychosis regardless of the severity of the disorder they earlier experienced. While this offers new and needed optimism, it raises several questions. How should we define and study the boundaries of recovery, especially as it is revealed as a deeply subjective process, and what are the parameters of clinical activities and therapies that best support recovery?

To explore these issues, this chapter will first offer an overview and critical discussion of how outcome has been conceptualized in psychosis and the rapid emergence of the concept of recovery. We will then discuss how research on

---

P. H. Lysaker (✉)
Department of Psychiatry, Indiana University School of Medicine, Indianapolis, IN, USA

Department of Psychiatry, Roudebush Veteran Affairs Medical Center, Indianapolis, IN, USA
e-mail: plysaker@iupui.edu

C. N. Wiesepape
Department of Psychology, Indiana State University, Terra Haute, IN, USA
e-mail: cwiesepape@sycamores.indstate.edu

J. A. Hamm
Eskenazi Health Midtown Community Mental Health, Indianapolis, IN, USA

College of Pharmacy, Purdue University, West Lafayette, IN, USA
e-mail: jay.a.hamm@gmail.com

B. L. Leonhardt
Eskenazi Health Midtown Community Mental Health, Indianapolis, IN, USA
e-mail: bethany.l.leonhardt@gmail.com

© The Author(s), under exclusive license to Springer Nature
Switzerland AG 2022
B. Carpiniello et al. (eds.), *Recovery and Major Mental Disorders*,
Comprehensive Approach to Psychiatry 2,
https://doi.org/10.1007/978-3-030-98301-7_7

outcome has posed the larger question of how to define recovery from psychosis and the potential that recovery is best seen as involving overlapping but separate sets of objective and subjective phenomenon. We will next focus on among the most subjective aspects of recovery, sense of self, and explore how research on metacognition offers ways to study the processes which may underpin the waning and waxing of an available sense of self for adults with psychosis. Next, we will discuss the implications for thinking about the general processes which are needed for interventions to promote recovery. Finally, we will present descriptions and supporting research for four specific emerging recovery-oriented interventions.

7.2 Historical Views of Outcome from Psychosis and the Emergence of the Concept of Recovery

Pessimistic views of outcome from serious mental illnesses are generally tied back to Kraepelin's [1] attempt to offer a definition of one form of psychosis on the basis of its features, course, and presumed etiology. Using the term Dementia Praecox, or precocious dementia, he asserted that a distinct psychiatric condition exists which is characterized by a progressive decline in mental functions, ultimately resulting in a metaphorical orchestra (the body) without a conductor (the mind). This view was based largely on the experience of case after case of persons with dismal outcomes that could not be explained by any current model or classification system (e.g., the negative outcomes were not the result of neurosyphilis). It was further asserted that this decline was fundamentally the result aberrant biological processes which were potentially metabolic in nature [2].

There are likely many reasons why Kraepelin's view came to be so broadly embraced in the United States and elsewhere. One admittedly disturbing possibility is that part of its appeal may have lain in its suggestion that the already observed poor outcomes for a group of institutionalized persons were inevitable. At the time when the ideas of Dementia Praecox were being circulated, psychiatric hospitals and sanitoriums in the United States were, and had long been, full of persons who had profoundly deteriorating courses of illness that often ended in death [2]. Kraepelin's view may, therefore, have provided a label that suggested terrible outcomes were largely unavoidable no matter what services were provided until the underlying causes were discovered and new treatments became available. Naturally, however, this view neglected the possibility that the limited gains noted in hospitals and sanitoriums across the century before Kraepelin were a function of the quality of living conditions and the treatments offered in these institutions. Indeed, one segment of those treatments was worse than ineffective and included interventions that were imposed without real informed consent and which were likely harmful. Examples of these included medicinal and mechanized emetics and hydrotherapies which could involve simulated drowning and forced baths [3, 4]. In a difficult sense, Kraepelin's view could thus be seen as a potential explanation for dismal outcomes, which avoided seeing whose poor outcomes may have been the result of inhumane treatment, and also saved the field from the responsibility of creating alternate treatments that could lead to positive outcomes.

During the same era, yet contrary to Kraepelin, Bleuler [5] proposed a more complex model of a singular form of psychosis. With an interest in integrating emerging views of the complexity of consciousness, Bleuler tried to replace the term dementia praecox with "schizophrenia." Bleuler suggested that in psychosis there was a rudimentary fragmentation of experience, or schism of the foundations of persons' sense of themselves in the world which results in a fundamental disconnection with the larger world [6]. While he held that these disturbances were likely of a biological origin, he noted that this was far from established as fact and allowed for the possibility, as we will discuss later, that treatment might address the psychological aspects of this condition. That is, the experience of fragmentation could be addressed in psychosocial treatment allowing for persons to achieve meaningful levels of wellness.

Though beyond the scope of this paper, the course of thought that proceeded Kraepelin and Bleuler has been circuitous to say the least. While there have been periods of interest in the unique lives of persons with psychosis [7, 8], the field has also largely been limited by a narrow focus on the oddness of experience or the otherness of persons with these conditions, a practice that has dissociated the diagnosed persons from their pain and assumed poor outcomes [6, 9]. Accordingly, for at least the first seven decades since these original formulations, the field largely continued to hold the idea that positive outcomes from psychosis are an anomaly and that the best outcomes include stability or merely a lack of worsening outcomes [10].

Rapidly, however, this changed when researchers began to seek out people who had once experienced significant psychiatric challenges and interviewed them later in their lives [11, 12]. Taking this approach, longitudinal research across Europe and North America found far more variability of outcomes than previous models would have suggested. When conducting long-term follows-ups, it was determined that many, if not most, persons who experienced psychosis had become well (e.g., [13, 14]). In addition to this work, a grassroots community based movement emerged in the 1980s and 1990s that began to challenge the idea that individuals with serious mental illness could not achieve a personally meaningful and fully acceptable quality of life. This movement, known as the recovery movement, was consistent with much earlier first-person accounts of recovery from serious mental illness [15], and argued for a broader and more individualized understanding of what represents recovery, and called for substantial reform to mental health services. One seminal expression of this can be found as Anthony [16] described recovery as: "…a deeply personal, unique process of changing one's attitudes, values, feelings, goals, skills, and/or roles… It is a way of living a satisfying, hopeful, and contributing life even with the limitations caused by illness."

As work accumulated in early part of the twenty-first century, recovery then moved from a controversial to a mainstream concept, with guidelines emerging for mental health treatment to emphasize recovery as the desired outcome [17]. Across varying settings, services began to be tasked with promoting recovery and identifying barriers to recovery. This has in turn spurred an entirely new set of research endeavors which has led to the identification of barriers to wellness, which are not biological in origin, including community exclusion [18, 19] and both external and internalized stigma [20].

7.2.1 The Challenge of Defining Recovery

The failure of the models suggesting that stability at most or decline at worst, is the generally expected outcome from psychosis, has engendered a far more optimistic outlook for persons diagnosed with psychosis. However, the idea that outcome is more than continuous disorder has raised a number of immediate questions. For one, while illness or disorder may be presumably defined by the presence of a discrete set of symptoms or dysfunctional behaviors, health is not as readily definable by the absence of those symptoms or behaviors. A person diagnosed can be said to be ill and remain ill, for example, because of persistent positive or negative symptoms. Yet recovery is more than the disappearance of those problematic experiences [21].

Decades of interviews with persons diagnosed with psychosis suggest that recovery involves the repair of a life that has been interrupted by mental illness [22–24]. Symptom remission or the attainment of a skill could be an important part of the repair of that interruption, but it cannot necessarily always be the whole story. Tempting as it may be to describe wellness in a manner analogous to remission from a chronic psychiatric condition in which there is a discrete site of pathology, recovery is far more complex, because it is a process that takes place in the world, involving relationships with both the world and oneself [11]. Recovery, because it is about a unique person's life, should be expected to vary considerably from person to person with the core of that recovery having meanings which are deeply subjective for each person.

Recovery for one person may mean to gain social status or a feeling of worth. For others recovery may be intimately tied to attaining housing and work. To recover from psychosis for others may involve the recapture of a sense of purpose, and that sense of purpose would naturally have to vary between persons. What makes up one person's purpose could be meaningless or noxious to another recovering person [25, 26].

7.2.2 Objective and Subjective Domains of Recovery

One way to approach the dilemma of how to define and measure health for persons diagnosed with psychosis is to consider that the definition of recovery is first a matter of who is measuring or describing it. Recovery may be thought of differently from the vantage point of a person living with it or others who know or live with the person living with it [11]. Thus, recovery can be conceptualized as having different dimensions which may in fact be potentially unrelated [27]. Early attempts to describe these different domains posited that recovery might be divided into objective and subjective forms of recovery [10, 28].

Objective domains of recovery: Objective forms of recovery include aspects of recovery that others might notice. These could include, for example, attaining work, enrolling in college, forming or renewing relationships, and other activities that could be definitively established and measured [29]. Other objective elements of recovery could include symptom remission, which can also be measured quantitatively [30]. An example of work that refers to a primarily objectively defined aspect of recovery includes Kane's [31] suggestion that recovery occurs after insight allows persons to accept pharmacological treatment, leading to symptom remission and enhanced function.

Research exploring objective domains of recovery have to date produced broadly varying results. As summarized by Leonhardt and colleagues [11, 12], symptom remission in studies of early psychosis ranged from 37 to 91.4%, with the follow-up periods within these studies ranging from a half year to a decade. The attainment of functional milestones has been reported in early psychosis to range from 29 to 58%, with 14–29.5% of those studied achieving both symptom remission and regaining acceptable levels of psychosocial function. A similar pattern has also been observed for adults with prolonged psychosis, with the rate of symptom remission varying between 37 and 89%, the attainment of acceptable psychosocial levels of function ranging from 21 to 53%, and with both symptom remission and the attainment of acceptable psychosocial function occurring in 13–27% of the sample. In these studies of prolonged psychosis, the follow-up periods lasted up to 20 years [11].

Subjective domains of recovery: Subjective domains of recovery in contrast to the objective domains involve experiences that are primarily observable only by the persons who have been diagnosed with psychosis. Examples of these include the attainment of a personally defined acceptable quality of life or the experience of again directing one's own life; things that others are not in a position to determine on their own. Recapturing a sense of purpose or a feeling that one's experiences and ideas could be valuable to others could similarly be described as subjective domains of recovery.

Research into the more subjective domains of recovery has had to utilize different tactics than what were employed by studies of objective domains of recovery. However, this has not meant that there is not objective measurement of subjective experience. One commonly used questionnaire to assess subjective recovery is the Recovery Assessment Scale (RAS) [32]. This instrument yields an overall estimate of the subjective experience of recovery and five potentially interrelated aspects: personal confidence and hope, goal and success orientation, willingness to ask for help, connection with others, and not feeling dominated by symptoms. Use of this instrument has led to work that has linked self-reported subjective recovery to a range of other factors, including emotional distress and perception of community involvement [33, 34].

Delving more deeply into the subjective qualities of recovery, others have studied recovery using qualitative methods and first-person accounts of mental illness.

Qualitative studies, definitionally, are interested in the quality and not quantity of experience and seek to identify participants' unique experiences of recovery from psychosis through formal interviews and then extract general themes. First-person accounts similarly are concerned with subjective experience as is unearthed in the personal narratives and reflections of individuals, rather than in their response to standard questions [35, 36].

One emerging attempt to synthesize work on the range of subjective experiences involved in recovery has been referred to as CHIME. This method suggests that there are discernable themes across subjective experiences of recovery which can be labeled as: connectedness, hope, identity, meaning in life, and empowerment [37]. In a recent thematic analysis, Ellison and colleagues [38] evaluated different reviews of recovery and found four of the CHIME elements commonly reoccurred: identity, empowerment, meaning in life, and hope. Earlier, McCarthy-Jones et al. [23] conducted a meta-synthesis of qualitative studies and also found alterations in sense of self, purpose and connection to others were common experiences. Other attempts at synthesis include a thematic analysis by Soundy and colleagues [39] that found the subjective experience of recovery was closely tied to ability to adjust to the experience of psychosis, to respond to the illness, and find social support.

While we have considered objective and subjective recovery separately here, research on their interaction suggests they may not represent phenomenon that should only be considered in isolation. For example, Hasson-Ohayon and colleagues [40] have demonstrated how the impact of a recovery-oriented intervention on objective outcomes can only be deeply understood in the context of the subjective experiences revealed in qualitative analyses. Thomas et al. [41] reported that estimates of social network were related to both objective and subjective outcomes, while the degree of self-efficacy mediated that relationship. Further, Shadami et al. [42] reported that subjectively appraised quality of life was a protective factor for rehospitalization and the burden of symptoms. Kukla and colleagues [43] similarly found that the subjective experience of recovery reduced the influence of symptoms on quality of life.

7.2.3   Recovery, the Self, and Metacognition

While distinguishing recovery objectively seen through the eyes of others from the subjective experience of recovery has been an important step, subjective aspects of recovery can occur at many levels. These can include how one appraises possibilities and quality of life. These can also involve a potently deeper realm of subjective, that is the person themselves [21]. Here we are referring to the experience of some diagnosed with psychosis, that to recover, is to recover a cohesive sense of themselves as being unique in the world. As a central part of the CHIME model, but also as noted broadly across very different research traditions, the loss of a coherent sense of self may characterize the onset of psychosis, while a return of a coherent sense of self may signal recovery [44]. Yet how is this most deeply subjective phenomenon to be conceptualized and formally studied?

To address this question we begin with an exploration of the processes that allow a sense of self to emerge within the flow of experience. In the simplest form, we do not know ourselves as we know other things in the world. We are not who we are because of our place in space or merely our appearance or even our physical properties. So how do I know myself and how could persons feel that their basic self has changed, been diminished, or returned?

In response to these dilemmas, William James proposed over a century and a quarter ago that self-experience is our instantaneous and evolving experience of ourselves as we experience the world [45]. Human beings, according to James, do not just have experiences of the world, but experience themselves experiencing the world. The self is not something we know through direct appraisal; we do not observe it like we would observe something as existing in a physical location in space. We interpret and respond to the world and we experience ourselves making those interpretations, and then responding to our experiences and ourselves accordingly.

Through the lens of James, recovering persons' sense of the recapture of a cohesive sense of self would be the recapturing of an experience of themselves experiencing the world. But how do we experience ourselves experiencing the world and what about that could we potentially measure? One empirical approach to both conceptualizing and studying how self-experience can wax and wane is rooted in the study of metacognition. In the integrated model of metacognition, metacognitive capacities are suggested to allow us to notice discrete elements or atoms of our experience of ourselves within the flow of life and then to reflect upon their relationship to one another [46–48]. Examples of what we might notice about ourselves experiencing the world could include a specific thought, feeling, or bodily state that arises in the moment. Concerning the relationship among these experiences we might reflect or notice patterns in how we think and understand what feeling arose when it did. We then might reflect further and discern something larger about ourselves.

Intact metacognitive capacities thus allow awareness of not only discrete mental experiences but also the larger whole of which they are a part [48]. Metacognitive capacities make it possible to synthesize discrete experiences into a more complex multi-faceted sense of a self which is then available to persons [24]. Conversely, metacognitive deficits or reductions in metacognitive capacity could leave persons with only a fragmented sense of the self. With diminished metacognitive capacity persons would be left with awareness of discrete aspects or atoms of experience but with limited ability to see how those aspects or atoms relate to and influence one another. Persons with significant metacognitive deficits might be able to notice a thought, emotion, or bodily state but not see any larger patterns or ideas about themselves which create the structure that allows us to have access to a continuous sense of who we are as unique persons over time [21]. With this in mind, it has been proposed that the loss of a coherent sense of self in psychosis could reflect the loss of metacognitive capacity, while the recovery of that sense of self could indicate a growth in metacognitive capacity [48, 49]. It has also been hypothesized that the general state of fragmentation that would ensure in the face of metacognition deficits corresponds closely to Blueler's [5] theoretical model of schizophrenia as rooted in the disorganization of thought, emotion, and desire [24].

Evidence supporting these hypotheses can be found in international studies which have compared quantitative assessments of metacognitive capacity within the personal narratives among groups with psychosis, other forms of mental and non-psychiatric adversity, and community members without any significant indication of mental illness. As expected, in these studies persons with more severe forms of psychosis, including schizophrenia, have tended to have the lowest levels of metacognitive function [24]. Other work has found that among persons with psychosis greater levels of impairment in metacognitive capacity are related to poorer function when assessed concurrently and prospectively [50]. Objective and subjective outcomes related to metacognitive capacity and recovery include social function [51], intrinsic motivation [52], self-compassion [53], emotional expression [54], empathy [55], and the ability to resist stigma [56] and use social support to move towards recovery [43]. More recent work has reported that changes in metacognitive capacity are correlated with changes in other essential features of psychosis including neurocognition and social cognition [57]. Finally, interventions that seek to improve metacognitive functioning have been observed to result in concurrent increases in subjective aspects of recovery related to self-experience among persons with psychosis, including an enhanced sense of personal agency and coherence [58–60].

To be clear, metacognition is not the self. Metacognition, though, is a potentially measurable process by which persons' availability to a sense of self could wax and wane, diminishing with onset of illness and returning with recovery. While this work is novel and awaiting more research, as we will see in the next section, it poses important implications about the possible essential elements of recovery-oriented treatment. For example, as has been observed, recovery does not take place in the theater of a single mind but is about participation in one's community through concrete activities [61]. One possibility is that with enhanced metacognitive capacities, persons may garner a better sense of how their thoughts, wishes, emotions, strengths, personal history, and values are related to one another in a larger whole, as well as how the same is true for others. This may then enable the emergence of a sense of agency and context which render certain things more personally meaningful than others, warranting some activities worthy of our risk and effort [62]. This path from fragmentation towards recovery over time as ignited by the growth in metacognition is portrayed in Fig. 7.1.

7.3   General Implications for Recovery-Oriented Practice

Turning to recovery-oriented practice, the task seems almost as dizzying as defining recovery itself. For the purposes of this chapter we suggest that much of recovery-oriented practice may follow from one larger insight, namely that a practice that promotes recovery cannot be defined by the content or delivery of a specific intervention. As noted by Leonhardt et al. [12], what follows from this literature is that

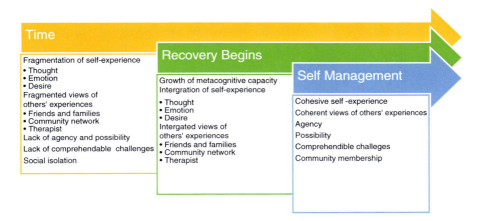

Fig. 7.1 The role of metacognition in the path from fragmentation towards recovery from psychosis

recovery-oriented interventions must be tailored to the unique way that an individual is choosing to understand and manage their psychiatric and social challenges. Regardless of whether a clinical intervention, for example, might be said to come from cognitive behavioral, humanistic, psychodynamic, or rehabilitative frameworks, its potential to promote recovery lies in how the recovering person is approached during the interventions and invited into a joint examination of the opportunities and dilemmas facing that person. In other words, recovery needs to be a matter of an overarching dialogue between the clinician and recovering person, as opposed to a clinician directing the recovering person or the clinician blindly going along with what the recovering person thinks.

Following Leonhardt and colleagues [12], such recovery-oriented interventions do share things in common and can be, to a degree, operationalized by their qualities. The first among these might be framed as requiring clinicians and practitioners to acknowledge and resist factors which limit recovering persons' ability to make their own sense of the opportunities and challenges they face. Factors which can limit recovering persons' ability to make meaning include externalized and internalized stigma which position recovering persons as unable to make their own decisions or as too unreliable to make their own decisions [63]. All stigma is not manifestly negative in content. Benevolent, but equally stigmatizing and dangerous beliefs can include practitioners, failing to see the whole person before them, sanitizing the aggressive or complex elements of the personalities of recovering person. Overly optimistic, patronizing, or sentimental ways of understanding recovering persons would seem to offer barriers to recovery deep as any other.

We believe, however, that the steps that come after the rejection of limiting factors, such as stigma or reactionary beliefs about recovery, may be complex. For one, many of the decisions that persons recovering from psychosis have to make can be frightening, given as noted above, that they involve risk. A person diagnosed with psychosis moving towards recovery must be an active participant in making decisions about their life. Those persons have to direct their own recovery, but there is always the looming possibility things may go badly. For example, a wish to reduce or discontinue antipsychotic medication may come with the risk of a rehospitalization. A decision to try to date or work may offer opportunities for failure and confirmation of negative thoughts about the self. There may even be deeper and less obvious risks. With the achievement of features of recovery, such as work and symptom remission, recovering persons may lose familiar features of the sick role they previously occupied or systems of meanings that came from positive symptoms [64]. Even beyond that, risk seems inevitable, since taking no risks certainly risks losing the potential for regaining much of what may have been lost or suspended during periods of psychosis and isolation. A life of dignity would always seem to involve risk and certainly that is as true for a recovering person.

What is needed then in recovery-oriented work is a sharing of those risks and joint reflection upon them. Clinicians here must neither be *the* decision maker or a passive supportive party. Instead, a non-hierarchical relationship is needed in which both parties jointly and openly discuss what is at issue. The experience of anxiety and fear as well as excitement of possibility should be shared. We do not dispute that there is a power differential inherent in clinical practice. Clinicians have expertise, but at issue is the use of that expertise. We suggest that in recovery-oriented practice that expertise is offered from the seat of a compassionate consultant willing to think with and share some of the risks with the consumer [65]. This is consistent with other work that emphasizes a continuous process in clinical work in which there is ongoing negotiation about the working alliance and the role of the clinician and recovering person within it [40].

A related thought about some processes of recovery-oriented practice is their focus cannot be merely on the amelioration of pain. As persons form an increasingly complex sense of themselves and what has transpired in their lives, distress may emerge and might even be expected [64]. This may present opportunities to affirm the resiliency of recovering persons and also to normalize deep pain as part of the human condition. It would seem essential for both partners in the dialogue to be able to accept the recovering person's pain without alarm, and with the expectation that the pain we all experience can be understood and endured in the context of compassionate connections with others. Echoing back to an earlier comment about the need to see the whole person, a clinician who is not attuned to the likelihood of the emergence of grief and loss that comes with recovery risks invalidating recovering persons' experiences, and undoing any previously empowering interventions.

Finally, if, as suggested by work on metacognition, the experience of fragmentation may complicate recovering persons' abilities to make sense of and decide what to do about the challenges they face, interventions may also need to be sensitive in some manner to the recovering person's current level of metacognitive capacity. In particular, efforts to arrive at a shared understanding with recovering persons may be unsuccessful if clinicians form ideas which are more complex than the recovering person can engage with. Indeed, interventions, regardless of their format, must be offered at levels that match how recovering persons integrate information and form ideas about themselves for shared meaning making to occur. For example, an intervention that involves helping persons to form goals and make plans could require different approaches given their capacities for metacognition at that moment. The complexity of interventions also then would be expected to change as persons experience changes in their metacognitive capacities [49]. Of note, the Metacognition Assessment Scale-Abbreviated [24] has been used for this purpose in different settings [60] though there is no reason to believe other approaches could not also be used.

7.4 Four Emerging Forms of Recovery Oriented Treatments

Finally, moving from general qualities of interventions we here turn to some of treatments currently being implemented. While there are certainly more than four forms of treatment that could be labeled as recovery oriented, we have chosen these given their fidelity to some of the core findings about recovery, because they illustrate how this work can range from more to less structured, and because they include work with individuals, families, and groups.

Open Dialogue: Predating the recovery movement, one of the most widely used forms of interventions focused on helping persons make sense of deciding how to manage the challenges of psychosis is Open Dialogue. Open dialogue calls for the rapid offering of group meetings involving the persons with the potential diagnosis and prominent members of their social network, which can include family friends and other key supports within the community [66, 67]. Open Dialogue is partially based on work suggesting human beings make meaning through dialogue and are indeed themselves the product of that dialogue [68]. Human beings in this model are complex collections of elements which may be contradictory, complimentary, and unrelated and dialogue requires the participation of these many different elements. The collapse of that dialogue is believed to result in a monologue which compromises persons' sense of agency [69] and which is believed to be common in psychosis [70]. Interventions are intended to either reestablish or repair collapsed dialogue.

Open in Open Dialogue refers to directly sharing ideas. Requirements for openness extend to clinicians as well, positing clinicians as joint meaning makers and not as experts directing the dialogue. Open dialogue is believed to allow persons in a social network to jointly develop a deeper and ongoing understanding of the complexities of psychosis and what would constitute effective adaption [71]. Research on the effects of this are mixed and research methodologies supporting this work have been criticized [72]. However, some recent reports have noted long-term evidence of effects on objective markers of recovery such as hospitalization [73]. A recent qualitative study also found that though some participants found the therapeutic dialogues to be confusing, they also felt understood by others during these encounters [74].

Cognitive Behavior Therapy for Psychosis (CBTp): CBTp is an adaptation of standard cognitive behavior therapy, which seeks to reflect with recovering persons about the relationship of their thoughts, feeling, and behaviors, to re-evaluate their beliefs about themselves and their distress, to monitor thoughts, feeling, and behaviors about their distress, and to ultimately find other ways of responding to that distress [75]. This treatment is believed to bring symptomatic relief when beliefs and behaviors which prolonged or exacerbated distress and dysfunction are replaced with more adaptive thoughts and behaviors.

Since its original application, CBTp has been applied to both helping persons reduce positive symptoms and more recently to formulating goals and finding ways to achieve them [76]. It has also been applied to negative self-beliefs [77]. CBTp in comparison to Open Dialogue is generally an individual form of psychotherapy with a prescribed length and content (e.g., 20–30 sessions, each of a specific length). CBTp is readily the most broadly studied intervention presented here with results of metanalysis showing its strongest effects involve reductions in positive symptoms [78, 79].

Metacognitive Reflection and Insight Therapy (MERIT). MERIT is a form of individual integrative psychotherapy for adults with psychosis developed by the authors [49, 60]. It is based on the research presented above suggesting deficits in metacognitive capacity limit persons' abilities to make sense of their challenges. In contrast to CBTp, it is not defined by a curriculum nor does it have a prescribed generic length. It is operationalized by eight core elements which should be present in each session. Most unique among these elements are the last two which require interventions match recovering persons' metacognitive capacity so that there can truly be joint reflection within session. Overall, these elements act as a guide for therapists and should each synergistically promote the development of metacognitive capacity. MERIT is believed to promote recovery by promoting the development of metacognitive capacity which then allows recovering persons to form more complex and evolving ides about themselves and others, leading to empowerment and self-directed recovery.

MERIT is the least studied of the interventions here with results of several randomized and open trials demonstrating acceptability to clinically meaningful gains in metacognitive capacity.[c.f. 60] Case reports have provided evidence that the treatment can be flexibly adapted in different setting to meet the needs of recovering persons with broadly varying needs [80]. Finally, qualitative analyses link MERIT to subjective changes in how persons think about themselves and their lives [58, 59].

Narrative Enhancement and Cognitive Therapy (NECT): NECT is a manualized form of group therapy, also contributed to by the authors, which seeks to reduce internalized stigma for adults with psychosis [81]. It consists of 20 sessions which can be divided into four phases: (1) introduction (1 week), (2) psychoeducation (3 weeks), (3) cognitive restructuring (8 weeks), and (4) narrative enhancement (8 weeks). The psychoeducation section introduces recovering persons to the idea of stigma and the cognitive restructuring section introduces participants to the ideas that thoughts and feelings and behavior interact. Narrative enhancement focuses on recovering persons telling and sharing personal narratives about themselves and the challenges and successes they have experienced in life. NECT is hypothesized to reduced self-stigma by helping recovering persons recognize stigma, see how stigmatizing beliefs negatively effects their lives and then through narrative work to find new and non-stigmatizing stories to tell about themselves and their lives.

NECT has been delivered and studied internationally. Randomized and open trials in the United States and Sweden have indicated NECT is acceptable to recovering persons and linked with clinically meaningful improvements in self-stigma [82, 83]. Findings from qualitative analyses have linked with multiple subjective aspects of recovery [27].

7.5   Reflections, Limitations, and Future Directions

In sum, recovery from psychosis is not an anomaly and is made up of a range of objective and subjective outcomes. Among the most subjective of these outcomes include the reclamation of a sense of self, which is potentially related to metacognition, or more specifically growth in persons abilities to form complex and evolving ideas of themselves and others. We have suggested that these insights suggest a need for the field to move away from thinking about isolated interventions and towards thinking about processes which engage with the recovering person in the processing of making meaning of the challenges they face. Finally, we have described four current attempts to offer interventions which are explicitly recovery oriented.

In considering these four interventions described, we are struck at how they themselves, by the stark differences between them, tell us something about the fuzzy and complex nature of recovery. CBTp is focused and structured, as is NECT. MERIT and Open Dialogue are far less structured and bound closely to theoretical models. In addition, MERIT and Open Dialogue explicitly seek to make sure meaning is made jointly. NECT and CBTp were engineered with particular end points, whereas MERIT and Open Dialogue were not. Each of these interventions also has its distinct limitations. MERIT, our own intervention, has the weakest research base and its method of action is notoriously difficult to measure. It also may be less feasible than other treatments which are shorter in duration. NECT, another treatment we are associated with, is focused only on one key outcome and its usefulness to recovering persons who do not have internalized stigma would seem minimal. CBTp, which has the strongest base, has focused primarily on positive symptoms, which are only a small portion of things which concern recovering persons. Open Dialogue, while rich theoretically does not seem to take into account the complexity of the barriers to dialogue which come with psychosis.

Of note, there are other broader limitations important to consider. Long-term longitudinal research is needed which includes both qualitative and quantitative assessments of various domains of recovery and other key phenomenon to understand how recovery unfolds for different persons. It is also important that this work be done in non-industrialized nations and includes participants who are notoriously difficult to recruit, those who refuse treatment. Work is also needed to more carefully parse apart the subjective experience of recovery and understand how often certain elements are at play and others not. Concerning practice, we have suggested overall processes, but it is unknown how these are best incorporated into practice. While we have explored how these processes may play a role in one form of metacognitively oriented psychotherapy, Metacognitive Reflection and Insight Therapy (MERIT) [49], it is unclear how their incorporation might differ in other approaches.

While little is known about the potential negative consequences of recovery-oriented treatment, it is possible that like any treatment, there could be undesirable consequences. If, as we have suggested, a healthy life calls for taking risks, some of those risks may not lead to what persons may have wanted or anticipated. Finally, we chose to present only four recovery-oriented treatments. Certainly, there are a host of newer and even some older revamped treatments which could potentially be called recovery oriented. Work is needed to better catalogue these and possibly even define different classes of such treatments according to their principals and proposed means of action.

References

1. Kraepelin E, Barclay RM, Robertson GM. Dementia praecox and paraphrenia. Edinburgh, UK: E&S Livingstone; 1919.
2. Noll R. American madness: the rise and fall of Dementia Praecox. Cambridge, MA: Harvard University Press; 2011.
3. Hinshaw S. Another kind of madness. New York, NY: St Martin's Press; 2017.
4. Whitaker R. Mad in America: bad science, bad medicine, and the enduring mistreatment of the mentally ill. New York, NY: Perseus Publishing; 2002.
5. Bleuler E. Dementia praecox or the group of schizophrenias. Zinkin J, trans. New York, NY: International Universities; 1950. Original work published 1911.
6. Katschnig H. Psychiatry's contribution to the public stereotype of schizophrenia: historical considerations. J Eval Clin Pract. 2018;24(5):1093–100.
7. Meyer A. The collected papers of Adolf Meyer. Baltimore, MD: John Hopkins Press; 1950.
8. Searles H. Collected papers on schizophrenia and related subjects. New York, NY: International Universities Press; 1965.
9. Hamm JA, Buck B, Lysaker PH. Reconciling the ipseity-disturbance model with the presence of painful affect in schizophrenia. Philos Psychiatr Psychol. 2015;22(3):197–208.
10. Lysaker PH, Buck KD. Is recovery from schizophrenia possible: an overview of concepts, evidence and clinical implications. Prim Psychiatry. 2008;15(6):60–6.
11. Leonhardt BL, Huling K, Hamm JA, Roe D, Hasson-Ohayon I, McLeod H, et al. Recovery and serious mental illness: a review of current clinical and research paradigms and future directions. Expert Rev Neurother. 2017;17(11):1117–30.
12. Leonhardt BL, Hamm JA, Lysaker PH. The recovery model in psychosis. In: Badcock J, Paulik-White, editors. Clinical introduction to psychosis: foundations for clinical and neuropsychologists. Elsevier; 2019. p. 113–34.
13. Ciompi L. The natural history of schizophrenia in the long term. Br J Psychiatry. 1980;136:413–20.
14. Harding CM, Brooks GW, Ashikaga T, Strauss JS, Breier A. The Vermont longitudinal study of persons with severe mental illness I: methodology, study sample, and overall status 32 years later. Am J Psychiatry. 1987;144(6):718–26.
15. Beers C. A mind that found itself. New York, NY: Longmans, Green; 1908.
16. Anthony WA. Recovery from mental illness: the guiding vision of the mental health service system in the 1990s. Psychosocial Rehabilitation Journal. 1993;16(4):11–23.

17. Substance Abuse and Mental Health Services Administration (SAMHSA). SAMHSA's working definition of recovery [Internet]. 2012. https://store.samhsa.gov/sites/default/files/d7/priv/pep12-recdef.pdf.
18. Jones N, Rosen C, Helm S, O'Neill S, Davidson L, Shattell M. Psychosis in public mental health: provider perspectives on clinical relationships and barriers to the improvement of services. Am J Orthopsychiatry. 2019;89(1):95–103.
19. Tanaka K, Davidson L, Craig TJ. Sense of clubhouse community belonging and empowerment. Int J Soc Psychiatry. 2018;64(3):276–85.
20. Yanos PT, Roe D, Lysaker PH. The impact of illness identity on recovery from severe mental illness. Am J Psychiatr Rehabil. 2010;13(2):73–93.
21. Lysaker PH, Kukla M, Leonhardt BL, Hamm JA, Schnackenberg MA, Zalzala AB, et al. Meaning, integration, and the self in serious mental illness: implications of research in metacognition for psychiatric rehabilitation. Am J Psychiatr Rehabil. 2020;43(4):275–83.
22. Andresen R, Caputi P, Oades L. Stages of recovery instrument: development of a measure of recovery from serious mental illness. Aust N Z J Psychiatry. 2006;40(11–12):972–80.
23. McCarthy-Jones S, Marriott M, Knowles R, Rowse G, Thompson AR. What is psychosis? A meta-synthesis of inductive qualitative studies exploring the experience of psychosis. Psychosis. 2013;5(1):1–16.
24. Lysaker PH, Zalzala AB, Ladegaard N, Buck B, Leonhardt BL, Hamm JA. A disorder by any other name: metacognition, schizophrenia, and diagnostic practice. J Humanist Psychol. 2019;59(1):26–47.
25. Davidson L, O'Connell M, Tondora J, Styron T, Kangas K. The top ten concerns about recovery encountered in mental health system transformation. Psychiatr Serv. 2006;57(5):640–5.
26. Silverstein SM, Bellack AS. A scientific agenda for the concept of recovery as it applies to schizophrenia. Clin Psychol Rev. 2004;28(7):1108–24.
27. Roe D, Meshiach-Eizernberg M, Lysaker PH. The relation between objective and subjective domains of recovery among persons with schizophrenia related disorders. Schizophr Res. 2011;131(1–3):133–8.
28. Resnick SG, Rosenheck RA, Lehman AF. An exploratory analysis of correlates of recovery. Psychiatr Serv. 2004;55(5):540–7.
29. Liberman RP, Kopelowicz A, Ventura J, Gutkind D. Operational criteria and factors related to recovery from schizophrenia. Int Rev Psychiatry. 2002;14(4):256–72.
30. Cassidy CM, Norman R, Manchanda R, Schmitz N, Malla A. Testing definitions of symptom remission in first-episode psychosis for prediction of functional outcome at 2 years. Schizophr Bull. 2010;36(5):1001–8.
31. Kane JM. Improving patient outcomes in schizophrenia: achieving remission, preventing relapse, and measuring success. J Clin Psychiatry. 2013;74(9):e18. https://doi.org/10.4088/JCP.12117tx1c.
32. Corrigan PW, Giffort D, Rashid F, Leary M, Okeke I. Recovery as a psychological construct. Community Ment Health J. 1999;35(3):231–9.
33. Jorgensen R, Zoffmann V, Munk-Jorgensen P, Buck KD, Jensen SO, Hasson I, et al. Relationships over time of subjective and objective elements of recovery in persons with schizophrenia. Psychiatry Res. 2015;228(1):14–9.
34. Garverich S, Prener CG, Guyer ME, Lincoln AK. What matters: factors impacting the recovery process among outpatient mental health service users. Psychiatr Rehabil J. 2021;44(1):77–86. https://doi.org/10.1037/prj0000407.
35. Hornstein GA. Agnes' jacket: a psychologist's search for the meanings of madness. New York, NY: Gildan Media, LLC; 2009.
36. Korsbek L. Corecovery: mental health recovery in a dynamic interplay between humans in a relationship. Am J Psychiatr Rehabil. 2016;19(3):196–205.
37. Leamy M, Bird V, Le Boutilier C, Williams J, Slade L. Conceptual framework for personal recovery in mental health: systematic review and narrative synthesis. Br J Psychiatry. 2011;199(6):445–52.

38. Ellison ML, Belanger LK, Niles BL, Evans LC, Bauer MS. Explication and definition of mental health recover: a systematic review. Admin Pol Ment Health. 2018;45(1):91–102.
39. Soundy A, Stubbs B, Roskell C, Williams SE, Fox A, Vancampfort D. Identifying the facilitators and processes which influence recovery in individuals with schizophrenia: a systematic review and thematic synthesis. J Ment Health. 2015;24(2):103–10.
40. Hasson-Ohayon I, Kravetz S, Lysaker PH. Special challenges of psychotherapy with persons with psychosis: intersubjective metacognitive model of agreement and shared meaning. Clin Psychol Psychother. 2017;24(2):428–40.
41. Thomas EC, Muralidharan A, Medoff D, Drapalski AL. Self-efficacy as a mediator of the relationship between social support and recovery in serious mental illness. Psychiatr Rehabil J. 2016;39(4):352–60.
42. Shadmi E, Gelkopf M, Garber-Epstein P, Baloush-Kleinman V, Doudai R, Roe D. Routine patient reported outcomes as predictors of psychiatric rehospitalization. Schizophr Res. 2017;192:119–23.
43. Kukla M, Lysaker PH, Roe D. Strong subjective recovery as a protective factor against the effects of positive symptoms on quality of life outcomes in schizophrenia. Compr Psychiatry. 2014;55(6):1363–8.
44. Lysaker PH, Lysaker JT. Schizophrenia and alterations in self-experience: a comparison of 6 perspectives. Schizophr Bull. 2010;36(2):331–40.
45. James W, Burkhardt F, Bowers F, Skrupskelis IK. The principles of psychology (1, 2). London: Macmillan; 1890.
46. Moritz S, Lysaker PH. Metacognition–what did James H. Flavell really say and the implications for the conceptualization and design of metacognitive interventions. Schizophr Res. 2018;201:20–6.
47. Lysaker PH, Dimaggio G. Metacognitive capacities for reflection in schizophrenia: implications for developing treatments. Schizophr Bull. 2014;40(3):487–91.
48. Lysaker PH, Keane J, Poirier-Culleton S, Lundin N. Schizophrenia, recovery and the self: an introduction to the special issue on metacognition. Schizophr Res Cogn. 2020;19:100167.
49. Lysaker PH, Klion R. Recovery, meaning making, and severe mental illness: a comprehensive guide to Metacognitive and Reflection Insight Therapy. New York, NY: Routledge; 2017.
50. Arnon-Ribenfeld N, Hasson-Ohayon I, Lavidor M, Atzil-Slonim D, Lysaker PH. The association between metacognitive abilities and outcome measures among people with schizophrenia: a meta-analysis. Eur Psychiatry. 2017;46:33–41.
51. Fisher MW, Dimaggio G, Hochheiser J, Vohs J, Phalen P, Lysaker PH. Metacognitive capacity is related to self-reported social functioning and may moderate the effects of symptoms on interpersonal behavior. J Nerv Ment Dis. 2020;208(2):138–42.
52. Luther L, Bonfils KA, Firmin RL, Buck KD, Choi J, Dimaggio G, et al. Is metacognition necessary for the emergence of motivation in schizophrenia? A necessary condition analysis. J Nerv Ment Dis. 2017;205(12):960–6.
53. Hochheiser J, Lundin N, Lysaker PH. The independent relationships of metacognition, mindfulness, and cognitive insight to self-compassion in schizophrenia. J Nerv Ment Dis. 2020;208(1):1–6.
54. Austin SF, Lysaker PH, Jansen JE, Trauelsen AM, Nielsen HL, Pedersen MB, et al. Metacognitive capacity and negative symptoms in first episode psychosis: evidence of a prospective relationship over a 3-year follow-up. J Exp Psychopathol. 2019;10(1)
55. Bonfils KA, Lysaker PH, Minor KS, Salyers MP. Metacognition, personal distress, and performance-based empathy in schizophrenia. Schizophr Bull. 2019;45(1):19–26.
56. Nabors LM, Yanos PT, Roe D, Hasson-Ohayon I, Leonhardt BL, Buck KD, et al. Stereotype endorsement, metacognitive capacity, and self-esteem as predictors of stigma resistance in persons with schizophrenia. Compr Psychiatry. 2014;55(4):792–8.
57. Kukla M, Lysaker PH. Metacognition over time related to neurocognition, social cognition, and intrapsychic foundations in psychosis. Schizophr Res Cogn. 2020;19:100149.

58. de Jong S, Hasson-Ohayon I, van Donkersgoed R, Aleman A, Pijnenborg GHM. A qualitative evaluation of the effects of metacognitive reflection and insight therapy: 'living more consciously'. Psychol Psychother. 2019;93(2)
59. Lysaker PH, Kukla M, Belanger E, White DA, Buck KD, Luther L, et al. Individual psychotherapy and changes in self-experience in schizophrenia: a qualitative comparison of patients in metacognitively focused and supportive psychotherapy. Psychiatry. 2015;78(4):305–16.
60. Lysaker PH, Gagen EC, Klion R, Zalzala AB, Vohs J, Faith LA, et al. Metacognitive reflection and insight therapy: a recovery-oriented treatment approach for psychosis. Psychol Res Behav Manag. 2020;13:331–41.
61. Drake RE, Whitley R. Recovery and severe mental illness: description and analysis. Can J Psychiatr. 2014;59(5):236–42.
62. May R. The contributions of existential psychotherapy. In: May R, Angel E, Ellenberger H, editors. Existence: a new dimension in psychiatry and psychology. Oxford, UK: Basic Books; 1958. p. 37–91.
63. Firmin R, Lysaker PH, Luther L, Yanos PT, Leonhardt BL, Breier A, et al. Internalized stigma in adults with early phase vs prolonged psychosis. Early Interv Psychiatry. 2019;13(4):745–51.
64. Buck KD, Roe D, Yanos PT, Buck B, Fogely R, Grant M, et al. Challenges to assisting with the recovery of personal identity and wellness for persons with serious mental illness: considerations for mental health professionals. Psychosis. 2013;5(2):134–43.
65. Hamm JA, Buck KD, Vohs J, Westerlund R, Lysaker PH. Interpersonal stance and dialogue in psychotherapy for schizophrenia: a supervisory approach. Clin Superv. 2016;35(1):42–62.
66. Seikkula J, Alakare B, Aaltonen J. Open dialogue in psychosis I: an introduction and case illustration. J Constr Psychol. 2001;14:247–65.
67. Seikkula J, Alakare B, Aaltonen J. Open dialogue in psychosis II: a comparison of good and poor outcome cases. J Constr Psychol. 2001;14:267–84.
68. Bakhtin M. Problems of Dostoyevsky's poetics. Emerson C, trans. Minneapolis, MN: University of Minnesota Press; 1985. (Original work published 1929).
69. Holma J, Aaltonen J. Narrative understanding in acute psychosis. Contemp Fam Ther. 1998;20(3):253–63.
70. Holma J, Aaltonen J. The sense of agency and the search for a narrative in acute psychosis. Contemp Fam Ther. 1997;19(4):463–77.
71. Seikkula J, Aaltonen J, Alakare B, Haarakangas K, Keranen J, Lehtinen K. Five-year experience of first episode nonaffective psychosis in open dialogue approach: treatment principles, follow-up outcomes, and two case studies. Psychother Res. 2006;16(2):214–28.
72. Freeman AM, Tribe RH, Stott JCH, Pilling S. Open dialogue: a review of the evidence. Psychiatr Serv. 2019;70(1):46–59.
73. Bergström T, Seikkula J, Alakare B, Mäki P, Köngäs-Saviaro P, Taskila JJ, et al. The family-oriented open dialogue approach in the treatment of first-episode psychosis: nineteen-year outcomes. Psychiatry Res. 2018;270:168–75.
74. Tribe RH, Freeman AM, Livingstone S, Stott JCH, Pilling S. Open dialogue in the UK: qualitative study. BJPsych Open. 2019;5(4):e49. https://doi.org/10.1192/bjo.2019.38.
75. Fowler D, Garety P, Kuipers E. Cognitive behaviour therapy for psychosis: theory and practice. Chichester, UK: Wiley; 1995.
76. Moritz S, Klein JP, Lysaker PH, Mehl S. Metacognitive and cognitive-behavioral interventions for psychosis: new developments. Dialogues Clin Neurosci. 2019;21(3):309–17.
77. Grant PM, Reisweber J, Luther L, Brinen AP, Beck AT. Successfully breaking a 20-year cycle of hospitalizations with recovery-oriented Cognitive Therapy for Schizophrenia. Psychol Serv. 2014;11(2):125–33.
78. Mehl S, Werner D, Lincoln TM. Does Cognitive Behavior Therapy for psychosis (CBTp) show a sustainable effect on delusions? A meta-analysis. Front Psychol. 2015;6:1450.
79. van der Gaag M, Valmaggia LR, Smit F. The effects of individually tailored formulation-based cognitive behavioural therapy in auditory hallucinations and delusions: a meta-analysis. Schizophr Res. 2014;156(1):30–7.

80. Hamm J, Lysaker PH. Integrative metacognitive psychotherapy for serious mental illness: applications to diverse clinical needs and its processes that promote recovery. Am J Psychother. 2018;71(4):122–7.
81. Yanos PT, Roe D, Lysaker PH. Narrative enhancement and cognitive therapy: a new group-based treatment for internalized stigma among persons with severe mental illness. Int J Group Psychother. 2011;61(4):576–95.
82. Hansson L, Lexen A, Holmen J. The effectiveness of narrative enhancement and cognitive therapy: a randomized controlled study of a self-stigma intervention. Soc Psychiatry Psychiatr Epidemiol. 2017;52(11):1415–23.
83. Yanos PT, Lysaker PH, Silverstein SM, Vayshenker B, Gonzales L, West ML, et al. A randomized controlled-trial of treatment for self-stigma among persons diagnosed with schizophrenia-spectrum disorders. Soc Psychiatry Psychiatr Epidemiol. 2019;54(11):1363–78.

Treatments and Recovery to Enhance Employment Outcomes for People with Schizophrenia and Other Major Mental Disorders: An Innovative Clinical and Organisational Model of Work Inclusion in Milan and Surrounding Area

8

Sonia Mazzardis, Andrea Quarenghi, Paola Fiorenza Rubelli, Barbara Sanna, and Claudio Mencacci

8.1 Introduction

This chapter is aimed at clinical and social workers who work in mental health services and deal with workplace inclusion for patients with schizophrenia and other major mental disorders. It is based on the guiding principles underlying the 2007 UN Convention on the Rights of People with Disabilities (specifically Article 8 and Article 27) [1], which focuses on raising awareness of the real contribution that people with disabilities make to the productive economy and on promoting specific programmes for workplace inclusion. However, to date, access to work opportunities and the social integration of people with mental disabilities have been only marginally successful, as a result of stereotypes and cultural prejudices and because of the lack of connections between the work and health services sectors.

Encouraging dialogue between different sectors and fostering a more nuanced view of disabled job applicants—understood as citizens, patients and workers—can promote a culture of inclusion and disseminate appropriate models of intervention, including at the organisational level.

S. Mazzardis · A. Quarenghi · P. F. Rubelli (✉) · B. Sanna
Department of Neuroscience and Mental Health, ASST Fatebenefratelli Sacco, Milan, Italy
e-mail: sonia.mazzardis@asst-fbf-sacco.it; quarenghi.andrea@asst-fbf-sacco.it;
paola.rubelli@asst-fbf-sacco.it; barbara.sanna@asst-fbf-sacco.it

C. Mencacci
Department of Neuroscience, Azienda Ospedaliera Fatebenefratelli e O, Milan, Italy
e-mail: claudio.mencacci@asst-fbf-sacco.it

© The Author(s), under exclusive license to Springer Nature
Switzerland AG 2022
B. Carpiniello et al. (eds.), *Recovery and Major Mental Disorders*,
Comprehensive Approach to Psychiatry 2,
https://doi.org/10.1007/978-3-030-98301-7_8

Following an analytical review of the most widespread models of inclusion for people with mental disorders in work settings, this chapter outlines the experiences of the Mental Health Department of the Fatebenefratelli Sacco Hospital. Since 2006 the department has carried out a project financed by regional funding based on a clinical and organisational model titled 'The application and dissemination in the Metropolitan City of Milan of operational models for the inclusion of people suffering from mental disorders'.

8.2 How to Improve Employment Outcomes for People with Schizophrenia and Other Major Mental Disorders. A Brief Introduction to the Main Models and Issues

Vocational rehabilitation for people with severe mental illness has a history spanning approximately 70 years, encompassing programme innovation and informal experimentation by many psychiatric rehabilitation programmes all over the world. Over the last three decades, a limited number of vocational rehabilitation approaches have proved to be the most effective in Europe and the United States in leading people into competitive employment [2, 3]. A modern approach to vocational rehabilitation focuses on eligibility, based on the patient's own choices, integration between mental health and employment services, competitive employment, and individualised and continuous job support [4]. Many different types of vocational rehabilitation programmes have been developed and implemented, but many researchers refer to two broad categories—pre-vocational training and supported employment—[5] according to expected outcomes. Some vocational programmes (i.e. hospital-based programmes, sheltered employment, psychosocial rehabilitation) consider work a means to achieving specific personal outcomes, such as better treatment compliance, symptom reduction, and improved quality of life. Vocational approaches, such as supported employment, include outcomes such as full-time competitive employment, the acquisition of job-related skills, percentage of time in paid employment (full-time or part-time, competitive or sheltered), total earnings, level of work (unskilled, skilled, etc.), job satisfaction, and job performance. *Pre-vocational training* or '*train and place*' refers to an approach focused on training and developing individual skills prior to seeking competitive employment. Systematic reviews have proved that pre-vocational training is less effective than supported employment in helping mentally ill people obtain competitive employment [6], although it is not clear to what extent different pre-vocational training approaches can affect patients' ability to re-enter the workforce or influence longer job tenure after placement[1] [6, 7]. *Supported Employment*, or '*place, then train*' focuses

---

[1] Some research findings indicate that cognitive deficits, rather than psychiatric symptoms or other clinical or demographic factors, seem to be the strongest clinical predictors of a poor response to supported employment [3]. Could 'pre-vocational training' be more effective for people with cognitive deficits and psychiatric conditions?

on getting people into competitive employment first, followed by training and support on the job [8]. Using a community-based approach, supported employment aims to facilitate the transfer of skills into real-world settings. The best-known model of supported employment is Individual Placement and Support (IPS). IPS uses a quick job search based on the patient's choices, matching their interest and skills with employment opportunities. Integration between the employment team and a multidisciplinary mental health team is emphasised as a means to facilitate finding a job. The mental health team and vocational specialists (VS) must share the values, aims and methods of the IPS model, as the VS and their clients must proceed together in an intensive job search for quick placement.

Nevertheless, there is no shared definition of what can be considered 'work' in terms of vocational rehabilitation. Approaches to VR differ between countries [9]: important cultural factors influence approaches to disability [10] and consequently to disability services and their goals. Can only competitive employment in integrated settings be considered successful? The modern job market and advanced welfare economies offer a great variety of opportunities (jobs in social enterprises, short-term placements, sheltered employment, etc.) that can hardly be defined as unsuccessful. Bachrach [11] asserts that the differences in interests, skills, talents, physical abilities and limitations of people with severe mental illnesses fit more appropriately within a broad definition of 'work'.

There is broad consensus on the effectiveness of supported employment models; however, ratings regarding the integration of people with mental illness in the labour market remain unsatisfactory. In recent years, researchers have tried to understand why, in spite of being supported by good scientific evidence, IPS has not been widely implemented in clinical practice [12]. Many studies have attempted to identify the critical factors affecting the development of IPS in Mental Health Services, and a number of issues have emerged:

- Inconsistent knowledge of IPS among healthcare professionals, and inability of some healthcare and employment support services to work together [13].
- Beliefs held by medical care teams regarding the value of IPS [14], fears that it will lead to relapses [15], or that all symptoms need to be addressed before any progress can be made [14], or employment—as an outcome—not being seen as a priority for recovery, or not a realistic one [13].
- Strategy of wider psychosocial approaches in the community agreed on at the local level between providers and commissioners, to support vocational specialist teams over longer periods [16].
- The role of employment support specialists, who are more effective when working directly with clients, employment services and agencies, and employers, and indirectly with care coordinators [12].
- Cost issues and lack of funding, particularly with regard to supporting IPS services over time and maintaining quality, in a context of increased demands on secondary services in national health systems [16].

- The importance for services and clients of having direct and fast access to job opportunities, as local unemployment rates, work labour characteristics, local policies and welfare regimes impact the effectiveness of IPS [17, 18].

In conclusion, the key issues that need to be addressed to increase the effectiveness of a supported employment service in the community seem to be (1) having an evidence-based vocational rehabilitation approach, (2) managing the implementation of the service at the local level, (3) sustainability over time, (4) having common views, beliefs and shared practices, from the vocational specialists to the medical teams and local stakeholders, and (5) being able to access job opportunities. Moreover, some studies highlight the importance of defining common inclusion criteria, which can influence the effectiveness of work inclusion programmes [17, 18].

8.3 Supporting Employment in an Advanced Welfare Context. Treatments, Recovery, Regulatory Changes and Methodological and Organisational Issues in the City of Milan

Based on observations in the city of Milan since the early 2000s, there appear to be widespread communication difficulties between the worlds of mental health and productive work, resulting in a cycle of non-cooperation. On the one hand, companies are wary of hiring individuals with mental illness and distrust care services. On the other hand, care services, and often the non-profit sector, give work experience a primary purpose of care and rehabilitation. These communication difficulties, combined with the economic situation in Milan over the last decade, have imposed a particularly complex framework of intervention on the city, characterised by the following critical points:

- A confused proliferation of opportunities, in a city network not connected by a genuine collaborative culture.
- Dispersal and fragmentation of resources that are not evenly accessible to patients.
- Professional skills not being optimised and utilised as part of a network.
- Lack of a method of care that would provide applicants with programmes to select, train for, support and maintain their jobs while respecting the health of the worker and the company's needs.
- Confusion between different types of work inclusion paths and actual employability of the person.

In addition to this complex picture, there are frequent and continuous changes in the legislative, administrative and organisational aspects that greatly influence the practices of job inclusion, and consequently the overall character of psychiatry services that the wider region of Lombardy offers patients in the area of vocational rehabilitation.

Over the last 20 years new labour policy scenarios at the European level have had a significant impact in Italy both on existing legislation and on the reorganisation of public employment services. Specifically, Law 68 from 1999 significantly changed the logic according to which the employment service for disabled people was managed: the concept of a disability quota was accompanied by that of 'targeted hiring', which was intended to be implemented through a set of agencies matching employers' needs to the individual characteristics of people with disabilities or other protected groups.

This was followed by national regulations that reorganised the institutional structure of social services and labour policies, empowering regions, provinces and municipalities in the planning and coordination of integrated social policies.

Further legislative change was implemented through a gradual increase in the application at the provincial level of Article 14 of legislative decree 276/03 [19]. This law makes it possible to shift part of the disability quota to social cooperatives, which carry out productive activities aimed at inserting people with physical or mental disadvantages into the labour system, in an attempt to foster a virtuous circle of introducing disabled people into companies.

Thanks to the multiplication at the national level of projects and good practices designed to facilitate inclusion in the workplace, a change in how work is conceived in mental healthcare has been possible: it is no longer seen as a substitute for care but as a means of fulfilment for the individual during a process of genuine recovery and social inclusion.

8.4 The Development of Regional Innovative Programme TR-106 Between 2009 and 2019 and Its Impact

In June 2004, the region of Lombardy issued the new Regional Plan for Mental Health in order to promote 'a community psychiatry that operates in a context rich in resources and opportunities, with treatment programmes based on effective and evaluable models, across a territory conceived as a large, functional whole—not a rigidly delimited area—with the possibility of integrating various services, including health and social, public, private and non-profit services, and to collaborate with the informal existing network, in a real opening to civil society'.

It is within this context that the region of Lombardy financed the TR-106 Regional Innovative Programme (PIR) in 2006. The purpose of the programme is 'the promotion of a permanent network for the work inclusion of psychiatric patients' and to establish an innovative way of supporting, reorganising and optimising the network to implement the measures taken by the ASL (Local Health Authority) of Milan to facilitate inclusion in the workplace. The PIR originated at the Sacco Hospital; since 1997 a second-level specialised service (ALA-Sacco) belonging to the Mental Health Department (DSM) of the Luigi Sacco Hospital has dealt with the evaluation, design and delivery of sustainable pathways towards work inclusion for patients of psychiatric services. The ALA-Sacco intervention methodology considers the therapeutic value of the paths themselves as a foundation and the integrated management with the referents of care (health) and work (companies) to be fundamental. The culture within the ALA-Sacco has always been to orient itself towards the larger territory, involving different DSMs.[2] The PIR fits into this experience, focusing on the study of a networked organisation system that can respond to some of the patients' and their families' essential needs on their path towards the workplace, as well as the needs and priorities of companies. The first choice was to involve all the DSMs of the city of Milan, which have thus become effective partners in the project, both in terms of sharing aims and in an equable use of resources and tools. In addition to the DSM of the Sacco Hospital, the following were therefore involved: DSM Niguarda Hospital, DSM Policlinico Hospital, DSM Fatebenefratelli Hospital, DSM San Paolo Hospital, DSM San Carlo Hospital.

At the same time, a technical committee was set up that involved DSMs as well as local stakeholders, including municipal and provincial labour inclusion services, business associations and trade unions.

The key objectives have been (and remain):

- To contribute to maintaining a coordinated network of services between health services and businesses, which responds to all the opportunities in the area for the person with mental illness, who is simultaneously a citizen, a patient and a worker.
- To promote efficient and effective responses capable of combining individualised support and coordinated overview, translatable into evaluable outcomes.
- To apply problem-solving to the nodes of the network that prevent the use of resources.

The organisational model has therefore been created through the construction of operational products that can respond to different emerging needs on work inclusion paths, including assessment and monitoring tools and sustainable agreements between different agencies. These agreements were approved by all heads of department, giving rise to new and monitored procedures between services. The connections between the different network actors were made possible thanks to the creation by the project of a specific professional role: that of the *network coach*. In the literature we find the figure of the vocational specialist, who supports patients in finding and keeping jobs [13]. The *network coach*, on the other hand, is a specialist trained to match the needs of the individual

---

[2]The Department of Mental Health (DSM) is the set of facilities and services that are responsible for taking charge of the demand related to the care and protection of mental health within the territory defined by the local health authority (ASL). The DSM includes day care services (Mental Health Centres—CSM), semi-replacement services (Day Centres—CD), Residential services (separate residential facilities (SRs) in therapeutic-rehabilitation and socio-rehabilitative residences), Hospital Services (Diagnostic and Care Psychiatric Services (SPDC) and Day Hospitals—DH).

candidate with the network of local opportunities. This figure actively collaborates to develop the network systems in the constant process of innovation that the healthcare and social contexts require. The complexity of this intervention requires that the *network coach* be supported by a cross-territorial functional team, which has the task of being guarantor of inter-institutional agreements as well as of the clinical value of the intervention. The focus is therefore not on the coach-patient pair, but on the directing of network skills that the coach and patient go through and nurture together. If it were centred on the coach-patient pair, the quality of the relationship would be optimised but energy would be wasted, since the operator would have to build and rebuild a network suited to each candidate. Furthermore, this system does not promote equity in the usability of the services by candidates because it is too closely tied to each individual's subjective skills. The establishment of a team of cross-territorial coaches has, instead, promoted:

- The optimisation of resources
- The creation of a culture of cooperation fed by constant exchanges

In the Milanese experience, the group performs a needs analysis and plans, designs and builds ad hoc procedural tools with managerial figures who act as guarantors of the process by collaborating with the network coach. The organisational system also enables the systematic collection of data, so that evaluation systems consistent with the range of indicators agreed with the region and local health authorities can be applied.

For these reasons, the PIR promoted by ALA-Sacco has primarily favoured centralised management, supported by the principle of subsidiarity, which was expressed in the creation of a technical working group that included all the subjects involved in the Milan ASL workplace inclusion group; the working group was supported and enhanced by the Milan ASL. The three overarching objectives of the working group were to:

- Intervene in existing relationship models
- Build consensus and cooperation
- Solve problems collaboratively [20]

In order for the network to be participatory, the following innovative organisational tools were adopted:

- A model (see Fig. 8.1), inspired by that of Mills [21], divided into clusters. This organisational structure enables networking, with regard to agreed objectives and actions, between services. The aim is to create targeted opportunities for job applicants, supported by a staff of operators who specialise in mediation between the different languages of the social and work sectors (network coach). This organisation enables work centres (*Poli Lavoro*) to support the process and allows for the creation of these in the DSM, where they were not yet present. By

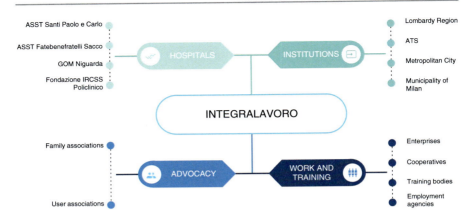

Fig. 8.1 Network of contacts with public institutions and non-profit sector

work centre we mean an agency inside the Department of Mental Health that specialises in evaluating, managing and maintaining patients in the department during the workplace inclusion process.
- The implementation of a method for building agreements based on mutual trust, between the DSM and institutions, inspired by the ORGI method [22], a problem-solving model for organisations that includes holding meetings to express needs, formulate questions, construct intervention hypotheses, distribute actions between entities and verify interventions.
- Network devices: three types of network devices have been identified. They are characterised and differentiated according to the level of involvement of the network subjects, degree of structuring of work processes and long-term expendability (technical work groups, platforms and procedures).
- Process consultancy in order to promote and maintain organisational development.

Network platforms are the network devices that involve different agencies and services in a specific area that can also include multiple work processes; in the last 8 years they have reached a good degree of structuring, with both operational and institutional agreements in place. They can also be supported by online IT tools. The programme has activated the following platforms (see Fig. 8.2):

- ALA-Sacco Information System (SIAL)
- Integralavoro [23]
- Informative Training Groups

SIAL is a candidate assessment tool that collects and correlates personal data and clinical and functional information related to the individual and their previous work experience, and also tracks the project phases of the patient's career path. It is a web-based platform, accessible to all operators at the work centres in the city of Milan, built based on the DSM's previous experience of workplace inclusion. The SIAL was designed to share the assessment of patients referred by their psychiatric

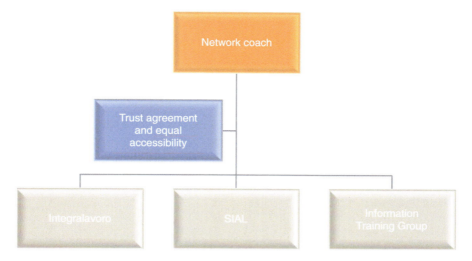

Fig. 8.2 Network platforms

team. This tool was devised to identify homogeneous and comparable placement criteria that are currently shared, to guarantee both the candidate's welfare and congruity with the needs of the production context. In addition to this objective, the system is designed to perform data analysis, which enables epidemiological observation and an assessment of the effectiveness and efficiency of our interventions.

Closely connected to this platform is Integralavoro, which is a point of reference for training and employment needs and opportunities for our clients and the world of work. Integralavoro is also a board composed of one delegate for each work centre of the Milan ASL.

The Integralavoro platform has set itself the goal of sharing experiences, good practices and professionalism from all the DSM's poles in Milan. Here, too, a web-based platform was chosen to facilitate communication between operators working at the different DSMs and to make it possible to share the available workstations. This platform also includes resources obtained from the programmatic agreements and procedures made available online by all the organisations that deal with job placement for members of disadvantaged groups.

Integralavoro has therefore become the heart of the PIR, which over time has taken on the function of connecting, monitoring and therefore evaluating the functioning of the operating practices agreed with the network actors. This governance, which is simultaneously centralised and participatory, makes it possible to collect and disseminate information regarding trends in opportunities found online and to build innovative strategies from time to time in relation to changes in the territory.

The most recently created platform is that of Informative Training Groups, designed to offer patients who are candidates for a work project the opportunity to acquire specific skills to start or stay on workplace inclusion paths. The training groups at work are cross-territorial interventions, built in collaboration with the DSM of the city of Milan based on the departments' experiences. Admission and evaluation criteria for each group were determined based on shared placement criteria. Most groups intentionally carried out the activity in a location outside the place of treatment, allowing users to experiment in new contexts.

8.5 Sample Description and Outcome

Between 2012 and 2019, every year the PIR TR-106 collected the data of clients in the care of all the work centres of the city who, for various reasons, benefited from the platforms and resources made available by the programme (see Table 8.1). The total number of admissions to the PIR TR-106 programme of people with psychiatric diagnoses between 2012 and 2019 is 2142 (60.8% males). The mean age in the final sample was 45 years (SD = 9.4).

Table 8.1 Client characteristics

Client characteristics (Total admissions to the programme between 2012 and 2019 = 2142)
Mean age: 45 years. (DS: +/− 9)
Distribution by age (%):   – 18–24[a]: 3%   – 25–34; 27.4%   – 35–44: 36.4%   – 45–54: 27.7%   – 55–64: 5.5%
Sex (%):   – Female: 39.2%   – Male: 60.8%
Diagnoses (%):   – Schizophrenia and other psychotic disorders: 39.0%   – Personality disorders: 25.3%   – Mood disorders: 22.2%   – Neurotic disorders: 9.3%   – Others: 4.4%
Job hiring per year: – 2012: 7.9%   – 2013: 11.6%   – 2014: 15%   – 2015: 17%   – 2016: 10.5%   – 2017: 20.3%   – 2018: 22.7%   – 2019: 22.8%
Hospitalisation (mean): 4.08%   Drop out (mean): 1.37%

[a] For the population aged 18–24 a separate project for workplace inclusion has been developed

8 Treatments and Recovery to Enhance Employment Outcomes for People... 127

Table 8.2 Clients with schizophrenia or other psychotic disorders

Total admissions with diagnoses F20-29 between 2012 and 2019 = 836
Mean age: 45 years (DS: +/− 9)
Distribution by age (%):   − 18-24[a]: 3%   − 25–34: 28.9%   − 35–44: 36.8%   − 45–54: 25.1%   − 55–64: 6.1%
Sex (%):   − Female: 37.3%   − Male: 62.7%
Job hiring per year: − 2012: 7.4%   − 2013: 9.2%   − 2014: 12.1%   − 2015: 11.8%   − 2016: 13.1%   − 2017: 21.3%   − 2018: 21.4%   − 2019: 28.7%
Hospitalisation (mean): 4.18%   Drop-out (mean): 1.31%

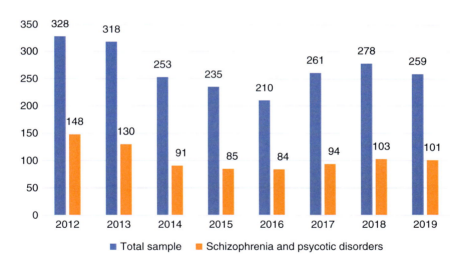

Fig. 8.3 Sample distribution per year (n)

Although the programme is not aimed at a specific diagnostic category, our sample does contain a preponderance of clients with schizophrenia or other psychotic disorders (see Table 8.2).

Most of these clients have gone through the programme for many years (see Fig. 8.3).

The programme wants the evaluation of its impact to focus on the process rather than on outcomes. As can be seen in the two tables, the more the programme is rooted in the territory, the more the outcome in terms of hiring has improved, both for the general population and for patients with schizophrenia. The more the network system has taken hold, the more hiring has increased. Drop-out and hospitalisations are, respectively, 1.3% and 4% in cluster F20-29.

8.6 Perspectives, Critical Issues and Conclusions

Work inclusion is a fundamental aspect of the care pathway for patients in the care of the territorial services of the Departments of Mental Health, as an integral part of healthcare and advanced rehabilitation that aims to promote a sense of personal self-efficacy and subjective well-being [24–27].

The programme has promoted and supported an organisational network model that provides, from a cross-territorial and city perspective, central and participatory management, as well as a coordinated and effective overall vision shared by health institutions, social institutions and the world of work, which:

- Provides access for individuals with psychic discomfort to all the resources the territory can offer in terms of workplace inclusion.
- Favours the optimisation of the opportunities already available in terms of integration, homogenisation and appropriateness of interventions.

The objective of the programme, in terms of detection of outcomes, is to evaluate both the candidate and the system. With both aims in mind, we can say that the PIR had an impact on the following aspects:

- Reduction of the fragmentation of interventions for workplace inclusion for people with mental illness in territorial services and consequent reduction of costs.
- Reduction of the heterogeneity of the services offered by the Mental Health Departments to patients in terms of usability and accessibility of the resources the territory has at its disposal to favour social inclusion and more appropriate interventions.
- Transitioning from a culture of competition between services to a culture of sharing, while prioritising the well-being of the candidate.

These results, obtained over time—due to the very nature of the programme, which proposes a community and participatory approach—require constant monitoring and review in the face of continuous changes at the organisational (new institutional arrangements at the territorial level), legislative (updates to labour policies) and workplace levels (characterised by rapid transformations that are often out of sync with treatment times).

We would like to emphasise here how difficult it is to work towards methodological and cultural changes with working groups that are accustomed to using self-referential methodological systems, and how deeply enriching it is to eventually achieve changes, defined by the contributions of the different actors. The cultural change that this perspective requires is challenging: trust must be established between the DSM and the world of work. However, we believe that trust must first be established when pooling resources and optimising skills within public services before it can be demanded in the world of work.

Genuine and mutual integration between the business world and the healthcare community can be achieved by enhancing governance and safeguarding public health services and promoting constant dialogue between health, social and labour policies.

The network system, as it has been conceptualised, can be flexibly applied to deal with states of discomfort that are widespread in the world of work and thus be supportive to companies and workers, even in connection with welfare systems.

References

1. United Nations Convention on the Rights of Persons with Disabilities. https://www.un.org/esa/socdev/enable/rights/convtexte.htm.
2. Bond GR, Becker DR, Drake RE, Rapp CA, Meisler N, Lehman AF, et al. Implementing supported employment as an evidence-based practice. Psychiatr Serv. 2001;52(3):313–22.
3. Bond GR, Drake RE, Becker DR. An update on randomized controlled trials of evidence-based supported employment. Psychiatr Rehabil J. 2008;31(4):280–90.
4. Drake RE, Bond GR, Becker DR. IPS supported employment: an evidence-based approach to supported employment. New York: Oxford University Press; 2012.
5. Bond GR, Boyer SL. Rehabilitation programs and outcomes. In: Ciardiello JA, Bell MD, editors. Vocational rehabilitation of persons with prolonged psychiatric disorders. Baltimore: Johns Hopkins University Press; 1988. p. 231–63.
6. Crowther R, Marshall M, Bond GR, Huxley P. Vocational rehabilitation for people with severe mental illness. Cochrane Database Syst Rev. 2001;2001(2):CD003080.
7. Tal A, Moran G, Rooth DO, Bendick M Jr. Using situation testing to document employment discrimination against persons with psychiatric disabilities. Employee Relat Law J. 2009;35(3):40–60.
8. Corrigan P, Steiner L, McCracken SG, Blaser B, Barr M. Strategies for disseminating evidence-based practices to staff who treat people with serious mental illness. Psychiatr Serv. 2001;52(12):1598–606.
9. Ross JC. Understanding vocational rehabilitation: a cross-sector perspective using case study methodology. Br J Occup Ther. 2012;75(6):263.
10. Pechak C, Thompson M. Disability and rehabilitation in developing countries. 2007. https://www.cugh.org/sites/default/files/105_Disability_and_Rehabilitation_in_Developing_Countries_FINAL_0.pdf.
11. Bachrach LL. Psychosocial rehabilitation and psychiatry in the treatment of schizophrenia—what are the boundaries? Acta Psychiatr Scand. 2000;(407):6–10.
12. Rinaldi M, Perkins R, Glynn E, Montibeller T, Clenaghan M, Rutherford J. Individual placement and support: from research to practice. Adv Psychiatr Treat. 2008;14(1):50–60.
13. Bevan SM, Guilford J, Steadman K, Taskila T, Thomas R, Moise A. Working with schizophrenia: pathways to employment, recovery & inclusion. 2013.
14. Shepherd G, Lockett H, Bacon J, Grove B. Establishing IPS in clinical teams—some key themes from a national implementation programme. J Rehabil. 2012;78(1):30–6.

15. Rinaldi M, Miller L, Perkins R. Implementing the individual placement and support (IPS) approach for people with mental health conditions in England. Int Rev Psychiatry. 2010;22(2):163–72.
16. Hutchinson J, Gilbert D, Papworth R, Boardman J. Implementing supported employment. Lessons from the making IPS work project. Int J Environ Res Public Health. 2018;5:1545.
17. Burns T, Catty J. IPS in Europe: the EQOLISE trial. Psychiatr Rehabil J. 2008;31(4):313–7.
18. Reme SE, Monstad K, Fyhn T, et al. A randomized controlled multicenter trial of individual placement and support for patients with moderate-to-severe mental illness. Scand J Work Environ Health. 2019;45(1):33–41.
19. Provincia di Milano. Cambiare passo. L'inserimento delle persone diversamente abili tra innovazione delle politiche e cambiamenti istituzionali. Milano: Franco Angeli; 2011.
20. Tosco L. Costruire modelli teorico-operativi, Animazione Sociale, A. 28, 2. ser., n. 121; 1998.
21. Mills Q. La rinascita dell'impresa. Come lavorare con successo nelle organizzazioni del futuro. Milano: Franco Angeli; 1993.
22. Schein EH. La consulenza di processo. Come costruire le relazioni d'aiuto e promuovere lo sviluppo organizzativo. Milano: Raffaello Cortina Editore; 2001.
23. www.integralavoro.com.
24. Walker C, Fincham B. Work and mental health in the UK. Chichester: Wiley-Blackwell; 2011.
25. Carozza P. Principi di riabilitazione psichiatrica. Per un sistema di servizi orientato alla guarigione. Milano: Francoangeli; 2006.
26. Farkas M, Anthony WA. Psychiatric rehabilitation interventions: a review. Int Rev Psychiatry. 22(2):114–29.
27. Davidson L, Strauss JS. Sense of self in recovery from severe mental illness. Br J Med Psychol. 1992;65(2):131–45.

Recovery-Oriented Psychopharmacological Interventions in Schizophrenia

9

Jasmina Mallet, Yann Le Strat, Caroline Dubertret, and Philip Gorwood

9.1 Introduction

9.1.1 Historical Aspects: From Chemical Contention to Remission and Recovery

During decades, schizophrenia was considered as a lifelong and debilitating illness with little or no hope of recovery [1]. The treatment of schizophrenia has dramatically changed since the discovery of psychoactive effects of chlorpromazine in the 1950s, giving new hopes for psychiatrists, patients, and families. The aims of clinicians were then to reduce agitation and aggressiveness, and to control positive symptoms (delusions, hallucinations).

Indeed, until recently, the major impact of antipsychotics was the reduction of symptoms, not necessarily correlated with the improvement of social functioning [2–4]. This was not an expected outcome. However, advances in pharmacological treatment and psychosocial interventions have heightened expectations for outcomes. We assisted to a progression of treatment goals from chemical containment to remission and, more recently, even recovery [5]. Recovery can be considered as

---

J. Mallet · C. Dubertret
Department of Psychiatry, University Hospital Louis Mourier (ap-hp), Colombes, France
e-mail: jasmina.mallet@aphp.fr; Caroline.dubertret@aphp.fr

Y. Le Strat
Department of Psychiatry and Addiction Medicine, Louis Mourier Hospital (ap-hp), Colombes, France
e-mail: yann.lestrat@aphp.fr

P. Gorwood (✉)
CMME, GHU Paris Psychiatrie et Neurosciences, Université Paris Cité, Paris, France
e-mail: p.gorwood@ghu-paris.fr

© The Author(s), under exclusive license to Springer Nature
Switzerland AG 2022
B. Carpiniello et al. (eds.), *Recovery and Major Mental Disorders*,
Comprehensive Approach to Psychiatry 2,
https://doi.org/10.1007/978-3-030-98301-7_9

131

both an outcome and a process. The combination of these two concepts offers the most complete framework to tend toward recovery [6]. It is now recognized that symptom reduction alone cannot be sufficient. Although rarely assessed, functionality, quality of life, empowerment, and reducing the internalized stigma are most meaningful to patients and their families and seem paramount when considering recovery as an outcome [7].

9.1.2 Clinical Recovery May Not Be Patient Recovery

Recovery is a complex entity and clinicians still debate to define it. It is more complex to define than remission. Recovery meaning "being cured" is maybe an unrealistic goal at the time of writing. It means different things to different people: clinical recovery is not patient recovery [6, 8]. Patients describe experiencing personal recovery despite ongoing symptoms of psychosis [9]. Thus recovery can occur even when psychotic symptoms are persistent [10]. Many consumer-based groups conceptualize recovery as a personal journey (i.e., a subjectively evaluated process dealing with symptoms over time), rather than a defined outcome (completely recovered vs persistent illness) [11]. Finally, the Remission in Schizophrenia Working Group (RSWG) regarded recovery as a more demanding and longer-term phenomenon than remission, stating that remission is necessary, but not sufficient, step toward recovery. The group did not define operational criteria for recovery, asking for more research on the longitudinal course of domains such as cognitive and psychosocial functioning, and their relationship to symptoms [1].

Regardless on how to define recovery, focusing on such a high demanding outcome helps to promote important aspects of the disease and unmet needs [12]. All clinicians agree that the reduction of symptoms is an important step toward recovery. Getting clinical remission at 6 months increased by 15 the chances to get functional remission 6 months later in a sample of 303 patients with schizophrenia followed up for a year [13]. Patients may emphasize the need for functional remission and quality of life. Reducing symptoms is easy to define, with clear cutoff at different assessment scales (such as for the PANSS [14]), but lacking sensitivity regarding the impact of co-morbidities, efficacy/efficiency, and phases of the disorder. Getting to symptomatic remission is a more clear-cut criteria [1] but time and impact are more difficult to assess. All these influences resulted in a comprehensive definition of recovery in schizophrenia, including remission of symptoms and functional improvement. The RSWG defined remission as improvements in core signs and symptoms to the extent that they are of such low intensity that they no longer interfere significantly with behavior [1]. Patients have to fulfill the symptomatic severity component of the criterion over a period of 6 months. The working group did not define operational criteria for recovery itself, but others have tried to define it, with a time criteria of at least 2 years [15].

Finally, several instruments have been developed, based on the experience of patients, to assess personal recovery [9] more or less related *to* functional remission. "Efficiency studies" should include those aspects, and outcome measures that

9 Recovery-Oriented Psychopharmacological Interventions in Schizophrenia

mainly focus on symptom remission should ideally be extended to other components of recovery. Various tools are now available to assess remission functional remission, with good psychometric properties and easiness to use [16, 17]. This led to the progressive incorporation of such outcome in clinical trials [18].

9.1.3 Psychopharmacological Interventions Among Other Factors of Recovery

The high heterogeneity in determinants of recovery can be explained by the inherent composite nature of recovery. Recovery depends on many factors, including domains as different as family involvement [19] and psychopharmacological interventions.

People with schizophrenia do not inevitably experience deterioration over time. A large proportion of them has the potential to achieve long-term remission and functional recovery. Findings suggest that sufficient focus on recovery goal setting may have specific impact on motivation in schizophrenia patients, especially in first-episode patients [20]. The fact that some experience deterioration in functioning over time may reflect poor access or adherence to treatment. The effects of concurrent conditions (e.g., substance use disorders) and social and financial impoverishment have also been mentioned [21].

Today, four psychosocial treatments are available for individuals with schizophrenia: social skills training, cognitive behavioral therapy, cognitive remediation therapy, and social cognition training [22]. There is an impact of psychosocial therapies on social functioning [23]. Integrated therapies and social skills therapy have been shown to enhance social functioning, whereas cognitive behavioral therapy (CBT), family intervention therapy, and cognitive remediation therapy would not be as efficient.

A 20-year follow-up study on six patients having "recovered completely" showed that only two remained fully recovered, one partly, and one in remission. One experienced a deterioration of the course of illness, the other was deceased [24]. According to the last meta-analysis to date, the proportion of individuals with schizophrenia and related psychoses who met recovery is 13.5% and appears not to have increased over time [25], despite recent psychosocial approaches. More targeted and personalized pharmacological approaches are more than ever warranted. Early intervention is also paramount, observing that shorter DUP predicts recovery in FEP individuals followed during 2 years [26].

9.1.4 How to Assess Functional Remission

As mentioned in 1.2, assessing functional remission is more realistic than recovery when considering pharmacological interventions efficiency. In contrast to clinical symptoms, outcomes related to functional remission and recovery do not rely on reliable and simple metrics [6]. Different types of instruments enable the assessment of functional remission, with different approaches and different related pros and cons: self-report (with poor validity in severe patients), clinicians rating (biased by clinical symptoms and "feelings"), informant report (difficult, long, and not always possible), tests (on specific skills), and naturalistic studies (long and culture specific). The list of instruments is long (e.g., Global Assessment of Functioning scale (GAF), the Personal and Social Performance scale (PSP), the Functional Remission of General Schizophrenia scale (FROGS)…) [16, 17, 27–29].

9.1.5 The Place of Functional Remission/Recovery in Pharmacological Trials

Functional remission is not the most targeted endpoint in mega-trial wherein the primary endpoint may be quality of life, or all cause of discontinuation [30–32]. This is not an unsolvable issue, as there is a gap between efficacy and effectiveness. Efficacy is an intervention performance under highly controlled experimental circumstances, while effectiveness is an intervention performance in general clinical usage, e.g., observational studies that are more appropriate in clinical practice. Consequently, interventions in clinical practice (effectiveness/efficiency) tend to be less robust than interventions in registration studies (efficacy) [33] but could be, on the other hand, highly needed.

9.2 The Impact of Psychopharmacological Interventions on Recovery

Modifiable risk factors for poor outcomes in patients with schizophrenia include longer duration of untreated illness, comorbid substance abuse, early nonresponse to an antipsychotic, and the number of relapses that are related to nonadherence [34]. Recommendations from experts therefore include selecting most appropriate medications based on a balanced risk-benefit assessment, and the consideration of long-acting injections (LAI) is indeed an alternative to oral medications as reducing hospitalization [35] and mortality [36]. Targeting symptoms or specific functions may also be efficient, in a personalized approach [34].

9.2.1 The Positive Impact of Psychopharmacological Interventions

– **On psychotic or affective symptoms**

A recent meta-analysis showed that symptom severity only partially explained personal recovery [9]. Moreover, psychotic symptoms were moderately associated with personal recovery, while affective symptoms were more closely linked to personal recovery. This is in line with the results presented by Bobes et al. [37], in which thymic symptoms were correlated with recovery in a 1-year follow-up of 452 patients with RSWG remission (shorter DUP, premorbid adjustment, social cognitive abilities being also associated). Negative symptoms were also involved in functional remission and recovery and should represent a therapeutic target [38–40].

Other studies underline the impact of depressive symptoms that interfere with the chances to get functional remission [41, 42]. Low mood is also a strong predictor of low quality of life and suicidality [38]. Therefore, clinicians should pay attention to affective symptoms of patients, and privilege antipsychotics with efficiency on these symptoms. Depression occurring in a patient with schizophrenia should be treated by using an antipsychotic with antidepressant activity, or, after having addressed positive symptoms, by adding an antidepressant agent [38].

– **On cognitive functioning**

Cognitive functioning is considered as the most predictive factor of functional outcome in terms of social, occupational, and living status, medication adherence and ability to self-manage medication as well as relapse prevention [43, 44]. Impairments are not correlated to positive symptoms or negative symptoms, suggesting different underlying physiopathological pathways which can constitute a therapeutical target per se [43–46]. Past studies have demonstrated that the therapeutic effects of conventional antipsychotics are limited to positive symptoms of the illness, and that they have substantially less impact on cognitive impairments, whereas atypical antipsychotics may improve cognitive deficits [45], although the cognitive profiles of different compounds are not clearly defined. FGAs are generally associated with deficits in working memory, processing speed, and motor skills, perhaps due to a higher affinity for the dopamine D2 receptor, or because anticholinergics are often used in combination with these drugs. A high affinity for the cholinergic and the histaminergic receptors is also seen in low-potency FGAs, with antagonistic cholinergic effects being correlated with decreases in attention, memory, and executive functions. It has been demonstrated that anticholinergic burden has a negative impact on the outcomes of psychosocial treatment. This negative effect would be mediated through impaired cognitive capacity [47], even if not systematically confirmed [48].

Second-generation antipsychotics (SGAs) receptor profiles are more diverse, and the group is more heterogeneous than FGAs. Atypical antipsychotics could potentially have an impact on cognitive functions through different paths. First, they have a differential action on gene expression in brain. Antipsychotics induce gene expression in many brain areas and improve neuroplasticity [49]. Atypical antipsychotics have a different regional expression profile and intensity of C-FOS compared to conventional antipsychotic drugs, in particular in brain areas such as the prefrontal cortex [49–51]. Neurophysiological compounds may also be impacted by the use of antipsychotics. The P50 is an early component of auditory-evoked potentials and a measure of sensory gating deficits. The P50 ratio reflects a neurophysiological substrate associated mostly with executive functioning [52]. Subjects with schizophrenia (and some of their first-degree relatives) present deficits in sensory gating, with P50 ratios being generally greater than 50%.

Treatment with typical neuroleptics does not reverse this deficit. However, previous studies have shown that treatment with clozapine, an atypical neuroleptic, ameliorates this deficit in clinically responsive patients. P50-evoked potential recordings were obtained from 132 patients with schizophrenia and 177 healthy comparison subjects. Eighty-eight patients were being treated with atypical neuroleptics (clozapine, olanzapine, risperidone, and quetiapine). Thirty-four patients were taking typical neuroleptics, and ten were unmedicated. Improvement in P50 gating appears to be the greatest in patients treated with clozapine [53].

The use of cognitive tests can also shed light on the differential impact of various medications. Findings suggest that neurocognition affects social cognition and that poorer social cognition leads to social discomfort at work, which in turn leads to poorer rehabilitation outcomes [54]. There is a scarcity of data concerning the impact of medications on social cognition (emotion recognition, theory of mind, attribution style, social perception), and at the time of writing it is not possible to draw any conclusions on the impact of current medication (antipsychotics) or other recent treatment (e.g., oxytocin) [55, 56]. However, among the social cognitive functions, the theory of mind (ToM), the ability to infer the mental states of others, shows the strongest link with everyday functioning in schizophrenia [57], and is a mediator between neurocognition and functioning. ToM is thus an important treatment target to promote functional recovery. A recent meta-analysis suggests that a deficit in any neurocognitive function could be associated with a negative impact on ToM performance [58].

Two meta-analyses converge toward a superiority of SGA against FGA when considering global cognition [59, 60], while a more recent one only detected trends when considering cognitive subtests [61]. An early study showed that treatment with risperidone appears to exert a more favorable effect on verbal working memory than treatment with a conventional neuroleptic (haloperidol) [62]. This beneficial effect appeared to be partially mediated by the antagonism of the $5\text{-}HT_{2A}$ receptor. Verbal working memory is a component of theoretical interest because of its link to prefrontal activity and, of practical interest, because of its link to psychosocial rehabilitation toward recovery. Verbal memory also predicted functional recovery in two recent naturalistic studies on FEP patients [48, 63], and was also the mediator of the negative effect of dopaminergic receptor blockade burden on functioning [48]. In the latter study, the 2-year dopaminergic receptor blockade burden of antipsychotic drugs significantly correlated to a poorer psychosocial functioning, in contrast to O'Reilly et al. [47]. Recent studies all support the idea of maintaining low doses in the early stages of the disease in terms of the benefit-to-risk ratio [48].

More specifically, partial agonists could represent a more valuable option to improve cognition than other SGAs [64]. A recent study demonstrated a relationship between the D2/3 receptor occupancy by aripiprazole and working-memory performance in patients with schizophrenia [65], which suggest the same cognitive profile for other partial agonists [66]. RCTs and prospective studies are definitely warranted to conclude on the potential superiority of partial agonists over other atypical antipsychotics in preserving and improving cognitive functions.

9.2.2 The Problem of Adherence

Despite new antipsychotics' discovery in the past decades, the proportion of patients who achieve remission is still low. Moreover, the average time to obtain remission increases with the number of successive episodes [67]. Non-adherence is common in schizophrenia whereas adherence is a paramount key to symptomatic and functional recovery [68], as increasing rate of relapses prevents recovery [69]. Discontinuation rates are ranging from 44% within 1 year after first episode [70] to as high as 74% over longer periods [71, 72]. Afterward, relapse rates are high following cessation of oral antipsychotics or partial adherence [73]. The lack of treatment adherence increased healthcare costs and is responsible of considerable disease exacerbation [74].

On the one hand, one way to increase adherence when observance is an issue is to propose long-acting antipsychotics.

9.2.2.1 The Impact of Side Effects on Adherence and Well-Being

On the other hand, another evident way to increase adherence is to diminish the impact of side effects on well-being. Antipsychotics are responsible for many side effects with different impact on patients' well-being. These side effects are correlated with adherence levels. Around 80% of patients will relapse within the first 5 years of onset, partly due to medication discontinuation. When patients are asked what impairs their quality of life the most, they rank the following side effects from most to least impairing: weight gain, somnolence or insomnia, concentration difficulties, memory loss, and disordered thoughts [75]. The potential for these side effects should be kept in mind when choosing medication, especially early in the illness, and clinicians should always employ a "first do not harm" approach [38]. Knowing that relapses are correlated with persistent cognitive deficits and severe impairment of social functioning [76], diminishing side effects is an objective per se.

A study reported the impact of each side effect on complete adherence in a sample of 876 schizophrenia patients, of whom 86.2% reported a side effect [77]. Participants who reported complete adherence were approximately half as likely to report a hospitalization for mental health reasons or other reasons, compared with participants reporting poor adherence. Specific side effects were found to be associated with reduced adherence; EPS or agitation reduced adherence by approximately 43%. Weight gain and metabolic side effects reduced adherence by 36%. Prolactin elevation and endocrine dysfunction reduced adherence by 31%. Sexual side effects also reduced adherence by 31%. Sexuality is an important dimension and can impact quality of life and patient's defined recovery. A recent review has highlighted the neurobiology of schizophrenia in the context of the understanding of sexuality functioning [78]. Data are scarce but converge toward the preferential use of atypical antipsychotics as first-line treatments, both in drug naive patients and in patients under FGAs. This sexual side effect is largely underpinned by hyperprolactinemia, which can cause long-term complications (e.g., osteoporosis, cardiovascular diseases) [79] impacting patient well-being. Finally, sedation and cognitive impairment reduced adherence by 30%, and gastrointestinal side effects by 21%. Sedation also interferes with cognition, social and vocational functioning [80].

In a sample of 1825 patients diagnosed with a psychotic disorder, 77% reported medication side effects, 61% reported impairment in their daily life as a result of medication side effects, and 30% reported moderate or severe impairment in their daily life as a result of medication side effects [81].

Side effects affect quality of life through small shifts in functional status and, if not addressed early, can cause long-term subjective distress and contribute to chronic health complications [82, 83]. When considering international guidelines, APA guidelines recommend choosing a medication that offers good clinical response without intolerable side effects, while NICE guidelines recommend regular monitoring of side effects based on the side-effect profile of the prescribed antipsychotic [84, 85]. Patients who experience serious side effects may decide that the adverse effects outweigh the benefits of medication.

9.2.2.2 Using Different Pharmacological Approaches to Diminish Side Effects

The best-known mechanism for antipsychotics is the D2 receptor blockade. Howes and colleagues reviewed the evidence for the major implication of dopamine in the emergence of schizophrenia [86, 87]. They proposed a "dopamine hypothesis" with a framework that links risk factors, including pregnancy and obstetric complications, stress and trauma, drug use, and genetic vulnerability, to increased presynaptic striatal dopaminergic function. It explains how a complex array of pathological conditions may converge neurochemically to cause psychosis through aberrant salience and lead to the occurrence of schizophrenia. However, it is important to remember that second-generation antipsychotics, and particularly partial agonists, also bind a range of other receptors, contributing to their efficacy [66]. Conversely, the blockade of such receptors can also lead to specific side effects. Determining the optimal level of intrinsic activity at the receptor is crucial to avoid an activity close to agonism (potential lack of efficacy, side effects such as nausea, vomiting, insomnia, and motor effects) or, on the contrary, closer to antagonism (and potential increased risk of extrapyramidal symptoms and raised prolactin levels) [88]. Few studies explore if using atypical antipsychotics increases adherence. Significantly greater adherence to atypical antipsychotics at 6 months was observed compared with conventional antipsychotics, but difference at the end of 1 year is not significant [89].

9.2.2.3 Using Long-Acting Injectable Antipsychotics to Enhance the Potential for Recovery

Tiihonen et al. [35] have demonstrated in a large nationwide cohort that the use of LAI antipsychotics in the early stages of schizophrenia was associated with a significantly lower risk of rehospitalization than use of oral formulations of the same compounds. It is not surprising when adherence with oral antipsychotics would be around 70% according a meta-analysis computing data from Electronic Adherence

Monitoring, lower than the 80% threshold used widely to define satisfactory adherence [90].

In a more recent cohort study, the authors showed that long-acting injectable antipsychotic medications (along with clozapine) were the pharmacologic treatments with the highest rates of prevention of relapse in schizophrenia (all stages included). The risk of rehospitalization was about 20–30% lower during long-acting injectable treatments compared with equivalent oral formulations [91].

In a naturalistic study following 13,087 subjects with schizophrenia, in the 1 year following discharge, patients in the LAIs group had a significantly lower rehospitalization rate and a significantly lengthened time to rehospitalization than those in the oral antipsychotics group. Rehospitalization rate and time to rehospitalization were not significantly different in patients receiving FGA-LAIs or SGA-LAIs. A significantly higher percentage of patients treated with FGA-LAIs received anticholinergic agents than those treated with SGA-LAIs [92].

There would be no relevant difference when comparing LAI between them (for the review of recent RCT, see Peters et al. [93]).

When focusing on recovery, in a recent meta-analysis of 26 RCT, long-acting injectable atypical antipsychotics were beneficial for recovery of psychosocial function in comparison with placebo [94]. The magnitude of superiority over oral antipsychotic treatment was small but psychosocial function was not included as primary outcome a priori. Severe psychopathology (including cognitive impairment) at baseline predicted poor psychosocial function and suggest that clinicians may stratify patients who may benefit from more intensive psychosocial therapies in adjunction to pharmacological treatment.

9.2.3 Using Antipsychotic Polypharmacy to Diminish the Risk of Hospitalization

Against current guidelines, the use of antipsychotic polypharmacy may represent a valuable option to decrease the risk of hospitalization and improve recovery. The use of antipsychotic polypharmacy raises concern due to the lack of evidence for its efficacy and safety. This question has been addressed in a large observational study using within-individual analyses, in a nationwide cohort including all patients with schizophrenia [95]. Patients had the lowest risk of psychiatric or all-cause hospitalization (i.e., relapses) when they received combination therapy with clozapine plus aripiprazole, which was significantly superior to clozapine, which was the monotherapy associated with the best outcomes. The authors suggest that rational antipsychotic polypharmacy seems to be feasible by using two particular antipsychotics with different types of receptor profiles, and that antipsychotic polypharmacy may be superior to monotherapy for maintenance treatment (which has not been examined with RCTs).

9.2.4 Shared Decision-Making to Improve Adherence and Empowerment

In recent years, clinical decision-making has evolved toward a more patient-inclusive approach and the concept of empowerment. Shared decision-making (SDM) could improve adherence, self-efficacy, and empowerment for patients, leading to a virtuous circle toward recovery [96]. It is also an increasingly ethical imperative that may reinforce therapeutic alliance, treatment satisfaction, and adherence. More than half of the patients who use mental health services say they are not involved in decisions about their treatment [97]. Using patient-reported adverse effect reporting is one way to improve adherence and minimize adverse effects via more appropriate medication selection and adjustment [98]. SDM also requires a specific training for clinicians, based on motivational approaches, and is rarely implemented in mental health settings whereas a recent study showed encouraging results in an acute psychiatric ward [99]. However, in this study, the effects of the intervention diminished after discharge, probably because the psychiatrists were not trained in the SDM. In a meta-analysis of 11 RCT, the implementation of SDM appeared to have small beneficial effects on indices of treatment-related empowerment [97]. Involving patients in the choice of therapy is not sufficient to increase pharmacological adherence if, at the same time, there is no constant work of comparison and communication with the reference psychiatric team. SDM can be particularly effective for LAI prescription, since patient can have prejudices and unjustified fears related to the LAI formulation, which the doctor must help resolving. Recommendations and positional statements in proposing LAI antipsychotics using SDM style have been proposed in Fiorillo et al. [96].

9.2.5 Recent Pharmacological Advances

9.2.5.1 Partial Agonists at the D2 Receptor

- **Pharmacology**

    As previously mentioned, clinicians should prefer an antipsychotic with antidepressant activity when confronted to a depressive dimension in patients (that interfere with the chance to achieve recovery). There are several mechanisms that might, at least in part, explain antidepressant efficacy of SGAs: blockade of neurotransmitter receptors other than dopamine, blockade of monoamine transporters, effects on sleep, decrease in cortisol levels, and increase in neurotrophic growth factors [100].

    However, many side effects reported with SGAs could lead to diminished treatment adhesion and also inhibit the clinician from prescribing such treatment [101]. D_2 partial agonism became a new approach, stabilizing dopamine function while mitigating side effects [66]. Aripiprazole was the first D_2 partial agonist to be approved for the treatment of schizophrenia and as an augmenting agent in major depression. However, some side effects (such as activation, agitation, and akathisia) have been ascribed to its high level of intrinsic activity at the D_2 receptor [102]. This led to the development of other molecules such as brexpiprazole and cariprazine.

Concerning pharmacologic properties, aripiprazole, brexpiprazole, and cariprazine all exhibit D_2 receptor partial agonism, but each displays a distinct receptor profile. Aripiprazole preferentially binds to D_2 receptors over D_3 receptors [103]. Cariprazine has an approximately tenfold higher affinity for human D_3 compared with human D_2 (S or L) receptors [104]. Brexpiprazole, a serotonin-dopamine activity modulator, is a partial agonist at 5-HT_{1A} and dopamine D_2 receptors and antagonist at 5-HT_{2A} and noradrenaline α_{1B} and α_{2C} receptors, all at similar potency. Brexpiprazole shows a lower intrinsic activity at the D_2 receptor compared with aripiprazole, and a greater affinity at the 5-HT_{2A} receptor compared with aripiprazole [105]. These properties would result in less akathisia and extrapyramidal symptoms. Finally, brexpiprazole and cariprazine bind less strongly to H_1 receptors than aripiprazole, suggesting a lower antihistaminic activity resulting in less sedation, somnolence, and weight gain.

Finally, several properties of aripiprazole are probably not yet known for brexpiprazole and cariprazine: possible absence of long-term dopamine-related neurochemical adaptations (involving a lack of dopamine super sensitivity and treatment resistance) and specific changes of the neuronal transcriptome in relevant biological functions (for review, see de Bartolomeis et al. [106]).

- **Summary of the efficacy and efficiency of D2 partial agonists on functional outcomes**

    Using the various scales briefly presented in the first part of this chapter, some longitudinal studies have addressed the impact of pharmacological strategies using D2 partial agonists on functional outcomes (for more information on side effects, efficacy, and other outcomes please refer to Mallet et al. [66]). The PSP mean score increased over 12 weeks of treatment with oral aripiprazole, and this effect was maintained over an additional 38 weeks with the same oral antipsychotic [107]. A 26 weeks, double-blind study compared the PSP mean score with cariprazine ($n = 227$) vs risperidone ($n = 227$) and found better improvement with cariprazine ($P < 0.001$ at week 26) [108]. Another long-term study (20 weeks open-label, 26–72 weeks double-blind) compared cariprazine with placebo [109]. PSP total score improved during open-label cariprazine treatment. Subsequent double-blind cariprazine treatment exhibited no PSP score change (mean change: 0.0), whereas patients switched to placebo showed worsening (mean change: −7.2).

    Studies concerning brexpiprazole also demonstrate encouraging results concerning short- and long-term functioning. The pooled results of two short-term studies showed better improvement at week 6 in PSP total score with brexpiprazole 2 mg ($n = 343$) and 4 mg ($n = 342$) vs placebo ($n = 333$) ($P < 0.01$ and $P < 0.001$, respectively) [110]. The long-term efficacy of brexpiprazole has been tested in two recent studies. The first evaluated mean change from baseline in GAF score with brexpiprazole 1–4 mg ($n = 95$) vs placebo ($n = 102$) [111]. In this double-blind maintenance phase, patients with brexpiprazole showed an increasing functioning score, whereas patients with placebo showed worsening from week 12 to week 52 ($P < 0.001$). The other study was an open-label design in 1015 patients with PSP score as a secondary outcome. Patients with brexpiprazole ($n = 410$) at week 52 showed a mean improvement in PSP score of 7.7 points over the course of treatment to a total of 68.3 points. This is above the threshold for potentially clinically meaningful response in stabilized patients with schizophrenia (an increase of four to seven points) and close to functional remission (a total score of 70 points) [112].

Further studies are needed to more directly attribute the benefit of partial agonists on functioning.

9.2.5.2 Anti-inflammatory Strategies

Some subgroups of patients with schizophrenia have been associated with immune dysregulations and could lead to a stratification model that better reflects the individual's immune state [113]. These subgroups are based on the following relatively easy to determine clinical entry points: genetic liability to immune dysregulation, childhood maltreatment, metabolic syndrome, cognitive dysfunction, negative symptoms, and treatment resistance. For patients presenting cognitive dysfunction and/or negative symptoms, immune biomarkers seem relevant as treatment targets. Indeed, these two domains are relatively resistant to common antipsychotic strategies. Add-on strategies with minocycline or N-acetyl cysteine showed mixed results on cognition [113]. On the contrary, two recent meta-analysis of RCT showed positive results on negative symptoms with various agents: minocycline, N-acetylcysteine, and estrogens [113, 114]. Knowing that anti-inflammatory drugs also have an action on depressive dimension, particularly on anhedonia, their use could be useful in a recovery-oriented strategy. Indeed anhedonia is one of the strongest predictors of poor psychosocial functioning in depressive disorder [115] and, even if it has been poorly investigated in schizophrenia, it is at least related to quality of life [116]. Using specific anti-inflammatory agents may represent an important step toward personalized treatment, as they may be efficient on depression dimensions, cognitive dysfunctions and negative symptoms, three aspects of schizophrenia that interfere with the recovery process [9, 38, 39, 46].

9.2.5.3 Other Promising Pharmacological Agents

Recent encouraging data suggest potential efficacy for a variety of new agents for the treatment of total symptoms and/or specific symptom domains. There are currently no data on functional outcomes, but new pharmacological targets seem promising. Mechanisms of action under investigation were recently reviewed in Correll [117] and include dopamine D_3 antagonism/serotonin 5-HT_{1A} partial agonism; combined dopamine, serotonin, and glutamate modulation; phosphodiesterase 10A inhibition; trace amine-associated receptor-1 (TAAR1) agonism plus 5-HT_{1A} agonism; 5-HT_{2A} inverse agonism; sigma-2/5-HT_{2A} antagonism; D-amino acid oxidase (DAAO) inhibition; glycine transporter-1 inhibition; vesicular monoamine

9 Recovery-Oriented Psychopharmacological Interventions in Schizophrenia

transporter-2 antagonism; mu opioid antagonism added to olanzapine; and novel long-acting injectable antipsychotic formulations.

Other strategies could be useful to target specific domains involved in functioning. Among them cannabidiol and intranasal oxytocin have been the focus of recent studies. Cannabidiol (CBD) is a constituent of the *Cannabis* plant and, oversimplifying, may have opposite effects to THC, the primary psychoactive component of cannabis (which is a risk factor for schizophrenia, at least in vulnerable individuals [118, 119]). The pharmacological profile of CBD is very different and still under investigation. CBD has drawn increased attention of public health services and researchers as a potential treatment, existing data suggesting that it is safe, well tolerated, and with few adverse effects [120]. However, to date there is no evidence to conclude that CBD can improve cognition or functioning in schizophrenia patients (for a review of recent trials or observational studies, see Ghabrash et al. [121]).

Regarding intranasal oxytocin, findings have been inconsistent. A recent meta-analysis of double-blind RCTs examined the efficacy and tolerability of adjunctive intranasal oxytocin in the treatment of schizophrenia but focused on psychotic symptoms [122]. Although the meta-analysis in general did not show significant symptomatic improvement, high doses appeared to be efficacious and safe in improving total psychopathology and positive symptom scores. Based on current literature, the authors postulate that the improvement of positive symptoms may be partly attributed to the effects of oxytocin on decreasing paranoid ideation and fear, enhancing social interaction. Oxytocin could also significantly increase facial expressivity [123] and improve cognitive function (results of a small study by Ota et al. [124]). Further studies using objective outcome measures and proper designs are warranted to determine if oxytocin can improve functional impairment in schizophrenia.

9.3 Conclusion

Objectives of psychiatrists have moved from "immediate response of acute symptoms" to "stable recovery of functioning." Much more is expected (also by patients, carers, and relatives) than symptoms reduction, but defining relevant outcomes is a largely more complex task. In addition to providing the best possible clinical assessment and pharmacological treatment, psychiatrists could function as an effective leader of a treatment team, ideally in a coordinated specialty framework. Measuring progress on multiple effectiveness domains will help to evaluate the effectiveness of providing optimal individualized treatment. Changing treatment aims also has advantages: increase psychiatrists' duties, getting closer to political and patient's request and focus on new aspects of the disorder. Recovery means optimizing individual outcomes. Recent advances on pharmacotherapy that targets cognitive functions (including social component) and negative symptoms are promising, among them second-generation antipsychotics. Increasing adherence through diminishing side effect and preferring long-acting medications, using shared decision-making, can be helpful. Novel agents are needed to better address the multidimensional syndrome of schizophrenia.

In combination with pharmacotherapy, psychosocial interventions that target cognition, family environment, social skills, and vocational rehabilitation are likely to have the best outcome.

References

1. Andreasen NC, Carpenter WT, Kane JM, Lasser RA, Marder SR, Weinberger DR. Remission in schizophrenia: proposed criteria and rationale for consensus. Am J Psychiatry. 2005;162:441–9. https://doi.org/10.1176/appi.ajp.162.3.441.
2. Lambert M, Naber D, Schacht A, Wagner T, Hundemer H-P, Karow A, Huber CG, Suarez D, Haro JM, Novick D, et al. Rates and predictors of remission and recovery during 3 years in 392 never-treated patients with schizophrenia. Acta Psychiatr Scand. 2008;118:220–9.
3. Priebe S, McCabe R, Bullenkamp J, Hansson L, Lauber C, Martinez-Leal R, Rössler W, Salize H, Svensson B, Torres-Gonzales F, van den Brink R, Wiersma D, Wright DJ. Structured patient-clinician communication and 1-year outcome in community mental healthcare: cluster randomised controlled trial. Br J Psychiatry J Ment Sci. 2007;191:420–6. https://doi.org/10.1192/bjp.bp.107.036939.
4. Ventura J, Subotnik KL, Guzik LH, Hellemann GS, Gitlin MJ, Wood RC, Nuechterlein KH. Remission and recovery during the first outpatient year of the early course of schizophrenia. Schizophr Res. 2011;132:18–23.
5. Phahladira L, Luckhoff HK, Asmal L, Kilian S, Scheffler F, du Plessis S, Chiliza B, Emsley R. Early recovery in the first 24 months of treatment in first-episode schizophrenia-spectrum disorders. NPJ Schizophr. 2020;6:2. https://doi.org/10.1038/s41537-019-0091-y.
6. Emsley R, Chiliza B, Asmal L, Lehloenya K. The concepts of remission and recovery in schizophrenia. Curr Opin Psychiatry. 2011;24:114–21.
7. Warner R. Recovery from schizophrenia and the recovery model. Curr Opin Psychiatry. 2009;22:374–80. https://doi.org/10.1097/YCO.0b013e32832c920b.
8. Slade M, Amering M, Oades L. Recovery: an international perspective. Epidemiol Psichiatr Soc. 2008;17:128–37. https://doi.org/10.1017/s1121189x00002827.
9. Van Eck RM, Burger TJ, Vellinga A, Schirmbeck F, de Haan L. The relationship between clinical and personal recovery in patients with schizophrenia spectrum disorders: a systematic review and meta-analysis. Schizophr Bull. 2018;44:631–42. https://doi.org/10.1093/schbul/sbx088.
10. Bellack AS. Scientific and consumer models of recovery in schizophrenia: concordance, contrasts, and implications. Schizophr Bull. 2006;32:432–42. https://doi.org/10.1093/schbul/sbj044.
11. Harvey PD, Bellack AS. Toward a terminology for functional recovery in schizophrenia: is functional remission a viable concept? Schizophr Bull. 2009;35:300–6. https://doi.org/10.1093/schbul/sbn171.
12. Torres-González F, Ibanez-Casas I, Saldivia S, Ballester D, Grandón P, Moreno-Küstner B, Xavier M, Gómez-Beneyto M. Unmet needs in the management of schizophrenia. Neuropsychiatr Dis Treat. 2014;10:97–110. https://doi.org/10.2147/NDT.S41063.
13. Gorwood P, Bouju S, Deal C, Gary C, Delva C, Lancrenon S, Llorca P-M. Predictive factors of functional remission in patients with early to mid-stage schizophrenia treated by long acting antipsychotics and the specific role of clinical remission. Psychiatry Res. 2019;281:112560. https://doi.org/10.1016/j.psychres.2019.112560.
14. Kay SR, Fiszbein A, Opler LA. The positive and negative syndrome scale (PANSS) for schizophrenia. Schizophr Bull. 1987;13:261–76.
15. Liberman RP, Kopelowicz A. Recovery from schizophrenia: a concept in search of research. Psychiatr Serv. 2005;56:735–42. https://doi.org/10.1176/appi.ps.56.6.735.

9 Recovery-Oriented Psychopharmacological Interventions in Schizophrenia

16. Gorwood P, Mallet J, Lancrenon S. Functional remission in schizophrenia: a FROGS-based definition and its convergent validity. Psychiatry Res. 2018;268:94–101. https://doi.org/10.1016/j.psychres.2018.07.001.

17. Mallet J, Lancrenon S, Llorca P-M, Lançon C, Baylé F-J, Gorwood P. Validation of a four items version of the Functional Remission of General Schizophrenia scale (the mini-FROGS) to capture the functional benefits of clinical remission. Eur Psychiatry J Assoc Eur Psychiatr. 2018;47:35–41. https://doi.org/10.1016/j.eurpsy.2017.09.001.

18. Wunderink L, Nieboer RM, Wiersma D, Sytema S, Nienhuis FJ. Recovery in remitted first-episode psychosis at 7 years of follow-up of an early dose reduction/discontinuation or maintenance treatment strategy: long-term follow-up of a 2-year randomized clinical trial. JAMA Psychiat. 2013;70:913–20. https://doi.org/10.1001/jamapsychiatry.2013.19.

19. Yu BCL, Mak WWS, Chio FHN. Family involvement moderates the relationship between perceived recovery orientation of services and personal narratives among Chinese with schizophrenia in Hong Kong: a 1-year longitudinal investigation. Soc Psychiatry Psychiatr Epidemiol. 2020; https://doi.org/10.1007/s00127-020-01935-4.

20. Fulford D, Meyer-Kalos PS, Mueser KT. Focusing on recovery goals improves motivation in first-episode psychosis. Soc Psychiatry Psychiatr Epidemiol. 2020; https://doi.org/10.1007/s00127-020-01877-x.

21. Zipursky RB, Reilly TJ, Murray RM. The myth of schizophrenia as a progressive brain disease. Schizophr Bull. 2013;39:1363–72. https://doi.org/10.1093/schbul/sbs135.

22. Kern RS, Glynn SM, Horan WP, Marder SR. Psychosocial treatments to promote functional recovery in schizophrenia. Schizophr Bull. 2009;35:347–61.

23. Patterson TL, Leeuwenkamp OR. Adjunctive psychosocial therapies for the treatment of schizophrenia. Schizophr Res. 2008;100:108–19. https://doi.org/10.1016/j.schres.2007.12.468.

24. Torgalsbøen A-K, Rund BR. Maintenance of recovery from schizophrenia at 20-year follow-up: what happened? Psychiatry. 2010;73:70–83. https://doi.org/10.1521/psyc.2010.73.1.70.

25. Jääskeläinen E, Juola P, Hirvonen N, McGrath JJ, Saha S, Isohanni M, Veijola J, Miettunen J. A systematic review and meta-analysis of recovery in schizophrenia. Schizophr Bull. 2013;39:1296–306. https://doi.org/10.1093/schbul/sbs130.

26. Wunderink L, Sytema S, Nienhuis FJ, Wiersma D. Clinical recovery in first-episode psychosis. Schizophr Bull. 2009;35:362–9. https://doi.org/10.1093/schbul/sbn143.

27. Endicott J, Spitzer RL, Fleiss JL, Cohen J. The global assessment scale. A procedure for measuring overall severity of psychiatric disturbance. Arch Gen Psychiatry. 1976;33:766–71.

28. Kawata AK, Revicki DA. Psychometric properties of the Personal and Social Performance scale (PSP) among individuals with schizophrenia living in the community. Qual Life Res Int J Qual Life Asp Treat Care Rehabil. 2008;17:1247–56. https://doi.org/10.1007/s11136-008-9400-z.

29. Llorca P-M, Lançon C, Lancrenon S, Bayle F-J, Caci H, Rouillon F, Gorwood P. The "Functional Remission of General Schizophrenia"(FROGS) scale: development and validation of a new questionnaire. Schizophr Res. 2009;113:218–25.

30. Fleischhacker WW, Keet IPM, Kahn RS, Steering Committee EUFEST. The European First Episode Schizophrenia Trial (EUFEST): rationale and design of the trial. Schizophr Res. 2005;78:147–56. https://doi.org/10.1016/j.schres.2005.06.004.

31. Jones PB, Barnes TRE, Davies L, Dunn G, Lloyd H, Hayhurst KP, Murray RM, Markwick A, Lewis SW. Randomized controlled trial of the effect on quality of life of second- vs first-generation antipsychotic drugs in schizophrenia: Cost Utility of the Latest Antipsychotic Drugs in Schizophrenia Study (CUtLASS 1). Arch Gen Psychiatry. 2006;63:1079–87. https://doi.org/10.1001/archpsyc.63.10.1079.

32. Swartz MS, Perkins DO, Stroup TS, McEvoy JP, Nieri JM, Haak DC. Assessing clinical and functional outcomes in the Clinical Antipsychotic Trials of Intervention Effectiveness (CATIE) schizophrenia trial. Schizophr Bull. 2003;29:33–43. https://doi.org/10.1093/oxfordjournals.schbul.a006989.

33. Gorwood P. Meeting everyday challenges: antipsychotic therapy in the real world. Eur Neuropsychopharmacol J Eur Coll Neuropsychopharmacol. 2006;16(Suppl 3):S156–62. https://doi.org/10.1016/j.euroneuro.2006.06.002.

34. Correll CU, Lauriello J. Using long-acting injectable antipsychotics to enhance the potential for recovery in schizophrenia. J Clin Psychiatry. 2020;81:MS19053AH5C. https://doi.org/10.4088/JCP.MS19053AH5C.
35. Tiihonen J, Haukka J, Taylor M, Haddad PM, Patel MX, Korhonen P. A nationwide cohort study of oral and depot antipsychotics after first hospitalization for schizophrenia. Am J Psychiatry. 2011;168:603–9. https://doi.org/10.1176/appi.ajp.2011.10081224.
36. Taipale H, Mittendorfer-Rutz E, Alexanderson K, Majak M, Mehtälä J, Hoti F, Jedenius E, Enkusson D, Leval A, Sermon J, Tanskanen A, Tiihonen J. Antipsychotics and mortality in a nationwide cohort of 29,823 patients with schizophrenia. Schizophr Res. 2018;197:274–80. https://doi.org/10.1016/j.schres.2017.12.010.
37. Bobes J, Ciudad A, Álvarez E, San L, Polavieja P, Gilaberte I. Recovery from schizophrenia: results from a 1-year follow-up observational study of patients in symptomatic remission. Schizophr Res. 2009;115:58–66. https://doi.org/10.1016/j.schres.2009.07.003.
38. Correll CU. Using patient-centered assessment in schizophrenia care: defining recovery and discussing concerns and preferences. J Clin Psychiatry. 2020a;81:MS19053BR2C. https://doi.org/10.4088/JCP.MS19053BR2C.
39. Guessoum SB, Le Strat Y, Dubertret C, Mallet J. A transnosographic approach of negative symptoms pathophysiology in schizophrenia and depressive disorders. Prog Neuro-Psychopharmacol Biol Psychiatry. 2020;99:109862. https://doi.org/10.1016/j.pnpbp.2020.109862.
40. Wunderink L, van Bebber J, Sytema S, Boonstra N, Meijer RR, Wigman JTW. Negative symptoms predict high relapse rates and both predict less favorable functional outcome in first episode psychosis, independent of treatment strategy. Schizophr Res. 2020;216:192–9. https://doi.org/10.1016/j.schres.2019.12.001.
41. Harvey PD, Twamley EW, Pinkham AE, Depp CA, Patterson TL. Depression in schizophrenia: associations with cognition, functional capacity, everyday functioning, and self-assessment. Schizophr Bull. 2017;43:575–82. https://doi.org/10.1093/schbul/sbw103.
42. Joseph J, Kremen WS, Franz CE, Glatt SJ, van de Leemput J, Chandler SD, Tsuang MT, Twamley EW. Predictors of current functioning and functional decline in schizophrenia. Schizophr Res. 2017;188:158–64. https://doi.org/10.1016/j.schres.2017.01.038.
43. Trapp W, Landgrebe M, Hoesl K, Lautenbacher S, Gallhofer B, Günther W, Hajak G. Cognitive remediation improves cognition and good cognitive performance increases time to relapse–results of a 5 year catamnestic study in schizophrenia patients. BMC Psychiatry. 2013;13:184.
44. Veselinović T, Scharpenberg M, Heinze M, Cordes J, Mühlbauer B, Juckel G, Habel U, Rüther E, Timm J, Gründer G, Bleich S, Borgmann M, Breunig-Lyriti V, Schulz C, Brüne M, Falkai P, Feyerabend S, Figge C, Frieling H, Gaebel W, Gallinat J, Handschuh D, Heller J, Kirchhefer R, Kirner A, Kowalenko B, Lautenschlager M, Wolff-Menzler C, Naber D, Prumbs K, Wobrock T. Disparate effects of first and second generation antipsychotics on cognition in schizophrenia—findings from the randomized NeSSy trial. Eur Neuropsychopharmacol. 2019;29:720–39. https://doi.org/10.1016/j.euroneuro.2019.03.014.
45. Hori H, Noguchi H, Hashimoto R, Nakabayashi T, Omori M, Takahashi S, Tsukue R, Anami K, Hirabayashi N, Harada S, Saitoh O, Iwase M, Kajimoto O, Takeda M, Okabe S, Kunugi H. Antipsychotic medication and cognitive function in schizophrenia. Schizophr Res. 2006;86:138–46. https://doi.org/10.1016/j.schres.2006.05.004.
46. Velligan DI, Mahurin RK, Diamond PL, Hazleton BC, Eckert SL, Miller AL. The functional significance of symptomatology and cognitive function in schizophrenia. Schizophr Res. 1997;25:21–31. https://doi.org/10.1016/S0920-9964(97)00010-8.
47. O'Reilly K, O'Connell P, Donohoe G, Coyle C, O'Sullivan D, Azvee Z, Maddock C, Sharma K, Sadi H, McMahon M, Kennedy HG. Anticholinergic burden in schizophrenia and ability to benefit from psychosocial treatment programmes: a 3-year prospective cohort study. Psychol Med. 2016;46:3199–211. https://doi.org/10.1017/S0033291716002154.
48. Ballesteros A, Sánchez Torres AM, López-Ilundáin J, Mezquida G, Lobo A, González-Pinto A, Pina-Camacho L, Corripio I, Vieta E, de la Serna E, Mané A, Bioque M, Moreno-Izco L, Espliego A, Lorente-Omeñaca R, Amoretti S, Bernardo M, Cuesta MJ, PEPs Group. The

longitudinal effect of antipsychotic burden on psychosocial functioning in first-episode psychosis patients: the role of verbal memory. Psychol Med. 2020:1–10. https://doi.org/10.1017/S003329172000080X.

49. Park SW, Lee CH, Cho HY, Seo MK, Lee JG, Lee BJ, Seol W, Kee BS, Kim YH. Effects of antipsychotic drugs on the expression of synaptic proteins and dendritic outgrowth in hippocampal neuronal cultures. Synap N Y N. 2013;67:224–34. https://doi.org/10.1002/syn.21634.

50. Gorwood P, Hamon MD, editors. Psychopharmacogenetics. Springer US; 2006. https://doi.org/10.1007/0-387-34577-2.

51. Scharfetter J. Pharmacogenetics of dopamine receptors and response to antipsychotic drugs in schizophrenia—an update. Pharmacogenomics. 2004;5:691–8. https://doi.org/10.1517/14622416.5.6.691.

52. Toyomaki A, Hashimoto N, Kako Y, Tomimatsu Y, Koyama T, Kusumi I. Different P50 sensory gating measures reflect different cognitive dysfunctions in schizophrenia. Schizophr Res Cogn. 2015;2:166–9. https://doi.org/10.1016/j.scog.2015.07.002.

53. Adler LE, Olincy A, Cawthra EM, McRae KA, Harris JG, Nagamoto HT, Waldo MC, Hall M-H, Bowles A, Woodward L, Ross RG, Freedman R. Varied effects of atypical neuroleptics on P50 auditory gating in schizophrenia patients. Am J Psychiatry. 2004;161:1822–8. https://doi.org/10.1176/ajp.161.10.1822.

54. Bell M, Tsang HWH, Greig TC, Bryson GJ. Neurocognition, social cognition, perceived social discomfort, and vocational outcomes in schizophrenia. Schizophr Bull. 2009;35:738–47. https://doi.org/10.1093/schbul/sbm169.

55. Kucharska-Pietura K, Mortimer A. Can antipsychotics improve social cognition in patients with schizophrenia? CNS Drugs. 2013;27:335–43. https://doi.org/10.1007/s40263-013-0047-0.

56. Yamada Y, Inagawa T, Sueyoshi K, Sugawara N, Ueda N, Omachi Y, Hirabayashi N, Matsumoto M, Sumiyoshi T. Social cognition deficits as a target of early intervention for psychoses: a systematic review. Front Psych. 2019;10:333. https://doi.org/10.3389/fpsyt.2019.00333.

57. Achim AM, Guitton M, Jackson PL, Boutin A, Monetta L. On what ground do we mentalize? Characteristics of current tasks and sources of information that contribute to mentalizing judgments. Psychol Assess. 2013;25:117–26. https://doi.org/10.1037/a0029137.

58. Thibaudeau É, Achim AM, Parent C, Turcotte M, Cellard C. A meta-analysis of the associations between theory of mind and neurocognition in schizophrenia. Schizophr Res. 2020;216:118–28. https://doi.org/10.1016/j.schres.2019.12.017.

59. Désaméricq G, Schurhoff F, Meary A, Szöke A, Macquin-Mavier I, Bachoud-Lévi AC, Maison P. Long-term neurocognitive effects of antipsychotics in schizophrenia: a network meta-analysis. Eur J Clin Pharmacol. 2014;70:127–34. https://doi.org/10.1007/s00228-013-1600-y.

60. Zhang J-P, Gallego JA, Robinson DG, Malhotra AK, Kane JM, Correll CU. Efficacy and safety of individual second-generation vs. first-generation antipsychotics in first-episode psychosis: a systematic review and meta-analysis. Int J Neuropsychopharmacol. 2013;16:1205–18. https://doi.org/10.1017/S1461145712001277.

61. Nielsen RE, Levander S, Kjaersdam Telleus G, Jensen SOW, Östergaard Christensen T, Leucht S. Second-generation antipsychotic effect on cognition in patients with schizophrenia—a meta-analysis of randomized clinical trials. Acta Psychiatr Scand. 2015;131:185–96.

62. Green MF, Marshall BD, Wirshing WC, Ames D, Marder SR, McGurk S, Kern RS, Mintz J. Does risperidone improve verbal working memory in treatment-resistant schizophrenia? Am J Psychiatry. 1997;154:799–804. https://doi.org/10.1176/ajp.154.6.799.

63. Jordan G, Lutgens D, Joober R, Lepage M, Iyer SN, Malla A. The relative contribution of cognition and symptomatic remission to functional outcome following treatment of a first episode of psychosis. J Clin Psychiatry. 2014;75:e566–72. https://doi.org/10.4088/JCP.13m08606.

64. Kim S-W, Shin I-S, Kim J-M, Lee J-H, Lee Y-H, Yang S-J, Yoon J-S. Effectiveness of switching to aripiprazole from atypical antipsychotics in patients with schizophrenia. Clin Neuropharmacol. 2009;32:243–9. https://doi.org/10.1097/WNF.0b013e31819a68b5.

65. Shin S, Kim S, Seo S, Lee JS, Howes OD, Kim E, Kwon JS. The relationship between dopamine receptor blockade and cognitive performance in schizophrenia: a [11C]-raclopride PET study with aripiprazole. Transl Psychiatry. 2018;8:87. https://doi.org/10.1038/s41398-018-0134-6.

66. Mallet J, Gorwood P, Le Strat Y, Dubertret C. Major Depressive Disorder (MDD) and schizophrenia—addressing unmet needs with partial agonists at the D2 receptor: a review. Int J Neuropsychopharmacol. 2019;22:651–64. https://doi.org/10.1093/ijnp/pyz043.
67. Lieberman JA. Atypical antipsychotic drugs as a first-line treatment of schizophrenia: a rationale and hypothesis. J Clin Psychiatry. 1996;57(Suppl 11):68–71.
68. Czobor P, Van Dorn RA, Citrome L, Kahn RS, Fleischhacker WW, Volavka J. Treatment adherence in schizophrenia: a patient-level meta-analysis of combined CATIE and EUFEST studies. Eur. Neuropsychopharmacol. J. Eur. Coll. Neuropsychopharmacol. 2015;25:1158–66. https://doi.org/10.1016/j.euroneuro.2015.04.003.
69. Carbon M, Correll CU. Rational use of generic psychotropic drugs. CNS Drugs. 2013;27:353–65. https://doi.org/10.1007/s40263-013-0045-2.
70. Kaplan G, Casoy J, Zummo J. Impact of long-acting injectable antipsychotics on medication adherence and clinical, functional, and economic outcomes of schizophrenia. Patient Prefer Adherence. 2013;7:1171–80. https://doi.org/10.2147/PPA.S53795.
71. Lieberman JA, Stroup TS, McEvoy JP, Swartz MS, Rosenheck RA, Perkins DO, Keefe RSE, Davis SM, Davis CE, Lebowitz BD, Severe J, Hsiao JK, Clinical Antipsychotic Trials of Intervention Effectiveness (CATIE) Investigators. Effectiveness of antipsychotic drugs in patients with chronic schizophrenia. N Engl J Med. 2005;353:1209–23. https://doi.org/10.1056/NEJMoa051688.
72. Valenstein M, Ganoczy D, McCarthy JF, Myra Kim H, Lee TA, Blow FC. Antipsychotic adherence over time among patients receiving treatment for schizophrenia: a retrospective review. J Clin Psychiatry. 2006;67:1542–50. https://doi.org/10.4088/jcp.v67n1008.
73. Alvarez-Jimenez M, Priede A, Hetrick SE, Bendall S, Killackey E, Parker AG, McGorry PD, Gleeson JF. Risk factors for relapse following treatment for first episode psychosis: a systematic review and meta-analysis of longitudinal studies. Schizophr Res. 2012;139:116–28. https://doi.org/10.1016/j.schres.2012.05.007.
74. Osterberg L, Blaschke T. Adherence to medication. N Engl J Med. 2005;353:487–97. https://doi.org/10.1056/NEJMra050100.
75. McIntyre RS. Understanding needs, interactions, treatment, and expectations among individuals affected by bipolar disorder or schizophrenia: the UNITE global survey. J Clin Psychiatry. 2009;70(Suppl 3):5–11. https://doi.org/10.4088/JCP.7075su1c.02.
76. Robinson D, Woerner MG, Alvir JM, Bilder R, Goldman R, Geisler S, Koreen A, Sheitman B, Chakos M, Mayerhoff D, Lieberman JA. Predictors of relapse following response from a first episode of schizophrenia or schizoaffective disorder. Arch Gen Psychiatry. 1999;56:241–7. https://doi.org/10.1001/archpsyc.56.3.241.
77. Dibonaventura M, Gabriel S, Dupclay L, Gupta S, Kim E. A patient perspective of the impact of medication side effects on adherence: results of a cross-sectional nationwide survey of patients with schizophrenia. BMC Psychiatry. 2012;12:20. https://doi.org/10.1186/1471-244X-12-20.
78. Adam RL, Sidi H, Midin M, Zakaria H, Das S, Mat KC. The role of atypical antipsychotics in sexuality: road to recovery in schizophrenia. Curr Drug Targets. 2018;19:1402–11. https://doi.org/10.2174/1389450118666170502130126.
79. Holt RIG, Peveler RC. Antipsychotics and hyperprolactinaemia: mechanisms, consequences and management. Clin Endocrinol. 2011;74:141–7. https://doi.org/10.1111/j.1365-2265.2010.03814.x.
80. Weiden PJ, Buckley PF. Reducing the burden of side effects during long-term antipsychotic therapy: the role of "switching" medications. J Clin Psychiatry. 2007;68(Suppl 6):14–23.
81. Morgan VA, Waterreus A, Jablensky A, Mackinnon A, McGrath JJ, Carr V, Bush R, Castle D, Cohen M, Harvey C, Galletly C, Stain HJ, Neil AL, McGorry P, Hocking B, Shah S, Saw S. People living with psychotic illness in 2010: the second Australian national survey of psychosis. Aust N Z J Psychiatry. 2012;46:735–52. https://doi.org/10.1177/0004867412449877.
82. Awad AG, Hogan TP. Subjective response to neuroleptics and the quality of life: implications for treatment outcome. Acta Psychiatr Scand Suppl. 1994;380:27–32.

83. Barnes TRE, Schizophrenia Consensus Group of British Association for Psychopharmacology. Evidence-based guidelines for the pharmacological treatment of schizophrenia: recommendations from the British Association for Psychopharmacology. J Psychopharmacol Oxf Engl. 2011;25:567–620. https://doi.org/10.1177/0269881110391123.
84. Kuipers E. Psychosis and schizophrenia in adults. NICE Guidelines; 2014.
85. Lehman AF. Schizophrenia practice guidelines. American Psychiatric Association; 2010.
86. Howes OD, Kambeitz J, Kim E, Stahl D, Slifstein M, Abi-Dargham A, Kapur S. The nature of dopamine dysfunction in schizophrenia and what this means for treatment. Arch Gen Psychiatry. 2012;69:776–86. https://doi.org/10.1001/archgenpsychiatry.2012.169.
87. Howes OD, Kapur S. The dopamine hypothesis of schizophrenia: version III—the final common pathway. Schizophr Bull. 2009;35:549–62. https://doi.org/10.1093/schbul/sbp006.
88. Citrome L, Eramo A, Francois C, Duffy R, Legacy SN, Offord SJ, Krasa HB, Johnston SS, Guiraud-Diawara A, Kamat SA, Rohman P. Lack of tolerable treatment options for patients with schizophrenia. Neuropsychiatr Dis Treat. 2015;11:3095–104. https://doi.org/10.2147/NDT.S91917.
89. Dolder CR, Lacro JP, Dunn LB, Jeste DV. Antipsychotic medication adherence: is there a difference between typical and atypical agents? Am J Psychiatry. 2002;159:103–8. https://doi.org/10.1176/appi.ajp.159.1.103.
90. Yaegashi H, Kirino S, Remington G, Misawa F, Takeuchi H. Adherence to oral antipsychotics measured by electronic adherence monitoring in schizophrenia: a systematic review and meta-analysis. CNS Drugs. 2020;34:579–98. https://doi.org/10.1007/s40263-020-00713-9.
91. Tiihonen J, Mittendorfer-Rutz E, Majak M, Mehtälä J, Hoti F, Jedenius E, Enkusson D, Leval A, Sermon J, Tanskanen A, Taipale H. Real-world effectiveness of antipsychotic treatments in a nationwide cohort of 29,823 patients with schizophrenia. JAMA Psychiat. 2017;74:686–93. https://doi.org/10.1001/jamapsychiatry.2017.1322.
92. Lin C-H, Chen F-C, Chan H-Y, Hsu C-C. Time to rehospitalization in patients with schizophrenia receiving long-acting injectable antipsychotics or oral antipsychotics. Int J Neuropsychopharmacol. 2019;22:541–7. https://doi.org/10.1093/ijnp/pyz035.
93. Peters L, Krogmann A, von Hardenberg L, Bödeker K, Nöhles VB, Correll CU. Long-acting injections in schizophrenia: a 3-year update on randomized controlled trials published January 2016-March 2019. Curr Psychiatry Rep. 2019;21:124. https://doi.org/10.1007/s11920-019-1114-0.
94. Olagunju AT, Clark SR, Baune BT. Long-acting atypical antipsychotics in schizophrenia: a systematic review and meta-analyses of effects on functional outcome. Aust N Z J Psychiatry. 2019;53:509–27. https://doi.org/10.1177/0004867419837358.
95. Tiihonen J, Taipale H, Mehtälä J, Vattulainen P, Correll CU, Tanskanen A. Association of antipsychotic polypharmacy vs monotherapy with psychiatric rehospitalization among adults with schizophrenia. JAMA Psychiat. 2019;76:499–507. https://doi.org/10.1001/jamapsychiatry.2018.4320.
96. Fiorillo A, Barlati S, Bellomo A, Corrivetti G, Nicolò G, Sampogna G, Stanga V, Veltro F, Maina G, Vita A. The role of shared decision-making in improving adherence to pharmacological treatments in patients with schizophrenia: a clinical review. Ann General Psychiatry. 2020;19:43. https://doi.org/10.1186/s12991-020-00293-4.
97. Stovell D, Morrison AP, Panayiotou M, Hutton P. Shared treatment decision-making and empowerment-related outcomes in psychosis: systematic review and meta-analysis. Br J Psychiatry J Ment Sci. 2016;209:23–8. https://doi.org/10.1192/bjp.bp.114.158931.
98. Robinson DG, Schooler NR, Correll CU, John M, Kurian BT, Marcy P, Miller AL, Pipes R, Trivedi MH, Kane JM. Psychopharmacological treatment in the RAISE-ETP study: outcomes of a manual and computer decision support system based intervention. Am J Psychiatry. 2018;175:169–79. https://doi.org/10.1176/appi.ajp.2017.16080919.
99. Hamann J, Holzhüter F, Blakaj S, Becher S, Haller B, Landgrebe M, Schmauß M, Heres S. Implementing shared decision-making on acute psychiatric wards: a cluster-randomized trial with inpatients suffering from schizophrenia (SDM-PLUS). Epidemiol Psychiatr Sci. 2020;29:e137. https://doi.org/10.1017/S2045796020000505.

100. Sagud M, Mihaljević-Peleš A, Begić D, Vuksan-Ćusa B, Kramarić M, Zivković M, Jakovljević M. Antipsychotics as antidepressants: what is the mechanism? Psychiatr Danub. 2011;23:302–7.

101. Thase ME. Adverse effects of second-generation antipsychotics as adjuncts to antidepressants: are the risks worth the benefits? Psychiatr Clin North Am. 2016;39:477–86. https://doi.org/10.1016/j.psc.2016.04.008.

102. Parikh NB, Robinson DM, Clayton AH. Clinical role of brexpiprazole in depression and schizophrenia. Ther Clin Risk Manag. 2017;13:299–306. https://doi.org/10.2147/TCRM.S94060.

103. Shapiro DA, Renock S, Arrington E, Chiodo LA, Liu L-X, Sibley DR, Roth BL, Mailman R. Aripiprazole, a novel atypical antipsychotic drug with a unique and robust pharmacology. Neuropsychopharmacol Off Publ Am Coll Neuropsychopharmacol. 2003;28:1400–11. https://doi.org/10.1038/sj.npp.1300203.

104. Kiss B, Horváth A, Némethy Z, Schmidt E, Laszlovszky I, Bugovics G, Fazekas K, Hornok K, Orosz S, Gyertyán I, Agai-Csongor E, Domány G, Tihanyi K, Adham N, Szombathelyi Z. Cariprazine (RGH-188), a dopamine D(3) receptor-preferring, D(3)/D(2) dopamine receptor antagonist-partial agonist antipsychotic candidate: in vitro and neurochemical profile. J Pharmacol Exp Ther. 2010;333:328–40. https://doi.org/10.1124/jpet.109.160432.

105. Maeda K, Sugino H, Akazawa H, Amada N, Shimada J, Futamura T, Yamashita H, Ito N, McQuade RD, Mørk A, Pehrson AL, Hentzer M, Nielsen V, Bundgaard C, Arnt J, Stensbøl TB, Kikuchi T. Brexpiprazole I: in vitro and in vivo characterization of a novel serotonindopamine activity modulator. J Pharmacol Exp Ther. 2014;350:589–604. https://doi.org/10.1124/jpet.114.213793.

106. de Bartolomeis A, Tomasetti C, Iasevoli F. Update on the mechanism of action of aripiprazole: translational insights into antipsychotic strategies beyond dopamine receptor antagonism. CNS Drugs. 2015;29:773–99. https://doi.org/10.1007/s40263-015-0278-3.

107. Fleischhacker WW, Baker RA, Eramo A, Sanchez R, Tsai L-F, Peters-Strickland T, Perry PP, McQuade RD, Johnson BR, Carson WH, Kane JM. Effects of aripiprazole once-monthly on domains of personal and social performance: results from 2 multicenter, randomized, double-blind studies. Schizophr Res. 2014;159:415–20. https://doi.org/10.1016/j.schres.2014.09.019.

108. Németh G, Laszlovszky I, Czobor P, Szalai E, Szatmári B, Harsányi J, Barabássy Á, Debelle M, Durgam S, Bitter I, Marder S, Fleischhacker WW. Cariprazine versus risperidone monotherapy for treatment of predominant negative symptoms in patients with schizophrenia: a randomised, double-blind, controlled trial. Lancet Lond Engl. 2017;389:1103–13. https://doi.org/10.1016/S0140-6736(17)30060-0.

109. Durgam S, Earley W, Li R, Li D, Lu K, Laszlovszky I, Fleischhacker WW, Nasrallah HA. Long-term cariprazine treatment for the prevention of relapse in patients with schizophrenia: a randomized, double-blind, placebo-controlled trial. Schizophr Res. 2016;176:264–71. https://doi.org/10.1016/j.schres.2016.06.030.

110. Correll CU, Skuban A, Hobart M, Ouyang J, Weiller E, Weiss C, Kane JM. Efficacy of brexpiprazole in patients with acute schizophrenia: review of three randomized, double-blind, placebo-controlled studies. Schizophr Res. 2016;174:82–92. https://doi.org/10.1016/j.schres.2016.04.012.

111. Fleischhacker WW, Hobart M, Ouyang J, Forbes A, Pfister S, McQuade RD, Carson WH, Sanchez R, Nyilas M, Weiller E. Efficacy and safety of brexpiprazole (OPC-34712) as maintenance treatment in adults with schizophrenia: a randomized, double-blind, placebo-controlled study. Int J Neuropsychopharmacol. 2017;20:11–21. https://doi.org/10.1093/ijnp/pyw076.

112. Forbes A, Hobart M, Ouyang J, Shi L, Pfister S, Hakala M. A long-term, open-label study to evaluate the safety and tolerability of brexpiprazole as maintenance treatment in adults with schizophrenia. Int J Neuropsychopharmacol. 2018;21:433–41. https://doi.org/10.1093/ijnp/pyy002.

113. Jeppesen R, Christensen RHB, Pedersen EMJ, Nordentoft M, Hjorthøj C, Köhler-Forsberg O, Benros ME. Efficacy and safety of anti-inflammatory agents in treatment of psychotic disorders—a comprehensive systematic review and meta-analysis. Brain Behav Immun. 2020;90:364–80. https://doi.org/10.1016/j.bbi.2020.08.028.
114. Çakici N, van Beveren NJM, Judge-Hundal G, Koola MM, Sommer IEC. An update on the efficacy of anti-inflammatory agents for patients with schizophrenia: a meta-analysis. Psychol Med. 2019;49:2307–19. https://doi.org/10.1017/S0033291719001995.
115. Vinckier F, Gourion D, Mouchabac S. Anhedonia predicts poor psychosocial functioning: results from a large cohort of patients treated for major depressive disorder by general practitioners. Eur. Psychiatry J. Assoc. Eur. Psychiatr. 2017;44:1–8. https://doi.org/10.1016/j.eurpsy.2017.02.485.
116. Ritsner MS, Arbitman M, Lisker A. Anhedonia is an important factor of health-related quality-of-life deficit in schizophrenia and schizoaffective disorder. J Nerv Ment Dis. 2011;199:845–53. https://doi.org/10.1097/NMD.0b013e3182349ce6.
117. Correll CU. Current treatment options and emerging agents for schizophrenia. J Clin Psychiatry. 2020b;81:MS19053BR3C. https://doi.org/10.4088/JCP.MS19053BR3C.
118. Mallet J. Place de la consommation de cannabis parmi les facteurs de vulnérabilité de la schizophrénie (Médecine). Paris: Paris Descartes; 2012.
119. Mallet J, Ramoz N, Le Strat Y, Gorwood P, Dubertret C. Heavy cannabis use prior psychosis in schizophrenia: clinical, cognitive and neurological evidences for a new endophenotype? Eur Arch Psychiatry Clin Neurosci. 2017;267(7):629–38. https://doi.org/10.1007/s00406-017-0767-0.
120. Wright M, Di Ciano P, Brands B. Use of cannabidiol for the treatment of anxiety: a short synthesis of pre-clinical and clinical evidence. Cannabis Cannabinoid Res. 2020;5:191–6. https://doi.org/10.1089/can.2019.0052.
121. Ghabrash MF, Coronado-Montoya S, Aoun J, Gagné A-A, Mansour F, Ouellet-Plamondon C, Trépanier A, Jutras-Aswad D. Cannabidiol for the treatment of psychosis among patients with schizophrenia and other primary psychotic disorders: a systematic review with a risk of bias assessment. Psychiatry Res. 2020;286:112890. https://doi.org/10.1016/j.psychres.2020.112890.
122. Zheng W, Zhu X-M, Zhang Q-E, Yang X-H, Cai D-B, Li L, Li X-B, Ng CH, Ungvari GS, Ning Y-P, Xiang Y-T. Adjunctive intranasal oxytocin for schizophrenia: a meta-analysis of randomized, double-blind, placebo-controlled trials. Schizophr Res. 2019;206:13–20. https://doi.org/10.1016/j.schres.2018.12.007.
123. Bradley ER, Woolley JD. Oxytocin effects in schizophrenia: reconciling mixed findings and moving forward. Neurosci Biobehav Rev. 2017;80:36–56. https://doi.org/10.1016/j.neubiorev.2017.05.007.
124. Ota M, Yoshida S, Nakata M, Yada T, Kunugi H. The effects of adjunctive intranasal oxytocin in patients with schizophrenia. Postgrad Med. 2018;130:122–8. https://doi.org/10.1080/00325481.2018.1398592.

Part II

Recovery in Mood Disorders

Predictors of Clinical Recovery in Bipolar Disorders

10

Giovanna Fico, Gerard Anmella, Andrea Murru, and Eduard Vieta

10.1 Introduction

Bipolar disorder is a clinical syndrome characterized by recurring acute mood episodes of depression, alternated with mania and/or hypomania alternating with depressive episodes with a prevalence in the general population of 2% [1]. The Diagnostic and Statistical Manual of Mental Disorders, fifth edition (DSM-5) [2], includes the category 'bipolar and related disorders', which encompasses bipolar I, bipolar II, and cyclothymic disorders [2]. Bipolar disorder is considered the second leading cause of disability-adjusted life-years in the WHO European Region [3], mainly because of its early onset and chronicity across the lifespan [4].

When untreated, bipolar disorders are characterized by recurrence rates of 50–90% and progressive increases in the frequency and severity of affective episodes [1]. It is estimated that more than 90% of individuals who experience a manic episode will have subsequent episodes [5].

Affective relapses have been linked to chronic disability and poorer-than-premorbid functioning, in many cases with a progressive deteriorating course [6]. Hence, for a long time, the primary clinical goal in the management of bipolar disorders was to treat affective acute episodes and avoid re-hospitalizations. As a result, treatment typically focused on symptom reduction and relapse prevention, without considering further problems. Later on, the presence of neurocognitive impairment during phases of euthymia came to light [7, 8], along with cognitive deficiencies during subsyndromal depressive phases [9]. These deficiencies showed a great impact on functioning, which includes other fundamental issues such as living

---

G. Fico · G. Anmella · A. Murru · E. Vieta (✉)
Bipolar and Depressive Disorders Unit, Institute of Neuroscience, Hospital Clinic, University of Barcelona, IDIBAPS, CIBERSAM, Barcelona, Catalonia, Spain
e-mail: gfico@clinic.cat; anmella@clinic.cat; amurru@clinic.cat; evieta@clinic.cat

© The Author(s), under exclusive license to Springer Nature Switzerland AG 2022
B. Carpiniello et al. (eds.), *Recovery and Major Mental Disorders*, Comprehensive Approach to Psychiatry 2,
https://doi.org/10.1007/978-3-030-98301-7_10

environment, relationships, work, and education [10]. Previous studies showed that the majority of patients achieve symptomatic recovery but less than half achieve functional recovery within 24 months of a first manic/mixed episode [11].

Currently, given the fact that bipolar disorder can have an impact on everyday life activities, work productivity, interpersonal relationships, and quality of life [12–14], treating bipolar disorders implies a more comprehensive and integrative approach to control acute episodes and prevent relapses, as well as improving inter-episodic residual symptoms, in order to improve global functioning [15]. Thus, in the last decade, the treatment target in clinical and research settings has focused not only on clinical remission, but also on functional recovery and, more recently, in personal recovery, by also integrating patients' well-being and quality of life [15].

In this respect, the conceptualization of *recovery* as a new medical model for psychiatry came forward [16], including symptomatic recovery (resolution of symptoms), also called remission, and functional recovery, the ability to return to an adequate level of functioning [16].

This chapter will review the definition of recovery, correlates and predictors of recovery, both symptomatic and functional, in bipolar disorder. In addition, we will briefly discuss the latest strategies to promote full functional recovery in patients with bipolar disorders, which is equivalent to resuming the life quality and ability that they had before the onset of illness.

10.2 Remission in Bipolar Disorders

10.2.1 Definition of Remission

The Diagnostic and Statistical Manual of Mental Disorders, 4th edition (DSM IV-TR) defined full remission as the absence of significant signs and symptoms of bipolar disorder for at least 2 months and partial remission as the persistence of some signs or symptoms in a patient who previously fulfilled all criteria for bipolar disorder [17].

In research, operationalized criteria for remission have been defined based on expert clinical consensus. For manic episodes, remission is defined as an endpoint scores of ≤ 16 on the Young Mania Rating Scale (YMRS) [18]. For bipolar depression, remission is defined as scores of ≤ 7 on the Hamilton Depression rating Scale (HAM-D), or ≤ 8 on the Montgomery-Åsberg Depression Rating Scale (MADRS) [18]. It should be underlined that conventional scales measure remission only from a specific affective pole. Hereby, a reduction of symptoms of depression or mania/hypomania might be viewed as a trend towards remission, while it may be related to a shift towards the opposite affective pole.

In this respect, previous evidence proposed the CGI-BP [19], a non-symptom-based instrument providing global measures of disease severity and improvement, as better candidate than symptom-based scales to capture clinical remission [20]. In particular, a score of 1 on its severity scale (CGI-S) has been used to indicate clinical remission [21].

10 Predictors of Clinical Recovery in Bipolar Disorders

Moreover, there is an intrinsic complexity in defining remission for bipolar disorder due to its pleomorphic clinical presentation, its frequent comorbidity with other psychiatric or medical disorders, and its functional impairment across multiple domains. When comorbidities are present, they increase the burden of illness and worsen the prognosis of bipolar disorder, preventing remission and overall recovery.

10.2.2 Treatment Strategies for Remission

Over the past decades the expanding pharmacopoeia and the development of psychosocial treatment strategies for bipolar disorder have provided clinicians with a large spectrum of opportunities to treat bipolar disorders.

There are a variety of pharmacological options available for management of acute affective episodes and preventing relapses, with polypharmacy being increasingly used [22]. Despite the variety of pharmacological and additional psychological therapies available to alleviate symptoms, only 62.1% of patients with bipolar disorder achieve symptomatic recovery within 1 year after the first episode of mania [23].

Several factors may influence the selection of a specific treatment in bipolar disorder, including patients' preference, medical or psychiatric comorbidities, specific key symptoms, such as thoughts of death, feelings of worthlessness, and/or aggressiveness [24], and previous response to treatments. During an acute affective episode, besides choosing the best treatment option among pharmacological and non-pharmacological ones, it is mandatory to evaluate the risk of suicide or aggressive behaviours, both self and hetero-directed.

Despite the remarkable increase in treatments for bipolar disorder, some patients still show inadequate response in acute manic or depressive episodes or in long-term preventive maintenance treatment. The definition itself of treatment-resistant bipolar disorder is still on debate, with no consensual definitions in the literature [25]. In some studies, treatment resistance in acute affective episodes is considered as the failure to respond to a specified number of treatments that are generally considered effective, while treatment resistance in maintenance treatment is typically defined as continued cycling despite adequate trials of previously demonstrated effective treatments [25]. A recent evidence-based expert panel defined treatment-resistant bipolar depression as the failure to reach sustained symptomatic remission for 8 consecutive weeks after two different treatment trials, at adequate therapeutic doses, with at least two recommended monotherapy treatments or at least one monotherapy treatment and another combination treatment [26]. Additionally, multi-therapy-resistant bipolar depression included to the previous definitions, the failure of at least one trial with an antidepressant, a psychological treatment and a course of electroconvulsive therapy [26]. Treatment-resistant patients show a clinical course that is characterized by frequent relapses and residual symptoms, causing significant disability and functional impairment [27].

Several evidence-based clinical guidelines for treating bipolar disorder [22, 28], including treatment-resistant bipolar disorder [29], provide detailed strategies for treating acute affective episodes of different polarities, and for maintenance treatment, as exposed below.

10.2.2.1 Acute Mania

Antipsychotic agents or mood stabilizers are the mainstream treatment for acute mania and hypomania [22]. Non-pharmacological strategies, such as electroconvulsive therapy, may also be used for patients with treatment-resistant or severe mania [30]. Treatment options for acute mania include lithium, valproate, others mood stabilizers, and atypical antipsychotics [31]. To date, there is no clear evidence that any of these categories of treatments is superior compared with the others. A network meta-analysis has shown that risperidone was more effective than aripiprazole and more effective than valproate in acute mania [32]. For patients with acute mania, if there is no response to a medication after 1–2 weeks, a different medication may be considered. When choosing between mono- or polytherapy, it should be noted that the best evidence comes from placebo-controlled trials in which patients' condition is milder than in clinical practice. Therefore, several considerations should be made for this clinical decision, such as the patient's previous history of response to treatment, the rapidity of response needed (polytherapy usually works faster), the severity of mania (better response rates with polytherapy), tolerability history (usually worse with polytherapy), the patient's preferences, and the long-term adherence (worse with polytherapy) [30]. The combination of an antipsychotic agent and a mood stabilizer, especially for severe mania, appears to be more efficacious than either medication alone.

Electroconvulsive therapy, as monotherapy or as an adjunctive treatment, has been reported to be effective for patients with treatment-resistant mania, aggressive behaviour or psychotic symptoms [33].

Although there is no clear consensus on the use of benzodiazepines in acute mania, they are usually prescribed to treat residual symptoms (e.g., anxiety, agitation, and insomnia). The long-term use of benzodiazepines is generally discouraged and is associated with several tolerability and safety concerns [34].

In sum, a personalized treatment is needed for acute mania, according to the different clinical presentations and clinical scenarios within the manic episode, and considering a long-term view with the objective of not only a symptomatic but also functional recovery. After remission from acute mania. Psychotherapy may be hard to provide during manic episodes; indeed, evidence has shown that psychosocial interventions have better outcomes when used after remission from acute mania, as well as psychoeducation strategies to ensure adherence to treatment [35].

10.2.2.2 Acute Bipolar Depression

Patients with bipolar disorder will spend at least half their lives with some degree of depressive symptomatology [36], with 20 years of follow-up studies showing a 3:1 predominance of depressive over (hypo)manic symptoms in bipolar disorder type I [37]. Although depressive episodes dominate the course of bipolar disorder, few studies have focused on the treatment of depression, with a little number of drugs currently approved by the FDA for the management of acute bipolar depressive episodes.

For this reason, other treatments, usually in combination (olanzapine with fluoxetine, lithium with lamotrigine, quetiapine with lamotrigine), are often used off

10 Predictors of Clinical Recovery in Bipolar Disorders

label in clinical practice. Among the drugs approved by FDA for bipolar depression, lurasidone was effective in a randomized controlled in patients from 10 to 17 years of age [38].

In a meta-analysis, cariprazine was effective as monotherapy for the treatment of acute episodes of bipolar depression [39]. Furthermore, recent evidence suggests possible, mild efficacy of dopamine-agonists [40] and non-steroidal anti-inflammatory drugs [41], and ketamine [42, 43] for the treatment of bipolar depression.

Conventional unimodal antidepressant medications have been limited in situations in which patients are nonresponsive to and/or intolerant of previous medications. This positioning reflects the concern that antidepressants may carry a higher risk of switches to the opposite polarity or acceleration of the cycling between them [44]. Thus, antidepressants are generally avoided in patients with bipolar disorder, especially type I, but they may be prescribed in addition to mood stabilizers [45]. Electroconvulsive therapy has proven effective for patients with treatment-resistant bipolar depression [46]. Among non-pharmacological treatments, evidence shows utility of using adjuvant psychotherapeutic approaches, such as psychoeducation, cognitive behavioural therapy (CBT), family-focused therapy, dialectical behavioural therapy, and mindfulness-based CBT [47]. Also, physical activity has been addressed as a possible beneficial factor for patients with bipolar depression even if evidence is still scarce [48]. Although, research on bipolar depression has increased over the last decade, its treatment and management is still an unmet need. Future studies will need to establish treatment efficacy in bipolar depression, to help develop personalized predictors or biomarkers of response, to finally optimize interventions for bipolar depression.

10.2.2.3 Mixed States

Mixed affective states in bipolar disorder are defined by co-occurrence of manic and depressive symptoms. While in DSM-IV-TR it was possible to diagnose a mixed episode if a patient presented with symptoms of depressive and manic/hypomanic episodes simultaneously, in DSM-5, instead, a 'mixed feature' specifier can be added to manic/hypomanic episodes or depressive episode in bipolar disorder, when at least three depressive symptoms are present in a manic episode or at least three manic symptoms occur during a depressive episode [49].

Mixed affective states are associated with a more severe course of illness, higher rates of suicide, more psychiatric comorbidities, such as personality disorders, and a greater risk of presenting with rapid cycling [50].

Even though more specific clinical definitions of mixed affective states have been developed, no drug treatment has been approved for their management. Recently, several guidelines were published: the World Federation of Societies of Biological Psychiatry (WFSBP) guidelines for the acute and long-term treatment of mixed episodes in bipolar disorder [51] and guidelines for recognition and treatment of mixed depression [52].

The vast majority of clinical trials have investigated the efficacy of atypical antipsychotics in monotherapy or in combination with mood stabilizers in manic and mixed bipolar patients, without reaching a clear consensus. Despite their heterogeneity, all guidelines agreed in interrupting an antidepressant monotherapy or adding mood-stabilizing medications. Indeed, evidence showed that antidepressant treatment in monotherapy may worsen mixed affective states [53].

A recent systematic review providing a critical synthesis and a comprehensive overview of guidelines on the treatment of mixed affective states showed that olanzapine seemed to have the best evidence for acute mixed hypo/manic/depressive states and maintenance treatment. Furthermore, in the same study it is reported that aripiprazole and paliperidone were possible alternatives for acute hypo/manic mixed states, while lurasidone and ziprasidone were useful in acute mixed depression. Valproic acid was recommended for the prevention of new mixed episodes, while clozapine and electroconvulsive therapy seemed to be effective in refractory mixed episodes [54, 55].

To date, there is no study in which the effect of psychotherapy specifically on mixed states has been investigated.

10.3 From Symptomatic to Functional Recovery

10.3.1 Maintenance Treatment of Bipolar Disorder

The maintenance treatment of bipolar disorder represents a major clinical challenge. Ideally, when the treatment of an acute affective episode is effective, the patient experiences symptomatic remission. Unfortunately, the intermediate and long-term prognosis of patients with bipolar disorder remains rather disappointing, being characterized by lifelong recurrent episodes and residual intra-episodic symptomatology, with almost half of patients experiencing a recurrence within 2 years and 70–90% within 5 years, while the lifetime recurrence rate is 95% [56–58]. Indeed, results from the Systematic Treatment Enhancement Program for Bipolar Disorder (STEP-BD), which combined psychosocial interventions with pharmacotherapy, indicated that about half of the patients with bipolar disorder who recovered from an index episode experienced a recurrence within 18 months of prospective follow-up [59]. Patients who do not achieve mood stabilization experience more frequent treatment changes, consult more frequently to emergencies units, and present significantly increased risks of life-threatening events as suicide attempts, as well as unwanted legal and interpersonal consequences such as hetero-aggressive acts [60].

The aims of maintenance treatment in bipolar disorders are preventing relapses, reducing subsyndromal symptoms, preventing cognitive decline and increase psychosocial functioning, ideally prolonging inter-episodic well-being [61]. Thus, maintenance treatment should be started immediately after the onset of illness, to improve the prognosis and assure a long-term clinical stability.

The current first-line pharmacological treatments used as maintenance treatment for bipolar disorder are mood stabilizers such as lithium, lamotrigine, valproate, and atypical antipsychotics such as olanzapine, quetiapine, aripiprazole, risperidone, and ziprasidone.

Lithium has 70 years of established clinical practice in preventing affective relapses [62]. Still today, lithium represents the first choice among the maintenance treatments in bipolar disorder [63, 64]. A network meta-analysis on the comparative efficacy and tolerability of different pharmacological treatments in the maintenance treatment of bipolar disorder showed that lithium was more efficacious than placebo in prevention of both manic and depressive relapses [65]. Also, in a multicentre, randomized, open-label trial including patients with bipolar disorder type I, both combination therapy with lithium plus valproate and lithium monotherapy were more likely to prevent relapse than is valproate monotherapy [66]. Moreover, lithium was also shown to reduce risk of suicide in patients with bipolar disorder [67].

A good clinical long-term management of bipolar disorder includes the monitoring of possibly emerging side effects during lithium treatment including renal failure, hypothyroidism, polydipsia, polyuria, tremors, and an increase in peripheral calcium and parathyroid hormone levels [68]. Clinicians should educate the patients to regular follow-ups, to avoid the risk of toxicity or its adverse effects [69].

Studies suggest that valproate has some efficacy in preventing affective relapses. However, valproate in combination was more effective/efficacious to prevent affective relapses than valproate monotherapy. Also, valproate was more acceptable than lithium, as it was associated with a lower risk for participants to treatment withdraw [70]. Carbamazepine, lamotrigine, olanzapine, quetiapine, paliperidone, asenapine, and cariprazine have also shown to be effective maintenance treatments for bipolar disorder.

Despite the growing evidence, unlike treatment trials for acute mood episodes, still few studies have been conducted on maintenance treatments for bipolar disorder. From a purely clinical point of view, when several treatment options are available, clinicians should evaluate not only the efficacy of the treatment in preventing mood episodes, but also the tolerability and long-term compliance, based on patient's characteristics and preferences. In this respect, monotherapy is initially recommended in order to enhance adherence and minimize side effects, but combination therapy is often necessary.

The inter-individual variability and precise characterization of bipolar disorder have led to the establishment of course specifiers in bipolar disorders, as the predominant polarity, defined as $\geq 2/3$ of lifetime episodes of a given polarity [71]. The marked clinical differences between predominantly manic and depressive bipolar patients justify that pharmacological maintenance treatment should be aligned according to the patient's polarity [72]. The polarity index (PI) is a useful metric to classify maintenance therapies and categorizes therapies as those with a predominant antimanic prophylactic profile and those with an antidepressant prophylactic profile [73]. International guidelines take into consideration the presence of a specific predominant polarity for maintenance drug choice in patients with bipolar disorder [22, 28, 29, 74, 75].

Despite pharmacological treatments remain the cornerstone to prevent relapses, they alone lead only a minority of patients to symptoms remission, with 40% of individuals typically experiencing recurrences at 1 year of follow-up [76, 77].

Furthermore, non-adherence to pharmacotherapy or drug-related adverse effects increase the probability of recurrence in mood episodes [78, 79]. Thus, adjunctive, evidence-based psychosocial treatments have been proposed and used effectively during the maintenance phase of treatment.

Adjunct psychosocial interventions have been shown to improve outcomes in bipolar disorder because they teach patients strategies to manage their mood instability. Evidence supporting the utility of psychotherapy to reduce the risk of relapse (as opposed to relieving acute affective episodes) in people with bipolar disorder has been particularly robust [47]. Available psychological interventions include psychoeducation, cognitive behavioural therapy, interpersonal and social rhythm therapy, dialectical behaviour therapy, mindfulness-based cognitive therapy, and family therapies such as family-focused therapy [35]. The choice of the psychological intervention may derive from the specific need to address illness courses characterized by predominance of relapse into either poles [80].

In the long-term management of bipolar disorder, other areas of future research include managing the leading cause of mortality, such as cardiovascular disease. The Nutrition, Exercise, and Wellness Treatment (NEW Tx) for overweight bipolar patients, is an 18-session, 20-week CBT-based treatment for lifestyle changes that also includes Motivational Interviewing techniques [81].

Clinicians should collect comprehensive information about patients' illness history, type of relapses, response to treatment, and medical comorbidities to develop a personalized treatment that should be re-adapted during the time, based on patients' needs.

10.3.2 Residual Symptoms

In the classical view, patients during inter-episodic periods are euthymic—that is to say in symptomatic remission. However, a large number of studies reported that patients who have suffered an acute affective episode continue presenting subsyndromal symptoms during remission periods [14, 21, 82]. These persistent symptoms can be defined as residual symptoms. Among residual symptoms, cognitive symptoms are reported to be the most common, with mood symptoms of both polarities, usually subsyndromal, being the second most common.

Other residual symptoms include sleep disorders, emotional dysregulation, and sexual dysfunction. The presence of residual symptoms has been linked to an overall negative impact on functional outcomes of patients with bipolar disorder [83, 84]. Residual symptoms appear to impact the natural course of bipolar disorder and represent potential predictors of long-term outcome and recovery. Depressive residual symptoms are associated with an increased risk of recurrence [85] and lower adherence to medication in bipolar patients [86] and, together with persistent cognitive deficits, are important predictors of functional impairment [9, 87, 88]. Moreover, residual depressive symptoms may worsen cognitive deficits, further affecting global functioning [89]. Residual manic symptoms may have a negative impact on financial issues, family stigma, interpersonal relationships, sexual

10 Predictors of Clinical Recovery in Bipolar Disorders

functioning, and occupational stigma [90]. Also, the intensity of residual symptoms and functional impairment in patients in remission is negatively related to the duration of euthymia [91].

Despite residual symptoms are consistently identified as predictors of worse functioning, in accordance with clinical practice and research evidence, there is still an open debate on finding a definition of residual symptoms in bipolar disorder. As for defining remission, given the heterogeneous nature of bipolar disorder, it is not surprising that previous studies tried to provide cut-offs to easily identify patients with residual symptoms: the International Task Force for bipolar disorder suggests that a Young Mania Rating Scale (YMRS) score of <8 or <5 should be used to define residual manic symptoms [18], while other studies have employed a threshold of YMRS score <7 [92, 93]. Similarly, remission for bipolar depression has been proposed as either a Hamilton Depression Rating Scale score (HAMD-17) of ≤ 7 or ≤ 5 [18], MADRS score of ≤ 7 or ≤ 5 or Bipolar Depression Rating Scale (BDRS) of ≤ 8 [94, 95].

In conclusion, it is mandatory to consider and implement the treatment of residual symptoms during euthymic phases of patients with bipolar disorder. Mood residual symptoms will require pharmacological treatments, but the role of other residuals symptoms, such as cognitive or sleep symptoms, should be not overlooked, since it can affect functioning and prevent full recovery.

10.4 Functional Recovery

A significant proportion of patients continue to experience substantial difficulties in different life aspects, even after clinical remission.

Patients do not search for only absence of symptoms, but rather for regain the quality of life and ability that they had before the illness onset, in their daily life, at work, with their family and friends. Thus, the focus in the management of bipolar disorder has moved from clinical remission to functional recovery [96]. Functional recovery has been defined as a deeply personal, unique process of changing one's attitudes, values, feelings, goals, skills, and/or roles, even with limitations caused by illness [97].

Most specifically, given the complexity and the multifaced nature of functional recovery, involving different aspects including the capacity to live independently, to enjoy leisure time, and to share life with a partner, it is often viewed as a process and not an outcome. Previous studies have indicated that the majority of patients with bipolar disorder achieve symptomatic recovery but less than half achieve functional recovery within 24 months of a first manic/mixed episode [11].

Indeed, bipolar disorder is associated with difficulties in psychosocial functioning—e.g. difficulties in occupational performance and social integration. Previous studies showed that less than half of the patients admitted for bipolar disorder returned to work after discharge; at 2 years, one-third of the patients demonstrated difficulties in work performance, and at 5 years even patients with 2-years clinical remission presented alterations in social functioning [98].

However, recovery rates are dependent on the criteria used to define recovery, the scales used to measure outcome, and the patient population studied [99].

Indeed, one of the major issues associated with functional recovery is the lack of consensus on the terminology and standards used to measure it [100]. Among the instruments used in psychiatry to address functional impairment, there are the global activity (GAF), the WHO Disability Assessment Schedule (WHODAS 2.0) [101], the Range of Impaired Functioning Tool (LIFE-RIFT) [102] or the Multidimensional Scale of Independent Functioning (MSIF) [103]. Most of these scales require quite a long time for administration and are not designed specifically to evaluate functional alterations in bipolar disorder or are self-reported questionnaires and their validity remains unclear. To this end, the Functioning Assessment Short Test (FAST) was developed for the clinical evaluation of functional impairment presented by patients suffering from mental disorders including bipolar disorder [104]. It is a highly reliable tool to evaluate the objective difficulties presented by patients in psychosocial functioning, an area which has also demonstrated sensitivity to changes in both the short and the long term.

In this line, a recent study has classified the patients into different groups according to the impairment shown in different domains of functioning in the FAST scale by using an exploratory cluster analysis [105]. In a study including 143 euthymic patients with bipolar disorder, only 30% showed in all the FAST areas (autonomy, occupational, cognitive, financial, interpersonal, and leisure), with almost 70% showing some kind of functional impairment. Three different patterns were observed: one group with no significant impairment in any of the assessed domains, a second one with mild impairment in different domains but severe impairment in occupational functioning, and the last one with severe impairment in most of the assessed domains. This study suggests a significant functional heterogeneity in patients with bipolar disorder regarding their functional profile, and proposes that they can be classified accordingly, ranging from patients showing a completely good functional performance, patients showing an intermediate functional performance, to patients with a severe impairment in multiple functional domains.

These data are consistent with other studies showing that around 60% of patients with bipolar disorder have functional impairments [106]. Furthermore, both functionally impaired groups in this study showed some kind of impairment which was associated with residual symptoms, including subsyndromal mood symptoms (depressive and manic) and cognitive performance, which seem to play an important role in psychosocial functioning. These patterns should be taken into consideration to develop more individualized interventions to restore, or improve, psychosocial outcomes.

Although among functional outcome affected in bipolar patients cognitive function has been considered a core feature of the illness, currently there is no Food and Drug Administration-approved pharmacological agent for the management of cognitive deficits in bipolar disorder. It has therefore been suggested that non-pharmacological interventions, such as cognitive remediation and non-invasive brain stimulation techniques, could also have a potential effect [107].

10 Predictors of Clinical Recovery in Bipolar Disorders

Also disease progression seems to be linked to a more difficult functional recovery. This goes in line with the neuroprogression theory in bipolar disorder, in which progressive changes in the central nervous system due to subsequent mood episodes are associated with cognitive dysfunction, which, in turn, seems to involve a functional disability and a worse clinical course [108]. The biochemical mechanisms of neuroprogression appear to include illness stage-related alterations in inflammatory cytokines, neurotrophins, and oxidative stress [109]. This model spawned the concept of staging in bipolar disorders, which presented as a way to categorize patients integrating multiple levels of information, including the clinical presentation, course, and illness severity, and allowed to define each patient's characteristics, severity, and prognosis in a more precise and individualized way. The model of clinical staging in bipolar disorder might contribute to precision psychiatry by allowing a more personalized treatment [110]. In fact, both psychological interventions and pharmacological treatments show a greater efficacy in the earlier stage of the disease [111].

10.4.1 The Pathway to Recovery in Bipolar Disorder: Functional Remediation

The term 'functional remediation' has been used to define an innovative strategy, developed in the Hospital Clinic of Barcelona, aimed at targeting the critical factors for functional recovery in bipolar disorders.

Functional remediation covers both cognition and functioning, including psychoeducation about cognitive deficits and their impact on daily life, providing strategies to manage cognitive deficiencies, such as in attention, memory, and executive functions. The family is also involved in the process to facilitate the practice of these strategies and for reinforcement [112].

The efficacy of functional remediation has been demonstrated in a multicentre, randomized, rater-blind clinical trial on euthymic bipolar patients comparing psychoeducation, functional remediation, and pharmacological treatment only (standard treatment). The primary outcome measure was improvement in global psychosocial functioning post-intervention and at 1 year, measured on the FAST from baseline to endpoint evaluation [112]. The results showed an improvement in the functioning of patients participating in the functional remediation group compared with those who receive only pharmacological treatment or psychoeducation. In addition, patients undergoing the functional remediation programme achieved significant improvement in occupational and interpersonal or social functioning compared with the standard treatment group. The efficacy of the functional remediation intervention programme was maintained at 1 year of follow-up.

The functional remediation programme, therefore, is a promising tool for achieving improvement in functional performance in euthymic bipolar patients.

In its current format, was developed for late-stage bipolar disorder, but with some modifications it could be tailored to enhance cognitive reserve [113], thus preventing cognitive disfunctions and functional impairment.

In clinical practice there is a need to reduce the impact of the disability of bipolar patients in order to the personal and societal burden of the disease. Functional remediation seems to be effective in promoting functional recovery in bipolar disorder.

New interventions that incorporate psychoeducation, functional remediation, and some content related to healthy life habits and mindfulness are being implemented [114]. Further studies will have to confirm the duration of the effects of the intervention and to identify the predictors of functional outcome in order to provide the most effective treatments or to individualize interventions.

10.5 Conclusions

Patients with bipolar disorders may experience serious impairments in psychosocial functioning and quality of life, despite adequate treatment. Numerous treatments are available for acute affective episodes, in most cases promoting symptomatic remission. Symptomatic remission does not necessarily lead to an acceptable level of functioning, defined as full recovery. Full recovery in bipolar disorder is mostly hampered by cognitive impairment and subclinical depressive symptoms, defined as residual symptoms. Moreover, with each successive illness episode, and the neurobiological effects of neuroprogression, residual symptoms increase, the stages of the disease advance, and the possibility of a functional recovery further declines. Functional remediation is an intervention based on neurocognitive training and psychoeducation that showed efficacy in improving functioning in both euthymic and patients with subsyndromal bipolar disorder. However, the ideal maintenance treatment for bipolar disorder is still to be found, and further studies should aim to find the optimal combinations of medications and psychosocial interventions for bipolar disorders at different stages, in the direction of a precision psychiatry and an integral holistic clinical recovery.

References

1. Carvalho AF, Firth J, Vieta E. Bipolar disorder. N Engl J Med. 2020;383(1):58–66.
2. APA. Diagnostic and statistical manual of mental disorders: DSM-5. Arlington, VA: American Psychiatric Association; 2013.
3. He H, Hu C, Ren Z, Bai L, Gao F, Lyu J. Trends in the incidence and DALYs of bipolar disorder at global, regional, and national levels: results from the global burden of disease study 2017. J Psychiatr Res. 2020;125:96–105.
4. Merikangas KR, Jin R, He J-P, Kessler RC, Lee S, Sampson NA, et al. Prevalence and correlates of bipolar spectrum disorder in the world mental health survey initiative. Arch Gen Psychiatry. 2011;68(3):241–51.
5. Müller-Oerlinghausen B, Berghöfer A, Bauer M. Bipolar disorder. Lancet (London, England). 2002;359(9302):241–7.
6. Kessing LV, Hansen MG, Andersen PK, Angst J. The predictive effect of episodes on the risk of recurrence in depressive and bipolar disorders—a life-long perspective. Acta Psychiatr Scand. 2004;109(5):339–44.

10 Predictors of Clinical Recovery in Bipolar Disorders

7. Martínez-Arán A, Vieta E, Colom F, Reinares M, Benabarre A, Gastó C, et al. Cognitive dysfunctions in bipolar disorder: evidence of neuropsychological disturbances. Psychother Psychosom. 2000;69:2–18.

8. Martínez-Arán A, Vieta E, Colom F, Torrent C, Sánchez-Moreno J, Reinares M, et al. Cognitive impairment in euthymic bipolar patients: implications for clinical and functional outcome. Bipolar Disord. 2004;6(3):224–32.

9. Bonnín CM, Martínez-Arán A, Torrent C, Pacchiarotti I, Rosa AR, Franco C, et al. Clinical and neurocognitive predictors of functional outcome in bipolar euthymic patients: a long-term, follow-up study. J Affect Disord. 2010;121(1–2):156–60.

10. Rosa AR, González-Ortega I, González-Pinto A, Echeburúa E, Comes M, Martínez-Àran A, et al. One-year psychosocial functioning in patients in the early vs. late stage of bipolar disorder. Acta Psychiatr Scand. 2012;125(4):335–41.

11. Tohen M, Hennen J, Zarate CMJ, Baldessarini RJ, Strakowski SM, Stoll AL, et al. Two-year syndromal and functional recovery in 219 cases of first-episode major affective disorder with psychotic features. Am J Psychiatry. 2000;157(2):220–8.

12. Michalak EE, Yatham LN, Lam RW. Quality of life in bipolar disorder: a review of the literature. Health Qual Life Outcomes. 2005;3(1):72. https://doi.org/10.1186/1477-7525-3-72.

13. Rosa AR, Franco C, Martinez-Aran A, Sanchez-Moreno J, Reinares M, Salamero M, et al. Functional impairment in patients with remitted bipolar disorder. Psychother Psychosom. 2008:390–2.

14. Tohen M, Bowden CL, Calabrese JR, Lin D, Forrester TD, Sachs GS, et al. Influence of sub-syndromal symptoms after remission from manic or mixed episodes. Br J Psychiatry. 2006;189(6):515–9. https://www.cambridge.org/core/article/influence-of-subsyndromal-symptoms-after-remission-from-manic-or-mixed-episodes/DB176EF66B0977711D33 1D1434A0E06A.

15. del Mar Bonnín C, Reinares M, Martínez-Arán A, Jiménez E, Sánchez-Moreno J, Solé B, et al. Improving functioning, quality of life, and well-being in patients with bipolar disorder. Int J Neuropsychopharmacol. 2019;22(8):467–77. https://doi.org/10.1093/ijnp/pyz018.

16. Schrank B, Slade M. Recovery in psychiatry. Psychiatr Bull. 2007;31(9):321–5. https://www.cambridge.org/core/article/recovery-in-psychiatry/1D707A2B60C5622D7028D79A84F7 9C2D.

17. American Psychiatric Association. Diagnostic and statistical manual of mental disorders (4th ed., Text Revision). Washington: Author; 2000.

18. Tohen M, Frank E, Bowden CL, Colom F, Ghaemi SN, Yatham LN, et al. The International Society for Bipolar Disorders (ISBD) Task Force report on the nomenclature of course and outcome in bipolar disorders. Bipolar Disord. 2009;11(5):453–73. https://doi.org/10.1111/ j.1399-5618.2009.00726.x.

19. Spearing MK, Post RM, Leverich GS, Brandt D, Nolen W. Modification of the Clinical Global Impressions (CGI) Scale for use in bipolar illness (BP): the CGI-BP. Psychiatry Res. 1997;73(3):159–71.

20. Berk M, Ng F, Wang WV, Calabrese JR, Mitchell PB, Malhi GS, et al. The empirical redefinition of the psychometric criteria for remission in bipolar disorder. J Affect Disord. 2008;106(1–2):153–8.

21. Vieta E, Sánchez-Moreno J, Lahuerta J, Zaragoza S. Subsyndromal depressive symptoms in patients with bipolar and unipolar disorder during clinical remission. J Affect Disord. 2008;107(1):169–74. http://www.sciencedirect.com/science/article/pii/S0165032707002893.

22. Yatham LN, Kennedy SH, Parikh SV, Schaffer A, Bond DJ, Frey BN, et al. Canadian Network for Mood and Anxiety Treatments (CANMAT) and International Society for Bipolar Disorders (ISBD) 2018 guidelines for the management of patients with bipolar disorder. Bipolar Disord. 2018;20(2):97–170.

23. Gignac A, McGirr A, Lam RW, Yatham LN. Recovery and recurrence following a first episode of mania: a systematic review and meta-analysis of prospectively characterized cohorts. J Clin Psychiatry. 2015;76(9):1241–8.

24. Anmella G, Gil-Badenes J, Pacchiarotti I, Verdolini N, Aedo A, Angst J, et al. Do depressive and manic symptoms differentially impact on functioning in acute depression? Results from a large, cross-sectional study. J Affect Disord. 2020a;261:30–9.
25. Gitlin M. Treatment-resistant bipolar disorder. Mol Psychiatry. 2006;11(3):227–40. https://doi.org/10.1038/sj.mp.4001793.
26. Hidalgo-Mazzei D, Berk M, Cipriani A, Cleare AJ, Di Florio A, Dietch D, et al. Treatment-resistant and multi-therapy-resistant criteria for bipolar depression: consensus definition. Br J Psychiatry. 2019;214(1):27–35.
27. Esan O, Osunbote C, Oladele O, Fakunle S, Ehindero C, Fountoulakis KN. Bipolar I disorder in remission vs. schizophrenia in remission: is there a difference in burden? Compr Psychiatry. 2017;72:130–5. http://www.sciencedirect.com/science/article/pii/S0010440X16303637.
28. Grunze H, Vieta E, Goodwin GM, Bowden C, Licht RW, Möller H-J, et al. The World Federation of Societies of Biological Psychiatry (WFSBP) guidelines for the biological treatment of bipolar disorders: update 2012 on the long-term treatment of bipolar disorder. World J Biol Psychiatry. 2013;14(3):154–219.
29. Fountoulakis KN, Grunze H, Vieta E, Young A, Yatham L, Blier P, et al. The International College of Neuro-Psychopharmacology (CINP) treatment guidelines for bipolar disorder in adults (CINP-BD-2017), Part 3: the clinical guidelines. Int J Neuropsychopharmacol. 2016;20(2):180–95. https://doi.org/10.1093/ijnp/pyw109.
30. Pacchiarotti I, Anmella G, Colomer L, Vieta E. How to treat mania. Acta Psychiatr Scand. 2020a;142:173–92.
31. Grande I, Vieta E. Pharmacotherapy of acute mania: monotherapy or combination therapy with mood stabilizers and antipsychotics? CNS Drugs. 2015;29(3):221–7.
32. Yildiz A, Nikodem M, Vieta E, Correll CU, Baldessarini RJ. A network meta-analysis on comparative efficacy and all-cause discontinuation of antimanic treatments in acute bipolar mania. Psychol Med. 2015;45(2):299–317.
33. Ciapparelli A, Dell'Osso L, Tundo A, Pini S, Chiavacci MC, Di Sacco I, et al. Electroconvulsive therapy in medication-nonresponsive patients with mixed mania and bipolar depression. J Clin Psychiatry. 2001;62(7):552–5. https://doi.org/10.4088/jcp.v62n07a09.
34. Bobo WV, Reilly-Harrington NA, Ketter TA, Brody BD, Kinrys G, Kemp DE, et al. Complexity of illness and adjunctive benzodiazepine use in outpatients with bipolar I or II disorder: results from the Bipolar CHOICE study. J Clin Psychopharmacol. 2015;35(1):68–74.
35. Salcedo S, Gold AK, Sheikh S, Marcus PH, Nierenberg AA, Deckersbach T, et al. Empirically supported psychosocial interventions for bipolar disorder: current state of the research. J Affect Disord. 2016;201:203–14. http://www.sciencedirect.com/science/article/pii/S0165032716303743.
36. Miller S, Dell'Osso B, Ketter TA. The prevalence and burden of bipolar depression. J Affect Disord. 2014;169:S3–11. http://www.sciencedirect.com/science/article/pii/S0165032714700035.
37. Judd LL, Akiskal HS, Schettler PJ, Endicott J, Maser J, Solomon DA, et al. The long-term natural history of the weekly symptomatic status of bipolar I disorder. Arch Gen Psychiatry. 2002;59(6):530–7.
38. DelBello MP, Goldman R, Phillips D, Deng L, Cucchiaro J, Loebel A. Efficacy and safety of lurasidone in children and adolescents with Bipolar I depression: a double-blind, placebo-controlled study. J Am Acad Child Adolesc Psychiatry. 2017;56(12):1015–25.
39. Pinto JV, Saraf G, Vigo D. Keramatian K, Chakrabarty T, Yatham LN. Cariprazine in the treatment of bipolar disorder: a systematic review and meta-analysis. Bipolar Disord. 2020;22(4):360–71.
40. Szmulewicz AG, Angriman F, Samamé C, Ferraris A, Vigo D, Strejilevich SA. Dopaminergic agents in the treatment of bipolar depression: a systematic review and meta-analysis. Acta Psychiatr Scand. 2017;135(6):527–38.
41. Rosenblat JD, Kakar R, Berk M, Kessing LV, Vinberg M, Baune BT, et al. Anti-inflammatory agents in the treatment of bipolar depression: a systematic review and meta-analysis. Bipolar Disord. 2016;18(2):89–101.

42. Kishimoto T, Chawla JM, Hagi K, Zarate CA, Kane JM, Bauer M, et al. Single-dose infusion ketamine and non-ketamine N-methyl-d-aspartate receptor antagonists for unipolar and bipolar depression: a meta-analysis of efficacy, safety and time trajectories. Psychol Med. 2016;46(7):1459–72.
43. Mccloud TL, Caddy C, Jochim J, Rendell JM, Diamond PR, Shuttleworth C, et al. Ketamine and other glutamate receptor modulators for depression in bipolar disorder in adults. Cochrane Database Syst Rev. 2015;(9):CD011611.
44. Pacchiarotti I, Bond DJ, Baldessarini RJ, Nolen WA, Grunze H, Licht RW, et al. The International Society for Bipolar Disorders (ISBD) task force report on antidepressant use in bipolar disorders. Am J Psychiatry. 2013;170(11):1249–62. https://www.ncbi.nlm.nih.gov/pubmed/24030475.
45. Nivoli AMA, Colom F, Murru A, Pacchiarotti I, Castro-Loli P, González-Pinto A, et al. New treatment guidelines for acute bipolar depression: a systematic review. J Affect Disord. 2011;129(1):14–26. http://www.sciencedirect.com/science/article/pii/S0165032710004039.
46. Ross EL, Zivin K, Maixner DF. Cost-effectiveness of electroconvulsive therapy vs pharmacotherapy/psychotherapy for treatment-resistant depression in the United States. JAMA Psychiat. 2018;75(7):713–22. https://doi.org/10.1001/jamapsychiatry.2018.0768.
47. Miklowitz DJ. Adjunctive psychotherapy for bipolar disorder: state of the evidence. Am J Psychiatry. 2008;165(11):1408–19. https://doi.org/10.1176/appi.ajp.2008.08040488.
48. Vancampfort D, Firth J, Schuch FB, Rosenbaum S, Mugisha J, Hallgren M, et al. Sedentary behavior and physical activity levels in people with schizophrenia, bipolar disorder and major depressive disorder: a global systematic review and meta-analysis. World Psychiatry. 2017;16(3):308–15. https://doi.org/10.1002/wps.20458.
49. Pacchiarotti I, Kotzalidis GD, Murru A, Mazzarini L, Rapinesi C, Valentí M, et al. Mixed features in depression: the unmet needs of diagnostic and statistical manual of mental disorders fifth edition. Psychiatr Clin North Am. 2020b;43(1):59–68. http://www.sciencedirect.com/science/article/pii/S0193953X19300991.
50. Vieta E, Valentí M. Mixed states in DSM-5: implications for clinical care, education, and research. J Affect Disord. 2013;148(1):28–36.
51. Grunze H, Vieta E, Goodwin GM, Bowden C, Licht RW, Azorin J-M, et al. The World Federation of Societies of Biological Psychiatry (WFSBP) guidelines for the biological treatment of bipolar disorders: acute and long-term treatment of mixed states in bipolar disorder. World J Biol Psychiatry. 2017;19(1):2–58.
52. Stahl SM. Mixed-up about how to diagnose and treat mixed features in major depressive episodes. CNS Spectr. 2017;22(02):111–5.
53. Akiskal HS, Benazzi F, Perugi G, Rihmer Z. Agitated "unipolar" depression re-conceptualized as a depressive mixed state: implications for the antidepressant-suicide controversy. J Affect Disord. 2005;85(3):245–58. http://www.sciencedirect.com/science/article/pii/S0165032704004343
54. Murru A. Electroconvulsive therapy in bipolar mixed states: an overlooked option. J Clin Psychiatry. 2015:e1149–50.
55. Verdolini N, Hidalgo-Mazzei D, Murru A, Pacchiarotti I, Samalin L, Young AH, et al. Mixed states in bipolar and major depressive disorders: systematic review and quality appraisal of guidelines. Acta Psychiatr Scand. 2018;138(3):196–222. https://doi.org/10.1111/acps.12896.
56. Angst J, Gamma A, Sellaro R, Lavori PW, Zhang H. Recurrence of bipolar disorders and major depression. Eur Arch Psychiatry Clin Neurosci. 2003;253(5):236–40. https://doi.org/10.1007/s00406-003-0437-2.
57. Keck PEJ, Calabrese JR, McIntyre RS, McQuade RD, Carson WH, Eudicone JM, et al. Aripiprazole monotherapy for maintenance therapy in bipolar I disorder: a 100-week, double-blind study versus placebo. J Clin Psychiatry. 2007;68(10):1480–91.
58. Perlis RH, Delbello MP, Miyahara S, Wisniewski SR, Sachs GS, Nierenberg AA. Revisiting depressive-prone bipolar disorder: polarity of initial mood episode and disease course among bipolar I systematic treatment enhancement program for bipolar disorder participants. Biol Psychiatry. 2005;58(7):549–53.

59. Perlis RH, Ostacher MJ, Patel JK, Marangell LB, Zhang H, Wisniewski SR, et al. Predictors of recurrence in bipolar disorder: primary outcomes from the Systematic Treatment Enhancement Program for Bipolar Disorder (STEP-BD). Am J Psychiatry. 2006;163(2):217–24. https://doi.org/10.1176/appi.ajp.163.2.217.
60. Murru A, Verdolini N, Anmella G, Pacchiarotti I, Samalin L, Aedo A, et al. A 12-month prospective study on the time to hospitalization and clinical management of a cohort of bipolar type I and schizoaffective bipolar patients. Eur Psychiatry. 2019;61:1–8.
61. Murru A, Pacchiarotti I, Verdolini N, Reinares M, Torrent C, Geoffroy PA, et al. Modifiable and non-modifiable factors associated with functional impairment during the inter-episodic periods of bipolar disorder. Eur Arch Psychiatry Clin Neurosci. 2017;268:749–55.
62. Nivoli AMA, Murru A, Vieta E. Lithium: still a cornerstone in the long-term treatment in bipolar disorder? Neuropsychobiology. 2010;62:27–35.
63. Anmella G, Vieta E, Hidalgo-Mazzei D. Commentary on: "Make lithium great again!". Bipolar Disord. 2020b;
64. Baldessarini R, Tondo L, Vázquez G. Lithium treatment for bipolar disorder. Bipolar Disord. Bipolar Disord; 2020.
65. Miura T, Noma H, Furukawa TA, Mitsuyasu H, Tanaka S, Stockton S, et al. Comparative efficacy and tolerability of pharmacological treatments in the maintenance treatment of bipolar disorder: a systematic review and network meta-analysis. Lancet Psychiatry. 2014;1(5):351–9.
66. Geddes JR, Goodwin GM, Rendell J, Morriss R, Alder N, Juszczak E, et al. Lithium plus valproate combination therapy versus monotherapy for relapse prevention in bipolar i disorder (BALANCE): a randomised open-label trial. Lancet. 2010;375(9712):385–95.
67. Goodwin FK, Fireman B, Simon GE, Hunkeler EM, Lee J, Revicki D. Suicide risk in bipolar disorder during treatment with lithium and divalproex. JAMA. 2003;290(11):1467–73. https://doi.org/10.1001/jama.290.11.1467.
68. Murru A, Popovic D, Pacchiarotti I, Hidalgo D, León-Caballero J, Vieta E. Management of adverse effects of mood stabilizers. Curr Psychiatry Rep. 2015;17(8):66.
69. Samalin L, Murru A, Vieta E. Management of inter-episodic periods in patients with bipolar disorder. Expert Rev Neurother. 2016b;16:659–70.
70. Cipriani A, Reid K, Young AH, Macritchie K, Geddes J. Valproic acid, valproate and divalproex in the maintenance treatment of bipolar disorder. Cochrane Database Syst Rev. 2013;2013(10):CD003196. https://pubmed.ncbi.nlm.nih.gov/24132760.
71. Colom F, Vieta E, Daban C, Pacchiarotti I, Sanchez-Moreno J. Clinical and therapeutic implications of predominant polarity in bipolar disorder. J Affect Disord. 2006;93(1–3):13–7.
72. Vieta E, Berk M, Schulze TG, Carvalho AF, Suppes T, Calabrese JR, et al. Bipolar disorders. Nat Rev Dis Prim. 2018;4:18008.
73. Popovic D, Reinares M, Goikolea JM, Bonnin CM, Gonzalez-Pinto A, Vieta E. Polarity index of pharmacological agents used for maintenance treatment of bipolar disorder. Eur Neuropsychopharmacol. 2012;22(5):339–46.
74. Goodwin GM, Haddad PM, Ferrier IN, Aronson JK, Barnes T, Cipriani A, et al. Evidence-based guidelines for treating bipolar disorder: revised third edition recommendations from the British Association for Psychopharmacology. J Psychopharmacol. 2016;30(6):495–553.
75. Malhi GS, Bassett D, Boyce P, Bryant R, Fitzgerald PB, Fritz K, et al. Royal Australian and New Zealand College of Psychiatrists clinical practice guidelines for mood disorders. Aust New Zeal J Psychiatry. 2015;49(12):1087–206.
76. Gitlin MJ, Swendsen J, Heller TL, Hammen C. Relapse and impairment in bipolar disorder. Am J Psychiatry. 1995;152(11):1635–40.
77. Murru A, Pacchiarotti I, Nivoli AMA, Bonnin CM, Patrizi B, Amann B, et al. Rates and clinical correlates of treatment non-adherence in schizoaffective bipolar patients. Acta Psychiatr Scand. 2012;125(5):412–8.
78. Colom F, Vieta E, Tacchi MJ, Sánchez-Moreno J, Scott J. Identifying and improving non-adherence in bipolar disorders. Bipolar Disord. 2005;7(Suppl 5):24–31.

10 Predictors of Clinical Recovery in Bipolar Disorders

79. Cuerda C, Velasco C, Merchán-Naranjo J, García-Peris P, Arango C. The effects of second-generation antipsychotics on food intake, resting energy expenditure and physical activity. Eur J Clin Nutr. 2014;68(2):146–52.
80. Popovic D, Reinares M, Scott J, Nivoli A, Murru A, Pacchiarotti I, et al. Polarity index of psychological interventions in maintenance treatment of bipolar disorder. Psychother Psychosom. 2013;82(5):292–8.
81. Sylvia LG, Salcedo S, Bernstein EE, Baek JH, Nierenberg AA, Deckersbach T. Nutrition, exercise, and wellness treatment in bipolar disorder: proof of concept for a consolidated intervention. Int J Bipolar Disord. 2013;1(1):24. https://pubmed.ncbi.nlm.nih.gov/24660139.
82. MacQueen GM, Marriott M, Begin H, Robb J, Joffe RT, Young LT. Subsyndromal symptoms assessed in longitudinal, prospective follow-up of a cohort of patients with bipolar disorder. Bipolar Disord. 2003;5(5):349–55. https://doi.org/10.1034/j.1399-5618.2003.00048.x.
83. Geoffroy PA, Boudebesse C, Bellivier F, Lajnef M, Henry C, Leboyer M, et al. Sleep in remitted bipolar disorder: a naturalistic case-control study using actigraphy. J Affect Disord. 2014;158:1–7.
84. Samalin L, Boyer L, Murru A, Pacchiarotti I, Reinares M, Bonnin CM, et al. Residual depressive symptoms, sleep disturbance and perceived cognitive impairment as determinants of functioning in patients with bipolar disorder. J Affect Disord. 2017;210:280–6.
85. De Dios C, Ezquiaga E, Agud JL, Vieta E, Soler B, García-López A. Subthreshold symptoms and time to relapse/recurrence in a community cohort of bipolar disorder outpatients. J Affect Disord. 2012;143(1):160–5. http://www.sciencedirect.com/science/article/pii/S0165032712004077.
86. Belzeaux R, Correard N, Boyer L, Etain B, Loftus J, Bellivier F, et al. Depressive residual symptoms are associated with lower adherence to medication in bipolar patients without substance use disorder: results from the FACE-BD cohort. J Affect Disord. 2013;151(3):1009–15.
87. Sanchez-Moreno J, Martinez-Aran A, Tabarés-Seisdedos R, Torrent C, Vieta E, Ayuso-Mateos JL. Functioning and disability in bipolar disorder: an extensive review. Psychother Psychosom. 2009;78(5):285–97. https://www.karger.com/DOI/10.1159/000228249.
88. Solé B, Bonnin CM, Torrent C, Balanzá-Martínez V, Tabarés-Seisdedos R, Popovic D, et al. Neurocognitive impairment and psychosocial functioning in bipolar II disorder. Acta Psychiatr Scand. 2012;125(4):309–17.
89. del Mar Bonnín C, González-Pinto A, Solé B, Reinares M, González-Ortega I, Alberich S, et al. Verbal memory as a mediator in the relationship between subthreshold depressive symptoms and functional outcome in bipolar disorder. J Affect Disord. 2014;160:50–4.
90. Samalin L, de Chazeron I, Vieta E, Bellivier F, Llorca P-M. Residual symptoms and specific functional impairments in euthymic patients with bipolar disorder. Bipolar Disord. 2016a;18(2):164–73.
91. Samalin L, Reinares M, de Chazeron I, Torrent C, Bonnin CM, Hidalgo-Mazzei D, et al. Course of residual symptoms according to the duration of euthymia in remitted bipolar patients. Acta Psychiatr Scand. 2016c;134(1):57–64. https://doi.org/10.1111/acps.12568.
92. Chengappa KNR, Baker RW, Shao L, Yatham LN, Tohen M, Gershon S, et al. Rates of response, euthymia and remission in two placebo-controlled olanzapine trials for bipolar mania. Bipolar Disord. 2003;5(1):1–5.
93. Tohen M, Zarate CAJ, Hennen J, Khalsa H-MK, Strakowski SM, Gebre-Medhin P, et al. The McLean-Harvard First-Episode Mania Study: prediction of recovery and first recurrence. Am J Psychiatry. 2003;160(12):2099–107.
94. Nierenberg AA, Keefe BR, Leslie VC, Alpert JE, Pava JA, Worthington JJ 3rd, et al. Residual symptoms in depressed patients who respond acutely to fluoxetine. J Clin Psychiatry. 1999;60(4):221–5.
95. Zimmerman M, Chelminski I, Posternak M. A review of studies of the Montgomery-Asberg Depression Rating Scale in controls: implications for the definition of remission in treatment studies of depression. Int Clin Psychopharmacol. 2004;19(1):1–7.
96. Vieta E, Torrent C. Functional remediation: the pathway from remission to recovery in bipolar disorder. World Psychiatry. 2016;15(3):288–9. https://pubmed.ncbi.nlm.nih.gov/27717267.

97. Barber ME. Recovery as the new medical model for psychiatry. Psychiatr Serv. 2012;63(3):277–9. https://doi.org/10.1176/appi.ps.201100248.
98. Dion GL, Tohen M, Anthony WA, Waternaux CS. Symptoms and functioning of patients with bipolar disorder six months after hospitalization. Hosp Community Psychiatry. 1988;39(6):652–7.
99. Martinez-Aran A, Vieta E, Torrent C, Sanchez-Moreno J, Goikolea JM, Salamero M, et al. Functional outcome in bipolar disorder: the role of clinical and cognitive factors. Bipolar Disord. 2007;9(1–2):103–13. https://doi.org/10.1111/j.1399-5618.2007.00327.x.
100. Harvey PD. Defining and achieving recovery from bipolar disorder. J Clin Psychiatry. 2006;67(Suppl 9):14–42.
101. Ayuso-Mateos JL, Ávila CC, Anaya C, Cieza A, Vieta E. Development of the International Classification of Functioning, Disability and Health core sets for bipolar disorders: results of an international consensus process. Disabil Rehabil. 2013;35(25):2138–46. https://doi.org/1 0.3109/09638288.2013.771708.
102. Leon AC, Solomon DA, Mueller TI, Turvey CL, Endicott J, Keller MB. The Range of Impaired Functioning Tool (LIFE–RIFT): a brief measure of functional impairment. Psychol Med. 1999;29(4):869–78. https://www.cambridge.org/core/article/range-of-impaired-functioning-tool-liferift-a-brief-measure-of-functional-impairment/4B166D2568EC06E57C A3A869B8485437.
103. Jaeger J, Berns SM, Czobor P. The multidimensional scale of independent functioning: a new instrument for measuring functional disability in psychiatric populations. Schizophr Bull. 2003;29(1):153–67. https://doi.org/10.1093/oxfordjournals.schbul.a006987.
104. Rosa AR, Sánchez-Moreno J, Martínez-Aran A, Salamero M, Torrent C, Reinares M, et al. Validity and reliability of the Functioning Assessment Short Test (FAST) in bipolar disorder. Clin Pract Epidemiol Ment Health. 2007;3:5.
105. Solé B, Bonnin CM, Jiménez E, Torrent C, Torres I, Varo C, et al. Heterogeneity of functional outcomes in patients with bipolar disorder: a cluster-analytic approach. Acta Psychiatr Scand. 2018;137(6):516–27. https://doi.org/10.1111/acps.12871.
106. MacQueen GM, Young LT, Joffe RT. A review of psychosocial outcome in patients with bipolar disorder. Acta Psychiatr Scand. 2001;103(3):163–70.
107. Solé B, Jiménez E, Torrent C, Reinares M, Bonnin CDM, Torres I, et al. Cognitive impairment in bipolar disorder: treatment and prevention strategies. Int J Neuropsychopharmacol. 2017;20(8):670–80. https://www.ncbi.nlm.nih.gov/pubmed/28498954.
108. Berk M. Neuroprogression: pathways to progressive brain changes in bipolar disorder. Int J Neuropsychopharmacol. 2009;12(4):441–5. https://doi.org/10.1017/S1461145708009498.
109. Morris G, Puri BK, Walker AJ, Maes M, Carvalho AF, Bortolasci CC, et al. Shared pathways for neuroprogression and somatoprogression in neuropsychiatric disorders. Neurosci Biobehav Rev. 2019;107:862–82. http://www.sciencedirect.com/science/article/pii/ S0149763419304889.
110. Salagre E, Dodd S, Aedo A, Rosa A, Amoretti S, Pinzon J, et al. Toward precision psychiatry in bipolar disorder: staging 2.0. Front Psych. 2018;9:641.
111. Tohen M, Vieta E, Gonzalez-Pinto A, Reed C, Lin D. Baseline characteristics and outcomes in patients with first episode or multiple episodes of acute mania. J Clin Psychiatry. 2010;71(3):255–61.
112. Torrent C, Bonnin CM, Martínez-Arán A, Valle J, Amann BL, González-Pinto A, et al. Efficacy of functional remediation in bipolar disorder: a multicenter randomized controlled study. Am J Psychiatry. 2013;170(8):852–9.
113. Forcada I, Mur M, Mora E, Vieta E, Bartrés-Faz D, Portella MJ. The influence of cognitive reserve on psychosocial and neuropsychological functioning in bipolar disorder. Eur Neuropsychopharmacol J Eur Coll Neuropsychopharmacol. 2015;25(2):214–22.
114. Reinares M. Psychotherapy for bipolar disorders: an integrative approach. Cambridge: Cambridge University Press; 2019. https://www.cambridge.org/core/books/psychotherapy-for-bipolar-disorders/39B0813F3749FDFB0B75426EEC627C04.

Psychosocial Recovery-Oriented Treatments in Bipolar Disorders

11

Caterina del Mar Bonnin, Laura Montejo, Anabel Martinez-Aran, Brisa Solé, Mercè Comes, and Carla Torrent

11.1 Psychosocial Functioning in Bipolar Disorder

Bipolar disorder (BD) is a mood disorder characterized by recurrent episodes of mania, hypomania, and depression separated by periods of euthymia affecting around 2.4% of the global population [1]. As a lifelong and recurrent illness, BD is associated with functional decline, cognitive impairment, and a reduction in quality of life (QoL) [2–4]. Psychosocial functioning is an essential component of a person's quality of life and includes social, psychological, and occupational domains. In 2001, a landmark review found that between 30 and 60% of adults with BD had significant impairments in occupational and social functioning during periods of euthymia [5]. A possible explanation for pervasive psychosocial dysfunction may be the illness itself or the high prevalence of comorbid mental disorders in BD [6].

Mental health comorbidities in BD are more likely to be multiple than singular, with the World Mental Health Survey reporting a 62% lifetime prevalence of 3 or more comorbidities when strict Diagnostic and Statistical Manual of Mental

C. del Mar Bonnin · L. Montejo · A. Martinez-Aran · B. Solé·M. Comes · C. Torrent (✉)
Bipolar and Depressive Disorders Unit, Hospital Clinic of Barcelona, Institute of Neurosciences, IDIBAPS, University of Barcelona, Barcelona, Catalonia, Spain

Biomedical Research Networking Center for Mental Health Network (CIBERSAM), Barcelona, Spain
e-mail: cbonnin@clinic.cat; lmontejo@clini.cat; AMARTIAR@CLINIC.CAT; bsole@clinic.cat; mcomes@clinic.cat; ctorrent@clinic.cat

© The Author(s), under exclusive license to Springer Nature Switzerland AG 2022
B. Carpiniello et al. (eds.), *Recovery and Major Mental Disorders*, Comprehensive Approach to Psychiatry 2, https://doi.org/10.1007/978-3-030-98301-7_11

Disorders-IV (DSM-IV) criteria were applied [1]. However, research into the psychosocial effects of multiple comorbidities in BD is limited, often due to lack of power in subgroup analyses [7]. Bennett et al. (2019) [8] published recently the first report that has demonstrated the negative impact of comorbid anxiety disorders and ADHD on psychosocial functioning in BD.

Earlier age at onset of BD is consistently linked with poorer clinical outcomes, including rapid cycling, greater number of mood episodes, and increased risk of suicide [9]. Some studies have linked psychosocial dysfunction with an early onset (<18 years), although this finding is not consistent [10]. The studies that have focused on patients with an early onset suggest that psychosocial impairment is due to earlier disruption in the development of interpersonal skills needed to build and maintain healthy relationships as patients grow older [11]. However, while younger age of onset is associated with an adverse course of illness in adulthood [9], how these may be related to psychosocial functioning has received little attention.

Given the complexity of this illness and its consequences, researchers and clinicians are not only focused on clinical remission but also functional recovery and, more lately, well-being too [12]. This emergent paradigm includes not only symptom recovery but also return to normal functioning and attainment of a meaningful life. In fact, in 1988, Dion and colleagues [13] already pointed out that factors other than symptoms were related to functioning of patients with BD and that treatment should target symptom amelioration as well as reduce a patient's disability [13]. It is known that even after the first manic episode, only 1 out of 3 patients regains psychosocial functioning at 1-year follow-up [14], suggesting that functional outcomes in BD are undoubtedly impaired from the very beginning and should become a priority in therapeutic interventions. Research into BD has often overlooked the role of psychosocial functioning; however, in the last decade, many efforts have been made to improve functioning and well-being in BD.

11.2 Defining and Measuring Psychosocial Functioning

Despite the importance of psychosocial functioning in BD there is not a clear consensus regarding its definition. In the Task Force for the International Society for Bipolar Disorders conducted by Tohen and colleagues in 2009 [15], different definitions of psychosocial functioning were examined but without reaching a consensus. The experts highlighted the definition provided by the International Classification of Functioning, Disability and Health (ICF) in which functioning comprises three different components: body structures and functions; activities and participation; and personal environmental factors. Moreover, the authors of these guidelines underlined that this construct was complex to measure and that besides the ICF, the Functioning Assessment Short Thest (FAST) scale [16] might also constitute a good approach to measure functioning [15]. Before these guidelines, there were other attempts to define psychosocial functioning. For instance, in 2000, Zarate and colleagues [17] suggested the assessment of psychosocial functioning should involve different behavioral domains such as the individuals' ability to function socially or occupationally, to live independently, and to engage in a romantic life, with functional recovery typically being defined as the restoration of normal role functioning in the domains under scrutiny [17]. This definition represented a breakthrough in the field because in that moment, psychosocial functioning was measured by means of the Global Assessment Functioning Scale (GAF), endorsed by several consecutive editions of the Diagnostic and Statistical Manual of Mental Disorders (DSM). GAF scale provides 1 single score without differentiating between the behavioral domains pointed by Zarate and colleagues [17]. Despite all, the GAF is still the most commonly used clinician rating scale to measure disability, at least in the United States [18]. In 2007, Rosa and colleagues [16] developed a tool to measure functioning, the already mentioned FAST scale. It was specifically created to measure the most common difficulties experienced by patients with BD. The rationale behind this scale is in line with the definition of functioning proposed by Zarate and colleagues in 2000 [17], mostly focused on the assessment of different behavioral domains. More specifically, the FAST targets the following areas: autonomy, occupational and cognitive functioning, financial issues, interpersonal functioning, and leisure time. In this regard, the FAST represented several advantages over the GAF, mainly that it assesses different behavioral domains, it does not rate the symptomatology, and it is specific for BD.

Currently, the DSM-5 no longer encourages the use of the GAF. Instead, the use of the World Health Organization Disability Assessment Schedule 2.0 (WHODAS 2.0) [19] is recommended. The WHODAS 2.0 allows the assessment of functioning and disability irrespective of diagnosis; that is, it can reflect difficulties due to any medical or psychiatric illness. In contrast, both the GAF and the FAST are limited to the impact of the psychiatric disease on functioning, excluding the medical or environmental limitations. The GAF, FAST, WHODAS 2.0, or ICF core sets specific for BD [20, 21] are clinical tools, either rater administered (GAF, FAST, ICF core sets) or self-administered (WHODAS 2.0), but other approaches exist. For instance, the UCSD Performance-based skills Assessment (UPSA) [22] is based on task performance and measures functional capacity, assessing the skills involved in community tasks such as comprehension and planning, finance, communication, mobility, and house management. Figure 11.1 represents an overview of some different scales available to measure functioning in BD during the last 40 years, starting in 1980, when the GAF was first endorsed by the DSM-III until the present.

The scales presented in Fig. 11.1 are just a little part of the big picture of the measurement of psychosocial functioning in BD. Nevertheless, it fairly represents the great variability that exists. It is likely that the way the researcher or clinician defines psychosocial functioning will determine the tool to measure it, but the reverse is true as well: the use of one tool or another implies how the concept of psychosocial functioning is understood. To overcome this bias, it would be ideal that psychosocial functioning could be measured taking into account three different perspectives: (1) a subjective view using a self-administered scale, such as the Sheehan

YEAR	SCALE/Measurement
1980	DSM-III starts endorsing FAST
2000	LIFE-RIFT (to assess functioning in affective disorders) (Leon et al, 2000)
2001	UPSA (Petterson et al, 2000)
2007	• FAST scale (Rosa et al, 2007) • ICF score tests for BD (Vieta et al, 2007) • Validation of the MSFI for BD (Bernset al, 2007)
2009	Validation of the SDS for BD (Arbuckle et al, 2009)
2013	DSM-5 starts endorsing WHODAS 2.0 and do not recommend the use of GAF anymore
2021	A measurement of functioning combining three perspectives is recommended: • A subjective assessment (using a self-administered scale) • A sem -objective assessment (using interviewer-rated scales) • An objective assessment using performance-based tools

Fig. 11.1 Chronology of Functioning measures

Disability Scale for BD (SDS) [23] or the WHODAS 2.0; (2) a semi-objective scale, using the FAST, GAF, or LIFE-RIFT [24], which are interviewer rated based on patients' answers; and finally (3) an objective scale, like the UPSA, which is performance based and measures functional capacity. Combining these three different approaches might help to disentangle all the variables associated with functional impairment observed in BD.

11.3 Variables Related with Psychosocial Functioning

Many variables have been associated with functional outcome in BD, including demographic, clinical, and neurocognitive factors.

Concerning the sociodemographic factors, it seems that male patients [25, 26] as well as older patients [26] show poorer functional outcomes. On the other hand, being married could represent a protective factor against functional impairment [27, 28]. Higher socioeconomic status, based on education and employment, has also been associated with better functional outcomes [28, 29].

Regarding the clinical variables, the presence of subsyndromal depressive symptoms has been consistently reported as the strongest factor associated with functional impairment [2, 25, 30–35]. Other clinical variables include history of psychosis, episode density, poor sleep quality, and longer illness duration [33, 34, 36–39]. Psychiatric comorbidity, particularly with substance use disorder (e.g., cannabis, alcohol) and personality disorders, can also negatively influence functional outcomes in patients with BD [40–44].

Finally, regarding neurocognitive variables, the evidence suggests that there are three or four discrete and coherent profiles, one cognitively intact and comparable to the general population, plus one or two subgroups presenting with selective moderate impairments, and a globally impaired subgroup with severe impairments across cognitive domains. Similar findings have been reported from studies with cross-diagnostic samples involving people with different diagnoses across the psychosis spectrum [45].

Verbal memory has been found to be a good predictor of functional outcome in several studies [10, 35, 46–48]. However, variables related to other neurocognitive areas have also been reported, including executive functions, processing speed, and attention [28, 49, 50]. It might be hypothesized that the neurocognitive variables influencing functional outcome in BD may vary depending on illness progression. For instance, patients in early stages of the disease seem to present a more selective profile of cognitive impairment, with some domains capable of improving 1 year after the first manic episode, including improvements in processing speed and executive functions [51]. In this line, at least two studies have found that first-episode patients who did not relapse during 1-year follow-up could improve their neurocognitive functioning [52, 53]; hence, preserving neurocognition from the very beginning of the illness might guarantee better functional outcomes.

11.4 Restoring Psychosocial Functioning

11.4.1 Pharmacological Interventions

Research on pharmacological and nonpharmacological treatments to restore functioning in BD is still immature. As previously mentioned, the link between functional outcomes and neurocognition is well recognized, which is why in recent years many efforts have improved cognition, including both pharmacological and psychological treatments. In fact, new trends in pharmacological treatments include focusing on restoring cognitive functioning rather than psychosocial functioning. Among the most promising medical treatments to improve cognition in BD are mifepristone [54], lurasidone [55], and erythropoietin, this last according to different studies improves verbal memory and learning in mood disorders [56, 57]. Given the link between neurocognition and psychosocial functioning, it is likely that the efforts directed to improve neurocognition will also improve functional outcome; however, so far, no studies on pharmacological treatments have addressed both issues at the same time. It is worth mentioning that the methodological recommendations for cognition trials by the Cognition Task Force from the International Society for Bipolar Disorders encourage the inclusion of a functional measure as a key secondary outcome [58]. In this regard, a tool to measure functional improvement that allows the researchers and clinicians to classify patients into different categories of functional performance could be useful to assess the efficacy of these treatments [59]. A very promising antidepressant is vortioxetine, a structural novel medication, which may have therapeutic effects on cognition. In a recent study, vortioxetine both as monotherapy and as adjunctive treatment performed better than SSRI monotherapy in improving psychosocial outcomes. Since functional assessments represent a broader construct, reflecting at the same time patients' symptomatic as well as their cognitive status, these improvements highlight a broad effect of vortioxetine across symptoms domains [60].

11.4.2 Psychological Interventions

In contrast to the area of pharmacological treatments, in the field of psychological interventions several efforts have been made lately to design therapies to restore psychosocial functioning in BD. Cognitive interventions have emerged as a new treatment option to promote functional recovery of patients with BD. The association between cognition and function has been extensively explored, with most evidence suggesting significant contributions of cognitive impairment to reduced functional capacities. The first attempt was an open trial using a program named Cognitive Rehabilitation [61]. The authors included a total of 18 patients with subsyndromal depressive symptoms and after 14 sessions of cognitive rehabilitation, patients improved cognitive performance and functional outcome. More interestingly, the findings showed that changes in executive function accounted, in part, for the improvements in occupational functioning. The first randomized controlled trial (RCT) implementing a similar therapy was conducted in 2013 by Torrent and colleagues [62]. The efficacy of functional remediation (FR) was proved in terms of improving functional outcomes in euthymic patients with moderate to severe functional impairment at baseline. Moreover, improvement in psychosocial functioning was maintained after 6 months' follow-up [63]. However, the impact of the intervention was low in terms of cognition. Contrary to other therapies labeled as "cognitive remediation," FR is specially centered on functional recovery, focusing on the training of neurocognitive skills that are useful for daily functioning. Hence, this approach might be suitable especially for patients in late stages of the illness and who present moderate to severe functional impairment. Currently, this approach has been adapted and being validated in other populations such as first-episode patients to assess its impact on psychosocial functioning as main outcome likewise in other measures such as neurocognition, depressive symptoms, psychological well-being, and cognitive complaints in order to become a tool that could diminish the impact that the new diagnosis has in patient's lives after the onset of psychosis, reducing sick leave and academic absenteeism improving their productivity and alleviating the academic and/or work difficulties they often experience.

Another preliminary study conducted in the Netherlands included 12 patients and replicated the positive results in functional outcome after receiving a shorter FR program [64]. However, not all the interventions targeting cognitive rehabilitation were found to improve functional outcome. For instance, another RCT conducted by Demant and colleagues (2015) [65] found no improvement on either cognition or functional outcome after a 12-week intervention. It is worth mentioning that these negative results might be explained by some methodological limitations of the trial, including the length of the intervention (too short) or the fact that patients were subsyndromic at study enrolment. Another study leaded by Lewandowski and colleagues (2017) [66] assessed the efficacy of an internet-based cognitive remediation program in patients with BD compared with an active control group both in neurocognition and community functioning. After treatment, patients who received the internet-based program improved cognitive performance in processing speed, visual learning and memory domains, and the composite score. These results were maintained over 6 months after finishing the intervention; however, the intervention was not associated with change in community functioning, although cognitive variation was associated with functional change across the sample.

Another program called action-based cognitive remediation (ABCR) is a manual-based restorative cognitive remediation program. The treatment duration is about 10 weeks with 2-h sessions twice a week. Each participant met with a therapist for a goal setting before the first session. The treatment includes computerized training, cognitive strategies together with practical activities to enable to transfer cognitive skills to everyday life. The sessions cover meta-cognition, visual and verbal working memory, attention, memory, and executive functions. In the first study investigating the effect of this program vs control treatment in patients with remitted BD, ABCR did not had a significant effect on the primary outcome, speed of complex cognitive processing. Nevertheless, there was an effect of ACBR vs control treatment on the secondary outcome, an executive functions measure of planning skills at treatment completion. Among the tertiary outcomes, there was an improvement on subjective functioning, and measures of verbal memory and spatial working [67].

In a naturalistic, open label non-controlled study the authors found that in patients with BD the global functioning improved by computerized working memory remediation, which was assessed by the FAST scale [68, 69]. In contrast, in a randomized clinical trial 39 patients with BD were randomized to either treatment as usual (TAU) or Cognitive Behavior Rehabilitation (CBR), an add-on treatment delivered in 12 weekly group sessions; the CBR intervention showed promising results in improving some of the commonly impaired cognitive domains without changes in functional and QoL scores. A longer follow-up may be necessary to detect chances in these domains [70].

A proof-of-concept, single-blind randomized trial recruited participants aged 18–65 with BD not currently experiencing an episode. Participants were assigned to receive Cognitive Remediation Therapy (CRT) in addition to treatment as usual (TAU) or TAU alone following completion of the baseline assessment. The four main feasibility outcomes were considered primary with equal weighting: trial feasibility, CRT intervention acceptability, cognitive outcomes, and functional outcomes. Despite a relatively small sample size ($N = 60$), large effects on cognition (working memory and executive functions), functioning, and goal attainment were observed, enduring for 3 months after the end of therapy. These results indicate high feasibility and acceptability of individual, therapist-led CRT using the established CIRCuiTS program, as a potential treatment to enhance cognition and functioning for BD. CIRCuiTS therapy was delivered using a combination of session types for all participants comprising: face-to-face and telephone sessions and practice together with independent practice sessions with computerized system [71].

It is difficult to measure the power of these current approaches in changing functioning, since very few studies have used psychosocial functioning as a primary outcome. The results of the first systematic review of the possible moderating effect of stage of illness on the impact of psychosocial treatments on functional outcomes in established BD suggest that psychosocial interventions are more effective for targeting general or social functioning in the earlier than later stage of BD [72]. In this line, in a multicenter, randomized, controlled trial patients at clinical risk for a serious mental illness presenting subthreshold bipolar symptoms with already impaired psychosocial functioning benefit from early group sessions of cognitive behavioral psychotherapy (CBT) [73]. Furthermore, two studies have been designed to examine the effectiveness of group psychotherapy on global adaptative function and neuropsychological functioning in early-stage bipolar disorder [74] and in young people at increased risk for developing a BD [75]; the results are expected in the near future.

11.5 Preventing Functional Decline

So far, there is no strong evidence regarding the prevention of functional decline in BD. The following section includes some targets and treatments that could address this issue and deserve to be further explored.

11.5.1 Addressing Subthreshold Depressive Symptoms

Between 20 and 50% of patients suffer inter-episodically or chronic residual depressive symptoms depending on the definition applied [76]. Subsyndromal depression interferes with role functioning in essential domains of normal life, such as work, duties at home, and maintaining relationships. In this regard, subthreshold depressive symptoms together with neurocognitive impairment might be one of the strongest predictors of functional outcome [2, 33, 35, 47, 77, 78]. However, the relationship between functional outcome and subthreshold depressive symptoms might not be linear and unidirectional; instead, they seem to influence one another [79]. Besides the implications in functional outcome, residual depressive symptoms are also a major cause of relapse [80, 81], consequently affecting psychosocial functioning and QoL [2]. The treatment of residual depressive symptoms during euthymia is an unmet need, but fortunately, clinical research has begun to investigate how to tackle them. One recent RCT proved that adjunctive extended-release quetiapine at a dose of 300 mg daily was significantly more effective than placebo in the treatment of subthreshold depressive symptoms [82], but no significant improvement was detected in functional outcome. One possible explanation is that the sample size was not powered enough to detect significant changes in this secondary outcome.

Regarding psychological interventions, a limited number of therapies have addressed subthreshold depressive symptoms as a primary outcome. To the best of our knowledge, only one pilot RCT study assessed the effect of Eye Movement Desensitization and Reprocessing therapy on this type of symptomatology. Specifically, patients in the treatment group showed a statistically significant improvement in depressive and hypomanic symptoms when compared with treatment as usual at 12-month follow-up; however, psychosocial functioning was not assessed [83]. Another multicenter study of Eye Movement Desensitization and Reprocessing with a bigger sample is underway with the objective to reduce symptoms and relapses and improve psychosocial functioning [84]. Regarding FR, secondary analyses showed that patients with subsyndromal symptoms could also improve psychosocial functioning after the therapy [85].

Other therapies include an approach testing the long-term efficacy of an intervention that combined cognitive behavior therapy (CBT) and psychoeducation, which has also been described to be effective in terms of symptoms and social-occupational functioning improvement [86]. Positive results in social functioning were also found with CBT [87]. Inder and colleagues (2015) [88] randomized a group of patients with BD to Interpersonal and Social Rhythm Therapy or specialist supportive care, and both groups improved in depressive/manic symptoms and social functioning. Finally, an intensive psychotherapy (family-focused treatment [FFT], Interpersonal and Social Rhythm Therapy (IPSRT), or CBT) in patients with BD during an acute depressive episode also showed beneficial functional outcomes [89]. The IPSRT Therapy contributes to reduce the levels of anxiety by helping patients to address their interpersonal deficits and improving their emotional dysregulation, and not just by managing affective symptoms. As expected, at the follow-up we observed an improvement of GAF score. This result emphasizes the importance of the interpersonal intervention in improving all aspects of patients' life, thus contributing to prevent mood shifts [90]. Another recent study shows that participants with recurrent mood disorders described improved functioning related to therapies that formulate their mood disorder in terms of a model, such as IPSRT with or without cognitive remediation. This supports the person in undertaking practical routines that can be integrated into daily life, focuses on communication and problem-solving skills, and engenders a sense of hope by working with the person to develop self-management strategies relevant to their specific symptom experiences [91].

Finally, positive results have also been reported on anxious and depressive symptoms using mindfulness-based cognitive therapy [92–94].

Although more research is needed, it might be hypothesized that treating sub-threshold depressive symptoms could be an indirect pathway to improve psychosocial functioning.

11.5.2 Enhancing Cognitive Reserve

Cognitive reserve (CR) is the capacity of the adult brain to endure neuropathology, minimizing clinical manifestations and allowing a successful accomplishment of cognitive tasks [95]. Genetics determine, to some extent, CR; however, environmental factors such as an active lifestyle, education, and brain stimulation (mental activities) can also influence it. In BD the most common ways to measure CR include years of education, premorbid Intelligence Quotient, and leisure activities.

So far, no interventions have tested whether improving CR enhances functioning, but some studies suggest that CR is a good predictor of both cognitive and psychosocial outcome in euthymic patients with BD [96, 97]. In a recent publication, the findings show that CR may be protective against cognitive impairment in both BD and major depressive disorder, and these effects were observed in euthymia and during depressive episodes of varying severity. These findings highlight the importance of investigating such variables in the neuropsychological evaluation of mood disorders, which may help to understand the cognitive heterogeneity within these populations [98]. Further, it could also play an important role in patients with first psychotic episode since CR has shown to predict psychosocial functioning 2 years after the first episode [99]. Hence, given the role of CR both in chronic patients and at early stages, this might constitute an area to explore and enhance to prevent functional decline [100]. In this regard, there is another ongoing trial by de la Serna et al. (2021) [101] that aims to enhance CR in child, adolescent, and young adult offspring of patients diagnosed with schizophrenia or BD; however, so far, no preliminary results are available.

In a study assessing cognitive impairment across four cognitive domains in 80 participants, the results show that individuals with cognitively impaired profiles demonstrate more cognitive decline after illness onset. Cognitive reserve may be one of the factors underlying cognitive variability across people with bipolar disorder. Patients in the intermediate and severe subgroups may be in greater need of interventions targeting cognitive difficulties [45].

11.5.3 Diet and Physical Exercise

"Nutritional Psychiatry" is an emerging area of research that has great potential as an adjunctive tool for the prevention and treatment of diverse neuropsychiatric disorders. Several nutrition-related aspects, such as obesity, dietary patterns, gut microbiome composition and gut permeability, bioactive food compounds, and nutrients can influence pathways implicated in the pathophysiology of mood disorders. A dietary pattern is composed of multiple nutrients and bioactive compounds that can theoretically modulate pathways associated with mood disorders. The Mediterranean diet, generally characterized by a higher intake of fruits, vegetables, legumes, nuts, whole grains, and good quality sources of protein (i.e., fish and/or seafood), have demonstrated benefits in cognitive performance and decreased risk of psychiatric disorders [102].

People with mood disorders have shown higher ratios of unhealthy lifestyle choices, including poor diet quality and suboptimal nutrition. Diet and nutrition impact on brain/mental health, but cognitive outcomes have been less researched in psychiatric disorders. Neurocognitive dysfunction is a major driver of social dysfunction and a therapeutic target in mood disorders, although effective cognitive-enhancers are currently lacking [103].

Obesity can also impact cognitive functioning [104] and, in turn, cognitive impairment could be a predictor of weight gain [105]. Hence, it seems that weight

11 Psychosocial Recovery-Oriented Treatments in Bipolar Disorders

increase and cognitive impairment can influence one another. Moreover, another study has found that increased body mass index (BMI) was associated with a more chronic course of the disease, longer duration of illness, and lower psychosocial functioning [106]. In line with this, Bond and colleagues (2010) [107] found that those patients who suffered a clinically significant weight gain (defined as gaining ≥7% of baseline weight over 12 months) had significantly poorer functional outcomes at 12-month follow-up, and, interestingly, functional impairment was independent from current mood symptoms.

Poor dietary habits and a sedentary lifestyle can increase physical and psychiatric morbidity, worsen psychosocial and cognitive functioning, and predict a poor pharmacological response. That is why clinicians treating individuals with BD face a dual challenge of treating not only patients' brains but also their bodies. Interventions targeting healthy habits (including nutrition and exercise) are expected to benefit patients with BD. One RCT examined the effects of a 20-week CBT intervention (NEW tx) for BD consisting of 3 modules: nutrition, exercise, and wellness [108]; patients who underwent the treatment showed improvements in nutritional habits, exercise, depressive symptoms, and overall functioning. Hence, this study provides preliminary evidence that improving nutrition and promoting an active lifestyle is associated with functional improvement and mood symptoms in patients with BD. Another previous study showed the efficacy of an intervention on healthy lifestyle, nutrition, and physical exercise on muscle mass index, particularly in women [109]. These lifestyle interventions are promising since they demonstrate that people with BD can engage and be successful in these types of therapies. Therapeutic mechanisms of action are still unknown but might include different pathways, for example, by reducing morbidity (i.e., depressive symptoms), which in turn would improve functional outcome [110], or by enhancing treatment effects, including the synergistic effects of exercise in combination with other treatments. For instance, in schizophrenia there is some preliminary evidence suggesting that cognitive remediation efficacy can be enhanced by aerobic exercise-induced BDNF upregulation [111, 112].

11.5.4 Multicomponent Programs

One advantage of this type of intervention is to tackle different areas to be improved at the same time, hence allowing a holistic treatment of patients, taking into account not only education on the illness but also how to improve healthy lifestyles and functional outcomes. Following the premise that no single psychosocial intervention might be sufficient to address the morbidity, the functional impairment and the consequences associated with severe mental illnesses [113], multicomponent programs, and care packages are being developed for patients with BD.

An example of this kind of treatment that has proven to be effective in BD is the Integrated Risk Reduction Intervention developed by Frank and colleagues (2015) [114]. More specifically, this program consists of 17 sessions grouped in different modules, including psychoeducation, training to improve sleep/wake patterns and social rhythm regularity, nutrition, physical activity, and healthy habits (smoking cessation). Results from this study showed that patients who followed the intervention significantly reduce their BMI. Moreover, 3 variables (C-reactive protein, total cholesterol, and instability of total sleep time) contributed to a combined moderator of faster decrease in BMI with Integrated Risk Reduction Intervention treatment.

Recently, the Bipolar Disorder and Depression Unit in Barcelona has developed an integrative approach consisting of therapeutic components of broader programs that the Barcelona Bipolar Disorders Program had previously developed and whose effectiveness had been proven separately, such as psychoeducation for patients [115], psychoeducation for family members [116], and FR [117]. In addition, an important emphasis is given to the promotion of a healthy lifestyle, and a module focused on mindfulness-based cognitive therapy has also been included. Therefore, some contents of psychoeducation for patients have been combined with a session for family members and complemented with aspects related to health promotion, mindfulness training, and strategies for cognitive and functional enhancement, always as adjunctive to pharmacological treatment. This integrative approach combines the main components of different treatments to cover broader therapeutic objectives, to improve the prognosis of the disease in both clinical and functional aspects, as well as the well-being and QoL of those who suffer from BD [118]. Due to the characteristics of the intervention (12 sessions of 90 min each), in case it shows its efficacy, it could be easily implemented in routine clinical care.

11.6 Personal Recovery: Well-Being and QoL

Subjective assessments and patient-reported outcomes are gaining ground in the field of BD [119, 120]. As in psychosocial functioning, the problem with subjective measures is the variability in the definitions and in the instruments to assess the subjective experience of these patients [119]. It is common that terms such as QoL, well-being, or life satisfaction are used as synonyms and interchangeable terms [119]. Moreover, the current lack of consensus between these construct definitions add uncertainty and complication to select an appropriate instrument to measure this dimension. Despite all, the subjective experience should always be taken into account since it can also impact on the course of the illness. Some studies indicate that the improvement in well-being provides a protective effect against recurrence [121], and it has also been found that low levels in QoL are associated with an increase in oxidative stress [122]. For this reason, it is important not only to evaluate objective outcomes (symptoms and functioning) but also to assess patients' subjective experience, since they can provide valuable information and might be an essential part to ensure better outcomes in BD.

11.6.1 Pharmacological Interventions

Rajagopalan et al. (2016) [123] tested the effects of lurasidone as monotherapy or as adjunctive to lithium/valproate on health-related QoL (HRQoL). They found that patients in both conditions increased HRQoL. However, this improvement was not independent of changes in depression, indicating that the effect of lurasidone on improving patient HRQoL may act through a reduction in depressive symptoms associated with BD. Similarly, Gonda and colleagues (2016) [124] found that patients enhanced both their work functional outcome and QoL after receiving prophylactic lamotrigine therapy at 6 months follow-up. In young patients (10–17 years old) with an acute episode of bipolar depression, it was found that those who received olanzapine/fluoxetine combination presented better QoL scores compared with those receiving placebo [125].

11.6.2 Psychological Interventions

Even though physical activity is not a psychological intervention itself, it is well known for increasing well-being and QoL; however, the impact of this kind of interventions has been less studied in the field of BD. Vancampfort and colleagues (2017) [126] proved the effect of 150 min/week of physical activity on physical, psychological, social, and environmental QoL; those patients who did not meet the established minimum (150 min) showed lower QoL outcomes.

Involving the family, O'Donnell and colleagues (2017) [127] tested the effect of 2 psychological interventions on QoL scores in a sample of adolescents with BD. They compared the efficacy of a FFT plus pharmacotherapy vs brief psychoeducation plus pharmacotherapy on self-related QoL over 2 years. They found the 2 groups did not differ in overall QoL scores at 24 months follow-up. However, adolescents who received the FFT had greater improvements in quality of family relationships and physical well-being compared with the brief psychoeducation program. Besides, internet-based approaches using smartphones are gaining traction [128, 129], a useful and attractive tool especially for the young population with BD [130]. So far, some preliminary studies using a mobile application (SIMPLe) have reported an improvement of biological rhythms [131] and increased QoL and well-being [129]. An important finding is that patients with BD and mild cognitive deficits do not present any limitation in using mental health apps [132].

There is much room for improvement in the field of subjective well-being and QoL. These abovementioned interventions may shed some light regarding the path to follow. Nevertheless, it is important to keep in mind that those patients who suffer from more depressive symptoms, irritability, and psychiatric comorbid conditions present lower QoL and functional outcomes [133, 134]; hence, all the strategies directed to reduce medical and psychiatric burdens might also be useful to increase patients' well-being and QoL. It is also worth mentioning that some authors defend that QoL not only depends on clinical remission but also relies on functional recovery [12]. In this line, poor QoL is also associated with poor occupational outcome, reduced academic attainment [135], and difficulties in activities of daily life [136]. Future studies should include subjective measures (such as QoL, well-being) to better understand the relationship with these clinical variables. Figure 11.2 represents a brief summary of the main interventions targeting cognition and functioning.

Intervention	Delivery method	Setting	Duration	Core therapy components
Compensatory cognitive remediation (Deckersbach et al, 2010)	Non-computerized training	Individual	50 min . Total 14 sessions	Training of cognitive skills with adaptative level of difficulty. Strategy learning focused on daily life management. Mood monitoring
Personalized restorative remediation (Preiss et al, 2013)	Computerized (CogniFit)	Individual	30 min three times per week for 8 weeks. Total 24 session	Traiing personalized bawsed on baseline evaluation. Cognitive tasks with adaptative level of difficulty.
Functional remediation (Torrent et al, 2013)	Pen-and-paper tasks and group activities	Group	90 min weekly for 21 weeks Total: 21 sessions	Education on cognitive deficits and training on strategies to manage cognitive difficulties.
Compensatory cognitive remediation (Demant et al, 2015)	Computerized (RehabCom)	Group	120 min weekly sessions for 3 months. Total 12 sessions	Psychoeducation and awareness of cognitive deficits. Computer practising and training of adaptative and compensatory strategies.
Functional remediation (Zyto et al, 2016)	Non-computerized individual training and group activities	Individual&Group	90 min weekly for 6 weeks & 45 min weekly for 6 weeks Total: 12 sessions	Personalized goal setting and strategy learning to cope with cognitive difficulties.
Neuroplasticity informed cognitive remediation (Lewandowsky et al, 2017)	Compujterized (BrainWorks)	Individual	45 min three times per week for 6 mponths (70 sessions)	Computer practising with games of adaptative difficulty level based on user performance. Bottom-up training
Compensatory cognitive remediation (Veeh et al, 2017)	Computerized (HappyNeuron Pro)	Individual&Group	90 minuts weekly for three months (12 sessions)	Computer tasks with adaptative difficulty level.
ABSR (Ott et al, 2020)	Combination (computerized and cognitive strategies)	Individual&Group	10 weeks with 2 hours session twice a week	Computerized training, cognitive strategies and practical activities to enable the transfer of cognitive skills to everyday life.
CIRCuiTS (Strawbridge et al, 2020)	Combination Computerized (Circuits program) and face-to-face, telephone and drop in sessions	Individual	3 sessions per week, target total 20-30 hours	Fundamental restorative cognitive processes and compensatory metacognitive skills.

Fig. 11.2 Main interventions targeting cognition and functioning in bipolar disorder

11.7 Conclusions

Different findings highlight that improvement in functioning depends on a set of influential factors that start with cognition. Neuropsychological assessment may help specify individual prognoses. Improving cognitive impairment for BD would alleviate long-term functional disability [137]. Regardless of the great variability in the assessment of psychosocial functioning, many efforts have successfully improved functional outcomes in BD. Currently, the interventions that have proven to be effective at enhancing functioning and/or QoL include lurasidone, lamotrigine, FR, some programs of cognitive remediation, ISPRT, and FFT, among others. These therapies have set the stage for developing further interventions to prevent functional decline and ensure well-being, because this is where we go. Ideally, future therapies should focus not only on restoring functional outcomes but also preventing functional decline and enhancing QoL and well-being. In this regard, those programs that target cognitive enhancement and promote healthy lifestyles (including healthy nutrition patterns and physical activity) are urgently needed, since they constitute a preventive tool for cognitive and functional decline. Although more studies are still needed, multicomponent therapies might be also a good option since they include different approaches to cover several areas at a time (symptoms, functioning, cognition, well-being, etc.). Finally, it is likely that the future will also include personalized treatments focusing on tailored interventions that may differ from one patient to another [138]; in this sense, the type and duration of interventions might differ from patients recently diagnosed, patients with a complex course of the illness and population at risk to develop a psychiatric disorder.

References

1. Merikangas KR, Jin R, He J-P, Kessler RC, Lee S, Sampson NA, et al. Prevalence and correlates of bipolar spectrum disorder in the world mental health survey initiative. Arch Gen Psychiatry. 2011;68(3):241–51.
2. Bonnín CM, Sánchez-Moreno J, Martínez-Arán A, Solé B, Reinares M, Rosa AR, et al. Subthreshold symptoms in bipolar disorder: impact on neurocognition, quality of life and disability. J Affect Disord. 2012;136(3):650–9. https://pubmed.ncbi.nlm.nih.gov/22051075/.
3. Martínez-Arán A, Vieta E, Reinares M, Colom F, Torrent C, Sánchez-Moreno J, et al. Cognitive function across manic or hypomanic, depressed, and euthymic states in bipolar disorder. Am J Psychiatry. 2004;161(2):262–70. http://www.ncbi.nlm.nih.gov/pubmed/14754775.
4. Michalak EE, Yatham LN, Lam RW. Quality of life in bipolar disorder: a review of the literature. Health Qual Life Outcomes. 2005;3:72. http://www.ncbi.nlm.nih.gov/pubmed/16288650.
5. MacQueen GM, Trevor Young L, Joffe RT. A review of psychosocial outcome in patients with bipolar disorder. Acta Psychiatr Scand. 2001;103:163–70.
6. Post RM, Altshuler L, Leverich GS, Frye MA, Suppes T, McElroy SL, et al. Relationship of clinical course of illness variables to medical comorbidities in 900 adult outpatients with bipolar disorder. Compr Psychiatry. 2015;56:21–8. http://www.ncbi.nlm.nih.gov/pubmed/25284280.
7. Sentissi O, Navarro JC, De Oliveira H, Gourion D, Bourdel MC, Baylé FJ, et al. Bipolar disorders and quality of life: the impact of attention deficit/hyperactivity disorder and substance

abuse in euthymic patients. Psychiatry Res. 2008;161(1):36–42. http://www.ncbi.nlm.nih.gov/pubmed/18786727.

8. Bennett F, Hodgetts S, Close A, Frye M, Grunze H, Keck P, et al. Predictors of psychosocial outcome of bipolar disorder: data from the Stanley Foundation Bipolar Network. Int J bipolar Disord. 2019;7(1):28. http://www.ncbi.nlm.nih.gov/pubmed/31840207.

9. Leverich GS, Post RM, Keck PE, Altshuler LL, Frye MA, Kupka RW, et al. The poor prognosis of childhood-onset bipolar disorder. J Pediatr. 2007;150(5):485–90. http://www.ncbi.nlm.nih.gov/pubmed/17452221.

10. Martinez-Aran A, Vieta E, Torrent C, Sanchez-Moreno J, Goikolea JM, Salamero M, et al. Functional outcome in bipolar disorder: the role of clinical and cognitive factors. Bipolar Disord. 2007;9(1–2):103–13.

11. Levy B, Manove E. Functional outcome in bipolar disorder: the big picture. Depress Res Treat. 2012;2012:949248. http://www.ncbi.nlm.nih.gov/pubmed/21961062.

12. Vieta E, Torrent C. Functional remediation: the pathway from remission to recovery in bipolar disorder. World Psychiatry. 2016;15(3):288–9. http://www.ncbi.nlm.nih.gov/pubmed/27717267.

13. Dion G, Tohen M, Anthony W, Waternaux C. Symptoms and functioning of patients with bipolar disorder six months after hospitalization. Hosp Community Psychiatry. 1988;39(6). https://pubmed.ncbi.nlm.nih.gov/3402925/.

14. Tohen M, Hennen J, Zarate CM, Baldessarini RJ, Strakowski SM, Stoll AL, et al. Two-year syndromal and functional recovery in 219 cases of first-episode major affective disorder with psychotic features. Am J Psychiatry. 2000;157(2):220–8. http://www.ncbi.nlm.nih.gov/pubmed/10671390.

15. Tohen M, Frank E, Bowden CL, Colom F, Ghaemi SN, Yatham LN, et al. The International Society for Bipolar Disorders (ISBD) Task Force report on the nomenclature of course and outcome in bipolar disorders. Bipolar Disord. 2009;11(5):453–73. http://www.ncbi.nlm.nih.gov/sites/entrez?Db=pubmed&DbFrom=pubmed&Cmd=Link&LinkName=pubmed_pubmed&LinkReadableName=RelatedArticles&IdsFromResult=19624385&ordinalpos=3&itool=EntrezSystem2.PEntrez.Pubmed.Pubmed_ResultsPanel.Pubmed_RVDocSum.

16. Rosa AR, Sánchez-Moreno J, Martínez-Aran A, Salamero M, Torrent C, Reinares M, et al. Validity and reliability of the Functioning Assessment Short Test (FAST) in bipolar disorder. Clin Pract Epidemiol Ment Health. 2007;3:5. http://www.ncbi.nlm.nih.gov/pubmed/17555558.

17. Zarate CA, Tohen M, Land M, Cavanagh S. Functional impairment and cognition in bipolar disorder. Psychiatry Q. 2000;71(4):309–29. http://www.ncbi.nlm.nih.gov/pubmed/11025910.

18. Von Korff M, Andrews G, Delves M. Assessing activity limitations and disability among adults. In: The conceptual evolution of DSM-5. Arlington, VA: American Psychiatric Publishing, Inc.; 2011. p. 163–88.

19. Ustün TB, Chatterji S, Kostanjsek N, Rehm J, Kennedy C, Epping-Jordan J, et al. Developing the World Health Organization Disability Assessment Schedule 2.0. Bull World Health Organ. 2010;88(11):815–23. http://www.ncbi.nlm.nih.gov/pubmed/21076562.

20. Vieta E, Cieza A, Stucki G, Chatterji S, Nieto M, Sánchez-Moreno J, et al. Developing core sets for persons with bipolar disorder based on the International Classification of Functioning. Disability and Health Bipolar Disord. 2007;9(1–2):16–24. http://www.ncbi.nlm.nih.gov/pubmed/17391346.

21. Ayuso-Mateos JL, Avila CC, Anaya C, Cieza A, Vieta E, Bipolar Disorders Core Sets Expert Group. Development of the International Classification of Functioning, Disability and Health core sets for bipolar disorders: results of an international consensus process. Disabil Rehabil. 2013;35(25):2138–46. http://www.ncbi.nlm.nih.gov/pubmed/23586666.

22. Patterson TL, Goldman S, McKibbin CL, Hughs T, Jeste DV. UCSD Performance-Based Skills Assessment: development of a new measure of everyday functioning for severely mentally ill adults. Schizophr Bull. 2001;27(2):235–45. http://www.ncbi.nlm.nih.gov/pubmed/11354591.

11 Psychosocial Recovery-Oriented Treatments in Bipolar Disorders 189

23. Arbuckle R, Frye MA, Brecher M, Paulsson B, Rajagopalan K, Palmer S, et al. The psychometric validation of the Sheehan Disability Scale (SDS) in patients with bipolar disorder. Psychiatry Res. 2009;165(1–2):163–74. http://www.ncbi.nlm.nih.gov/pubmed/19042030.

24. Leon AC, Solomon DA, Mueller TI, Turvey CL, Endicott J, Keller MB. The Range of Impaired Functioning Tool (LIFE-RIFT): a brief measure of functional impairment. Psychol Med. 1999;29(4):869–78. http://www.ncbi.nlm.nih.gov/pubmed/10473314.

25. Tohen M, Waternaux CM, Tsuang MT, Outcome in Mania. A 4-year prospective follow-up of 75 patients utilizing survival analysis. Arch Gen Psychiatry. 1990;47(12):1106–11. http://www.ncbi.nlm.nih.gov/sites/entrez?Db=pubmed&DbFrom=pubmed&Cmd=Link&LinkName=pubmed_pubmed&LinkReadableName=RelatedArticles&IdsFromResult=2244795&ordinalpos=3&itool=EntrezSystem2.PEntrez.Pubmed.Pubmed_ResultsPanel.Pubmed_RVDocSum.

26. Sanchez-Moreno J, Bonnin CM, González-Pinto A, Amann BL, Solé B, Balanzá-Martinez V, et al. Factors associated with poor functional outcome in bipolar disorder: sociodemographic, clinical, and neurocognitive variables. Acta Psychiatr Scand. 2018;138(2):145–54. http://www.ncbi.nlm.nih.gov/pubmed/29726004.

27. Kupfer DJ, Frank E, Grochocinski VJ, Cluss PA, Houck PR, Stapf DA. Demographic and clinical characteristics of individuals in a bipolar disorder case registry. J Clin Psychiatry. 2002;63(2):120–5. http://www.ncbi.nlm.nih.gov/pubmed/11874212.

28. Wingo AP, Baldessarini RJ, Holtzheimer PE, Harvey PD. Factors associated with functional recovery in bipolar disorder patients. Bipolar Disord. 2010;12(3):319–26. http://www.ncbi.nlm.nih.gov/pubmed/20565439.

29. Keck PE, McElroy SL, Strakowski SM, West SA, Sax KW, Hawkins JM, et al. 12-month outcome of patients with bipolar disorder following hospitalization for a manic or mixed episode. Am J Psychiatry. 1998;155(5):646–52. http://www.ncbi.nlm.nih.gov/pubmed/9585716.

30. Samalin L, de Chazeron I, Vieta E, Bellivier F, Llorca P-M. Residual symptoms and specific functional impairments in euthymic patients with bipolar disorder. Bipolar Disord. 2016;18(2):164–73. http://www.ncbi.nlm.nih.gov/pubmed/26946486.

31. Gitlin MJ, Mintz J, Sokolski K, Hammen C, Altshuler LL. Subsyndromal depressive symptoms after symptomatic recovery from mania are associated with delayed functional recovery. J Clin Psychiatry. 2011;72(5):692–7. https://pubmed.ncbi.nlm.nih.gov/20673560/.

32. Gutiérrez-Rojas L, Jurado D, Gurpegui M. Factors associated with work, social life and family life disability in bipolar disorder patients. Psychiatry Res. 2011;186(2–3):254–60. http://www.ncbi.nlm.nih.gov/pubmed/20647154.

33. Reinares M, Papachristou E, Harvey P, Mar Bonnín C, Sánchez-Moreno J, Torrent C, et al. Towards a clinical staging for bipolar disorder: defining patient subtypes based on functional outcome. J Affect Disord. 2013;144(1–2):65–71. http://www.ncbi.nlm.nih.gov/pubmed/22862890.

34. Murru A, Pacchiarotti I, Verdolini N, Reinares M, Torrent C, Geoffroy P-A, et al. Modifiable and non-modifiable factors associated with functional impairment during the inter-episodic periods of bipolar disorder. Eur Arch Psychiatry Clin Neurosci. 2018;268(8):749–55. http://www.ncbi.nlm.nih.gov/pubmed/28534186.

35. Bonnín CM, Martínez-Arán A, Torrent C, Pacchiarotti I, Rosa AR, Franco C, et al. Clinical and neurocognitive predictors of functional outcome in bipolar euthymic patients: a long-term, follow-up study. J Affect Disord. 2010;121(1–2):156–60. http://www.ncbi.nlm.nih.gov/pubmed/19505727.

36. Huxley N, Baldessarini RJ. Disability and its treatment in bipolar disorder patients. Bipolar Disord. 2007;9(1–2):183–96. http://www.ncbi.nlm.nih.gov/pubmed/17391360.

37. Sanchez-Moreno J, Martinez-Aran A, Gadelrab HF, Cabello M, Torrent C, Bonnin CM, et al. The role and impact of contextual factors on functioning in patients with bipolar disorder. Disabil Rehabil. 2010;32(Suppl 1):S94–104. http://www.ncbi.nlm.nih.gov/sites/entrez?Db=pubmed&DbFrom=pubmed&Cmd=Link&LinkName=pubmed_pubmed&LinkReadableName=RelatedArticles&IdsFromResult=20883145&ordinalpos=3&itool=EntrezSystem2.PEntrez.Pubmed.Pubmed_ResultsPanel.Pubmed_RVDocSum.

38. Etain B, Godin O, Boudebesse C, Aubin V, Azorin JM, Bellivier F, et al. Sleep quality and emotional reactivity cluster in bipolar disorders and impact on functioning. Eur Psychiatry. 2017;45:190–7. http://www.ncbi.nlm.nih.gov/pubmed/28957786.
39. Sanchez-Moreno J, Martinez-Aran A, Tabarés-Seisdedos R, Torrent C, Vieta E, Ayuso-Mateos JL. Functioning and disability in bipolar disorder: an extensive review. Psychother Psychosom. 2009;78(5):285–97. http://www.ncbi.nlm.nih.gov/sites/entrez?Db=pubmed&DbFrom= pubmed&Cmd=Link&LinkName=pubmed_pubmed&LinkReadableName=RelatedArticles& IdsFromResult=19602917&ordinalpos=3&itool=EntrezSystem2.PEntrez.Pubmed.Pubmed_ ResultsPanel.Pubmed_RVDocSum.
40. Sanchez-Moreno J, Martinez-Aran A, Colom F, Scott J, Tabares-Seisdedos R, Sugranyes G, et al. Neurocognitive dysfunctions in euthymic bipolar patients with and without prior history of alcohol use. J Clin Psychiatry. 2009;70(8):1120–7. http://www.ncbi.nlm.nih.gov/ pubmed/19758523.
41. Leen J, Soczynska JK, Gallaugher LA, Woldeyohannes HO, Alsuwaidan MT, Cha DS, et al. The effect of personality dimensions on functional outcomes in mood disorders. Adv Ther. 2013;30(7):671–83. http://www.ncbi.nlm.nih.gov/pubmed/23839119.
42. Icick R, Gard S, Barde M, Carminati M, Desage A, Guillaume S, et al. Physical and mental health burden in cases of bipolar disorder classified as current, former, or non-tobacco smokers. J Affect Disord. 2017;208:406–13. http://www.ncbi.nlm.nih.gov/pubmed/27810725.
43. Kizilkurt OK, Gulec MY, Giynas FE, Gulec H. Effects of personality functioning on the global functioning of patients with bipolar disorder I. Psychiatry Res. 2018;266:309–16. http://www. ncbi.nlm.nih.gov/pubmed/29598836.
44. Williams TF, Simms LJ. Personality traits and maladaptivity: unipolarity versus bipolarity. J Pers. 2018;86(5):888–901. http://www.ncbi.nlm.nih.gov/pubmed/29171877.
45. Tsapekos D, Strawbridge R, Mantingh T, Cella M, Wykes T, Young AH. Role of cognitive reserve in cognitive variability in euthymic individuals with bipolar disorder: cross-sectional cluster analysis. BJPsych open. 2020;6(6):e133. http://www.ncbi.nlm.nih.gov/ pubmed/33121561.
46. Jiménez-López E, Sánchez-Morla EM, Aparicio AI, López-Villarreal A, Martínez-Vizcaíno V, Rodriguez-Jimenez R, et al. Psychosocial functioning in patients with psychotic and non-psychotic bipolar I disorder. A comparative study with individuals with schizophrenia. J Affect Disord. 2018;229:177–85. http://www.ncbi.nlm.nih.gov/pubmed/29316520.
47. Bonnín CM, González-Pinto A, Solé B, Reinares M, González-Ortega I, Alberich S, et al. Verbal memory as a mediator in the relationship between subthreshold depressive symptoms and functional outcome in bipolar disorder. J Affect Disord. 2014;160:50–4. http://www.ncbi. nlm.nih.gov/pubmed/24709022.
48. Torres IJ, DeFreitas CM, DeFreitas VG, Bond DJ, Kunz M, Honer WG, et al. Relationship between cognitive functioning and 6-month clinical and functional outcome in patients with first manic episode bipolar I disorder. Psychol Med. 2011;41(5):971–82. http://www.ncbi.nlm. nih.gov/sites/entrez?Db=pubmed&DbFrom=pubmed&Cmd=Link&LinkName=pubmed_pub med&LinkReadableName=RelatedArticles&IdsFromResult=20810001&ordinalpos=3&itool =EntrezSystem2.PEntrez.Pubmed.Pubmed_ResultsPanel.Pubmed_RVDocSum.
49. Jaeger J, Berns S, Loftus S, Gonzalez C, Czobor P. Neurocognitive test performance predicts functional recovery from acute exacerbation leading to hospitalization in bipolar disorder. Bipolar Disord. 2007;9(1–2):93–102. http://www.ncbi.nlm.nih.gov/pubmed/17391353.
50. Mur M, Portella MJ, Martinez-Aran A, Pifarre J, Vieta E. Influence of clinical and neuropsychological variables on the psychosocial and occupational outcome of remitted bipolar patients. Psychopathology. 2009;42(3):148–56. http://www.ncbi.nlm.nih.gov/pubmed/19276630.
51. Torres IJ, Kozicky J, Popuri S, Bond DJ, Honer WG, Lam RW, et al. 12-month longitudinal cognitive functioning in patients recently diagnosed with bipolar disorder. Bipolar Disord. 2014;16(2):159–71. http://www.ncbi.nlm.nih.gov/pubmed/24636366.
52. Kozicky J-M, Torres IJ, Silveira LE, Bond DJ, Lam RW, Yatham LN. Cognitive change in the year after a first manic episode. J Clin Psychiatry. 2014;75(06):e587–93. http://article.psychiatrist.com/?ContentType=START&ID=10008687.

53. Demmo C, Lagerberg TV, Kvitland LR, Aminoff SR, Hellvin T, Simonsen C, et al. Neurocognitive functioning, clinical course and functional outcome in first-treatment bipolar I disorder patients with and without clinical relapse: a 1-year follow-up study. Bipolar Disord. 2018;20(3):228–37. http://www.ncbi.nlm.nih.gov/pubmed/29121444.
54. Watson S, Gallagher P, Porter RJ, Smith MS, Herron LJ, Bulmer S, et al. A randomized trial to examine the effect of mifepristone on neuropsychological performance and mood in patients with bipolar depression. Biol Psychiatry. 2012;72(11):943–9. http://www.ncbi.nlm.nih.gov/sites/entrez?Db=pubmed&DbFrom=pubmed&Cmd=Link&LinkName=pubmed_pubmed&LinkReadableName=RelatedArticles&IdsFromResult=22770649&ordinalpos=3&itool=Entrez System2.PEntrez.Pubmed.Pubmed_ResultsPanel.Pubmed_RVDocSum.
55. Yatham LN, Mackala S, Basivireddy J, Ahn S, Walji N, Hu C, et al. Lurasidone versus treatment as usual for cognitive impairment in euthymic patients with bipolar I disorder: a randomised, open-label, pilot study. Lancet Psychiatry. 2017;4(3):208–17. http://www.ncbi.nlm.nih.gov/pubmed/28185899.
56. Miskowiak KW, Ehrenreich H, Christensen EM, Kessing LV, Vinberg M. Recombinant human erythropoietin to target cognitive dysfunction in bipolar disorder: a double-blind, randomized, placebo-controlled phase 2 trial. J Clin Psychiatry. 2014;75(12):1347–55. http://www.ncbi.nlm.nih.gov/pubmed/25099079.
57. Miskowiak KW, Vinberg M, Macoveanu J, Ehrenreich H, Køster N, Inkster B, et al. Effects of erythropoietin on hippocampal volume and memory in mood disorders. Biol Psychiatry. 2015;78(4):270–7. https://www.sciencedirect.com/science/article/abs/pii/S0006322314009974.
58. Miskowiak KW, Burdick KE, Martinez-Aran A, Bonnin CM, Bowie CR, Carvalho AF, et al. Methodological recommendations for cognition trials in bipolar disorder by the International Society for Bipolar Disorders Targeting Cognition Task Force. Bipolar Disord. 2017;19(8):614–26. http://www.ncbi.nlm.nih.gov/pubmed/28895274.
59. Bonnín CM, Martínez-Arán A, Reinares M, Valentí M, Solé B, Jiménez E, et al. Thresholds for severity, remission and recovery using the functioning assessment short test (FAST) in bipolar disorder. J Affect Disord. 2018;240:57–62. https://doi.org/10.1016/j.jad.2018.07.045.
60. Nierenberg AA, Loft H, Olsen CK. Treatment effects on residual cognitive symptoms among partially or fully remitted patients with major depressive disorder: a randomized, double-blinded, exploratory study with vortioxetine. J Affect Disord. 2019;250:35–42. http://www.ncbi.nlm.nih.gov/pubmed/30826492.
61. Deckersbach T, Nierenberg AA, Kessler R, Lund HG, Ametrano RM, Sachs G, et al. RESEARCH: cognitive rehabilitation for bipolar disorder: an open trial for employed patients with residual depressive symptoms. CNS Neurosci Ther. 2010;16(5):298–307. http://www.ncbi.nlm.nih.gov/pubmed/19895584.
62. Torrent C, Bonnin CM, Martínez-Arán A, Valle J, Amann BL, González-Pinto A, et al. Efficacy of functional remediation in bipolar disorder: a multicenter randomized controlled study. Am J Psychiatry. 2013;170(8):852–9. http://www.ncbi.nlm.nih.gov/pubmed/23511717.
63. Bonnin CM, Torrent C, Arango C, Amann BL, Solé B, González-Pinto A, et al. Functional remediation in bipolar disorder: 1-year follow-up of neurocognitive and functional outcome. Br J Psychiatry. 2016;208(1):87–93. http://www.ncbi.nlm.nih.gov/pubmed/26541692.
64. Zyto S, Jabben N, Schulte PFJ, Regeer BJ, Kupka RW. A pilot study of a combined group and individual functional remediation program for patients with bipolar I disorder. J Affect Disord. 2016;194:9–15. http://www.ncbi.nlm.nih.gov/sites/entrez?Db=pubmed&DbFrom=pubmed&Cmd=Link&LinkName=pubmed_pubmed&LinkReadableName=RelatedArticles&IdsFromResult=26800305&ordinalpos=3&itool=EntrezSystem2.PEntrez.Pubmed.Pubmed_ResultsPanel.Pubmed_RVDocSum.
65. Demant KM, Vinberg M, Kessing LV, Miskowiak KW. Effects of short-term cognitive remediation on cognitive dysfunction in partially or fully remitted individuals with bipolar disorder: results of a randomised controlled trial. PLoS One. 2015;10(6):e0127955. http://www.ncbi.nlm.nih.gov/pubmed/26070195.

66. Lewandowski KE, Sperry SH, Cohen BM, Norris LA, Fitzmaurice GM, Ongur D, et al. Treatment to Enhance Cognition in Bipolar Disorder (TREC-BD): efficacy of a randomized controlled trial of cognitive remediation versus active control. J Clin Psychiatry. 2017;78(9):e1242–9. http //www.ncbi.nlm.nih.gov/pubmed/29045770.
67. Ott CV, Vinberg M, Kessing LV, Bowie CR, Forman JL, Miskowiak KW. Effect of action-based cognitive remediation on cognitive impairment in patients with remitted bipolar disorder: a randomized controlled trial. Bipolar Disord. 2020; http://www.ncbi.nlm.nih.gov/pubmed/33053258.
68. Lengvenyte A, Coppola F, Jaussent I, Courtet P, Olié E. Improved functioning following computerized working memory training (COGMED®) in euthymic patients with bipolar disorder and cognitive complaints: an exploratory study. J Affect Disord. 2020;262:414–21. http://www.ncbi.nlm.nih.gov/pubmed/31740107.
69. Sayegh L, Touré EH, Farquhar E, Beaulieu S, Renaud S, Rej S, et al. Group Cognitive Behavioral Analysis System of Psychotherapy (CBASP): a pilot study for bipolar depression. Front Psych. 2020;11:565681. http://www.ncbi.nlm.nih.gov/sites/entrez?Db=pubmed&DbFrom=pubmed&Cmd=Link&LinkName=pubmed_pubmed&LinkReadableName=RelatedArticles&IdsFromResult=33173513&ordinalpos=3&itool=EntrezSystem2.PEntrez.Pubmed.Pubmed_ResultsPanel.Pubmed_RVDocSum.
70. Gomes BC, Rocca CC, Belizario GO, Fernandes F, Valois I, Olmo GC, et al. Cognitive behavioral rehabilitation for bipolar disorder patients: a randomized controlled trial. Bipolar Disord. 2019;21(7):621–33. http://www.ncbi.nlm.nih.gov/pubmed/31025470.
71. Strawbridge R, Tsapekos D, Hodsoll J, Mantingh T, Yalin N, McCrone P, et al. Cognitive remediation therapy for patients with bipolar disorder: a randomised proof-of-concept trial. Bipolar Disord. 2020; http://www.ncbi.nlm.nih.gov/pubmed/32583630.
72. Tremain H, Fletcher K, Scott J, McEnery C, Berk M, Murray G. The influence of stage of illness on functional outcomes after psychological treatment in bipolar disorder: a systematic review. Bipolar Disord. 2020;22(7):666–92. http://www.ncbi.nlm.nih.gov/sites/entrez?Db=pubmed&DbFrom=pubmed&Cmd=Link&LinkName=pubmed_pubmed&LinkReadableName=RelatedArticles&IdsFromResult=32621794&ordinalpos=3&itool=EntrezSystem2.PEntrez.Pubmed.Pubmed_ResultsPanel.Pubmed_RVDocSum.
73. Leopold K, Bauer M, Bechdolf A, Correll CU, Holtmann M, Juckel G, et al. Efficacy of cognitive-behavioral group therapy in patients at risk for serious mental illness presenting with subthreshold bipolar symptoms: results from a prespecified interim analysis of a multicenter, randomized, controlled study. Bipolar Disord. 2020;22(5):517–29. http://www.ncbi.nlm.nih.gov/pubmed/32112496.
74. Stamm TJ, Zwick JC, O'Malley G, Sondergeld L-M, Hautzinger M. Adjuvant psychotherapy in early-stage bipolar disorder: study protocol for a randomized controlled trial. Trials. 2020;21(1):845. http://www.ncbi.nlm.nih.gov/pubmed/33050952.
75. Pfennig A, Leopold K, Martini J, Boehme A, Lambert M, Stamm T, et al. Improving early recognition and intervention in people at increased risk for the development of bipolar disorder: study protocol of a prospective-longitudinal, naturalistic cohort study (Early-BipoLife). Int J bipolar Disord. 2020;8(1):22. http://www.ncbi.nlm.nih.gov/pubmed/32607662.
76. Grunze H, Born C. The impact of subsyndromal bipolar symptoms on patient's functionality and quality of life. Front Psych. 2020;11:510. http://www.ncbi.nlm.nih.gov/pubmed/32595531.
77. Samalin L, Boyer L, Murru A, Pacchiarotti I, Reinares M, Bonnin CM, et al. Residual depressive symptoms, sleep disturbance and perceived cognitive impairment as determinants of functioning in patients with bipolar disorder. J Affect Disord. 2017;210:280–6. http://www.ncbi.nlm.nih.gov/pubmed/28068616.
78. Martinez-Aran A, Vieta E. Cognition as a target in schizophrenia, bipolar disorder and depression. Eur Neuropsychopharmacol. 2015;25(2):151–7. http://www.ncbi.nlm.nih.gov/pubmed/25661911.
79. Gitlin MJ, Miklowitz DJ. The difficult lives of individuals with bipolar disorder: a review of functional outcomes and their implications for treatment. J Affect Disord. 2017;209:147–54. http://www.ncbi.nlm.nih.gov/pubmed/27914248.

80. Vieta E, Garriga M. Adjunctive antidepressants in bipolar depression. The lancet. Psychiatry. 2016;3(12):1095–6. http://www.ncbi.nlm.nih.gov/sites/entrez?Db=pubmed&DbFrom=pubmed&Cmd=Link&LinkName=pubmed_pubmed&LinkReadableName=RelatedArticles&IdsFromResult=28100424&ordinalpos=3&itool=EntrezSystem2.PEntrez.Pubmed.Pubmed_ResultsPanel.Pubmed_RVDocSum.
81. Radua J, Grunze H, Amann BL. Meta-analysis of the risk of subsequent mood episodes in bipolar disorder. Psychother Psychosom. 2017;86(2):90–8. http://www.ncbi.nlm.nih.gov/sites/entrez?Db=pubmed&DbFrom=pubmed&Cmd=Link&LinkName=pubmed_pubmed&LinkReadableName=RelatedArticles&IdsFromResult=28183076&ordinalpos=3&itool=EntrezSystem2.PEntrez.Pubmed.Pubmed_ResultsPanel.Pubmed_RVDocSum.
82. Garriga M, Solé E, González-Pinto A, Selva-Vera G, Arranz B, Amann BL, et al. Efficacy of quetiapine XR vs. placebo as concomitant treatment to mood stabilizers in the control of subthreshold symptoms of bipolar disorder: results from a pilot, randomized controlled trial. Eur Neuropsychopharmacol. 2017;27(10):959–69. http://www.ncbi.nlm.nih.gov/pubmed/28882405.
83. Novo P, Landin-Romero R, Radua J, Vicens V, Fernandez I, Garcia F, et al. Eye movement desensitization and reprocessing therapy in subsyndromal bipolar patients with a history of traumatic events: a randomized, controlled pilot-study. Psychiatry Res. 2014;219(1):122–8. http://www.ncbi.nlm.nih.gov/pubmed/24880581.
84. Moreno-Alcázar A, Treen D, Valiente-Gómez A, Sio-Eroles A, Pérez V, Amann BL, et al. Efficacy of eye movement desensitization and reprocessing in children and adolescent with post-traumatic stress disorder: a meta-analysis of randomized controlled trials. Front Psychol. 2017;8:1750. http://www.ncbi.nlm.nih.gov/pubmed/29066991.
85. Sanchez-Moreno J, Bonnín C, González-Pinto A, Amann BL, Solé B, Balanzá-Martínez V, et al. Do patients with bipolar disorder and subsyndromal symptoms benefit from functional remediation? A 12-month follow-up study. Eur Neuropsychopharmacol. 2017;27(4):350–9. http://www.ncbi.nlm.nih.gov/sites/entrez?Db=pubmed&DbFrom=pubmed&Cmd=Link&LinkName=pubmed_pubmed&LinkReadableName=RelatedArticles&IdsFromResult=28126401&ordinalpos=3&itool=EntrezSystem2.PEntrez.Pubmed.Pubmed_ResultsPanel.Pubmed_RVDocSum.
86. González Isasi A, Echeburúa E, Limiñana JM, González-Pinto A. Psychoeducation and cognitive-behavioral therapy for patients with refractory bipolar disorder: a 5-year controlled clinical trial. Eur Psychiatry. 2014;29(3):134–41. http://www.ncbi.nlm.nih.gov/pubmed/23276524.
87. Lam DH, Watkins ER, Hayward P, Bright J, Wright K, Kerr N, et al. A randomized controlled study of cognitive therapy for relapse prevention for bipolar affective disorder: outcome of the first year. Arch Gen Psychiatry. 2003;60(2):145–52. http://www.ncbi.nlm.nih.gov/pubmed/12578431.
88. Inder ML, Crowe MT, Luty SE, Carter JD, Moor S, Frampton CM, et al. Randomized, controlled trial of Interpersonal and Social Rhythm Therapy for young people with bipolar disorder. Bipolar Disord. 2015;17(2):128–38. http://www.ncbi.nlm.nih.gov/pubmed/25346391.
89. Miklowitz DJ, Otto MW, Frank E, Reilly-Harrington NA, Kogan JN, Sachs GS, et al. Intensive psychosocial intervention enhances functioning in patients with bipolar depression: results from a 9-month randomized controlled trial. Am J Psychiatry. 2007;164(9):1340–7. http://www.ncbi.nlm.nih.gov/pubmed/17728418.
90. Steardo L, Luciano M, Sampogna G, Zinno F, Saviano P, Staltari F, et al. Correction to: efficacy of the interpersonal and social rhythm therapy (IPSRT) in patients with bipolar disorder: results from a real-world, controlled trial. Ann General Psychiatry. 2020;19(1):28. https://annals-general-psychiatry.biomedcentral.com/articles/10.1186/s12991-020-00278-3.
91. Crowe M, Inder M, Porter R, Wells H, Jordan J, Lacey C, et al. Patients' perceptions of functional improvement in psychotherapy for mood disorders. Am J Psychother. 2020;74:22–9. http://www.ncbi.nlm.nih.gov/pubmed/33302704.

92. Williams JMG, Alatiq Y, Crane C, Barnhofer T, Fennell MJV, Duggan DS, et al. Mindfulness-based Cognitive Therapy (MBCT) in bipolar disorder: preliminary evaluation of immediate effects on between-episode functioning. J Affect Disord. 2008;107(1–3):275–9. http://www.ncbi.nlm.nih.gov/sites/entrez?Db=pubmed&DbFrom=pubmed&Cmd=Link&LinkName=pubmed_pubmed&LinkReadableName=RelatedArticles&IdsFromResult=17884176&ordinalpos=3&itool=EntrezSystem2.PEntrez.Pubmed.Pubmed_ResultsPanel.Pubmed_RVDocSum.

93. Ives-Deliperi VL, Howells F, Stein DJ, Meintjes EM, Horn N. The effects of mindfulness-based cognitive therapy in patients with bipolar disorder: a controlled functional MRI investigation. J Affect Disord. 2013;150(3):1152–7. http://www.ncbi.nlm.nih.gov/pubmed/23790741.

94. Perich T, Manicavasagar V, Mitchell PB, Ball JR. The association between meditation practice and treatment outcome in Mindfulness-based Cognitive Therapy for bipolar disorder. Behav Res Ther. 2013;51(7):338–43. http://www.ncbi.nlm.nih.gov/pubmed/23639299.

95. Stern Y. Cognitive reserve☆. Neuropsychologia. 2009;47(10):2015–28. http://www.ncbi.nlm.nih.gov/pubmed/19467352.

96. Forcada I, Mur M, Mora E, Vieta E, Bartrés-Faz D, Portella MJ. The influence of cognitive reserve on psychosocial and neuropsychological functioning in bipolar disorder. Eur Neuropsychopharmacol. 2015;25(2):214–22. https://pubmed.ncbi.nlm.nih.gov/25172270/.

97. Anaya C, Martinez Aran A, Ayuso-Mateos JL, Wykes T, Vieta E, Scott J. A systematic review of cognitive remediation for schizo-affective and affective disorders. J Affect Disord. 2012;142(1–3):13–21. http://www.ncbi.nlm.nih.gov/pubmed/22840620.

98. Ponsoni A, Damiani Branco L, Cotrena C, Milman Shansis F, Fonseca RP. The effects of cognitive reserve and depressive symptoms on cognitive performance in major depression and bipolar disorder. J Affect Disord. 2020;274:813–8. https://pubmed.ncbi.nlm.nih.gov/32664019/.

99. Amoretti S, Bernardo M, Bonnin CM, Bioque M, Cabrera B, Mezquida G, et al. The impact of cognitive reserve in the outcome of first-episode psychoses: 2-year follow-up study. Eur Neuropsychopharmacol. 2016;26(10):1638–48. http://linkinghub.elsevier.com/retrieve/pii/S0924977X16301018.

100. Vieta E. [Personalised medicine applied to mental health: precision psychiatry]. Rev Psiquiatr Salud Ment 2015;8(3):117–118. http://www.ncbi.nlm.nih.gov/pubmed/25959401.

101. de la Serna E, Montejo L, Solé B, Castro-Fornieles J, Camprodon-Boadas P, Sugranyes G, et al. Effectiveness of enhancing cognitive reserve in children, adolescents and young adults at genetic risk for psychosis: study protocol for a randomized controlled trial Rev Psiquiatr Salud Ment. 2021. https://linkinghub.elsevier.com/retrieve/pii/S188898912100029X.

102. Bhering Martins L, Braga Tibães JR, Sanches M, Jacka F, Berk M, Teixeira AL. Nutrition-based interventions for mood disorders. Expert Rev Neurother. 2021; http://www.ncbi.nlm.nih.gov/pubmed/33487078.

103. Balanzá-Martínez V, Shansis FM, Tatay-Manteiga A, López-García P. Diet and neurocognition in mood disorders—an overview of the overlooked. Curr Pharm Des. 2020;26(20):2353–62. http://www.ncbi.nlm.nih.gov/pubmed/32188376.

104. Mora E, Portella MJ, Martinez-Alonso M, Teres M, Forcada I, Vieta E, et al. The impact of obesity on cognitive functioning in euthymic bipolar patients: a cross-sectional and longitudinal study. J Clin Psychiatry. 2017;78(8):e924–32. http://www.ncbi.nlm.nih.gov/pubmed/28994517.

105. Bond DJ, Torres IJ, Lee SS, Kozicky J-M, Silveira LE, Dhanoa T, et al. Lower cognitive functioning as a predictor of weight gain in bipolar disorder: a 12-month study. Acta Psychiatr Scand. 2017;135(3):239–49. http://www.ncbi.nlm.nih.gov/pubmed/27995622.

106. Calkin C, van de Velde C, Růzicková M, Slaney C, Garnham J, Hajek T, et al. Can body mass index help predict outcome in patients with bipolar disorder? Bipolar Disord. 2009;11(6):650–6. http://www.ncbi.nlm.nih.gov/pubmed/19689507.

107. Bond DJ, Kunz M, Torres IJ, Lam RW, Yatham LN. The association of weight gain with mood symptoms and functional outcomes following a first manic episode: prospective 12-month data from the Systematic Treatment Optimization Program for Early Mania (STOP-EM). Bipolar Disord. 2010;12(6):616–26. https://doi.org/10.1111/j.1399-5618.2010.00855.x.

108. Sylvia LG, Salcedo S, Bernstein EE, Baek JH, Nierenberg AA, Deckersbach T. Nutrition, exercise, and wellness treatment in bipolar disorder: proof of concept for a consolidated intervention. Int J bipolar Disord. 2013;1(1):24. http://www.ncbi.nlm.nih.gov/sites/entrez?Db=pubmed&DbFrom=pubmed&Cmd=Link&LinkName=pubmed_pubmed&LinkReadablEName=RelatedArticles&IdsFromResult=24660139&ordinalpos=3&itool=EntrezSystem2.PEntrez.Pubmed.Pubmed_ResultsPanel.Pubmed_RVDocSum.
109. Gillhoff K, Gaab J, Emini L, Maroni C, Tholuck J, Greil W. Effects of a multimodal lifestyle intervention on body mass index in patients with bipolar disorder: a randomized controlled trial. Prim Care Companion J Clin Psychiatry. 2010;12(5). http://www.ncbi.nlm.nih.gov/pubmed/21274359.
110. Ernst C, Olson AK, Pinel JPJ, Lam RW, Christie BR. Antidepressant effects of exercise: evidence for an adult-neurogenesis hypothesis? J Psychiatry Neurosci. 2006;31(2):84–92. http://www.ncbi.nlm.nih.gov/pubmed/16575423.
111. Nuechterlein KH, Ventura J, McEwen SC, Gretchen-Doorly D, Vinogradov S, Subotnik KL. Enhancing cognitive training through aerobic exercise after a first schizophrenia episode: theoretical conception and pilot study. Schizophr Bull. 2016;42(Suppl 1):S44–52. http://www.ncbi.nlm.nih.gov/pubmed/27460618.
112. Campos C, Rocha NBF, Lattari E, Nardi AE, Machado S. Exercise induced neuroplasticity to enhance therapeutic outcomes of cognitive remediation in schizophrenia: analyzing the role of brain derived neurotrophic factor. CNS Neurol Disord Drug Targets. 2017;16(6):638–51. http://www.ncbi.nlm.nih.gov/pubmed/28017130.
113. Kern RS, Glynn SM, Horan WP, Marder SR. Psychosocial treatments to promote functional recovery in schizophrenia. Schizophr Bull. 2009;35(2):347–61. http://www.ncbi.nlm.nih.gov/pubmed/19176470.
114. Frank E, Wallace ML, Hall M, Hasler B, Levenson JC, Janney CA, et al. An integrated risk reduction intervention can reduce body mass index in individuals being treated for bipolar I disorder: results from a randomized trial. Bipolar Disord. 2015;17(4):424–37. http://www.ncbi.nlm.nih.gov/pubmed/25495748.
115. Colom F, Vieta E, Martínez-Arán A, Reinares M, Goikolea JM, Benabarre A, et al. A randomized trial on the efficacy of group psychoeducation in the prophylaxis of recurrences in bipolar patients whose disease is in remission. Arch Gen Psychiatry. 2003;60(4):402. https://doi.org/10.1001/archpsyc.60.4.402.
116. Reinares M, Colom F, Sánchez-Moreno J, Torrent C, Martínez-Arán A, Comes M, et al. Impact of caregiver group psychoeducation on the course and outcome of bipolar patients in remission: a randomized controlled trial. Bipolar Disord. 2008;10(4):511–9. http://www.ncbi.nlm.nih.gov/sites/entrez?Db=pubmed&DbFrom=pubmed&Cmd=Link&LinkName=pubmed_pubmed&LinkReadableName=RelatedArticles&IdsFromResult=18452447&ordinalpos=3&itool=EntrezSystem2.PEntrez.Pubmed.Pubmed_ResultsPanel.Pubmed_RVDocSum.
117. Torrent C, Del Mar Bonnin C, Martínez-Arán A, Valle J, Amann BL, González-Pinto A, et al. Efficacy of functional remediation in bipolar disorder: a multicenter randomized controlled study. Am J Psychiatry. 2013;170(8):852–9.
118. Reinares M, Martínez-Arán A, Vieta E. Psychotherapy for bipolar disorders: an integrative approach. Cambridge: Cambridge University Press; 2020. p. 126. http://services.cambridge.org/us/academic/subjects/medicine/mental-health-psychiatry-and-clinical-psychology/psychotherapy-bipolar-disorders-integrative-approach?format=PB&isbn=9781108460095.
119. Morton E, Michalak EE, Murray G. What does quality of life refer to in bipolar disorders research? A systematic review of the construct's definition, usage and measurement. J Affect Disord. 2017;212:128–37. http://www.ncbi.nlm.nih.gov/pubmed/28160685.
120. Bonnín CM, Yatham LN, Michalak EE, Martínez-Arán A, Dhanoa T, Torres I, et al. Psychometric properties of the well-being index (WHO-5) spanish version in a sample of euthymic patients with bipolar disorder. J Affect Disord. 2018;228:153–9. http://www.ncbi.nlm.nih.gov/pubmed/29248821.

121. Keyes CLM, Dhingra SS, Simoes EJ. Change in level of positive mental health as a predictor of future risk of mental illness. Am J Public Health. 2010;100(12):2366–71. http://www.ncbi.nlm.nih.gov/pubmed/20966364.
122. Nunes CS, Maes M, Rocmruangwong C, Moraes JB, Bonifacio KL, Vargas HO, et al. Lowered quality of life in mood disorders is associated with increased neuro-oxidative stress and basal thyroid-stimulating hormone levels and use of anticonvulsant mood stabilizers. J Eval Clin Pract. 2018;24(4):869–78. http://www.ncbi.nlm.nih.gov/pubmed/29665163.
123. Rajagopalan K, Bacci ED, Ng-Mak D, Wyrwich K, Pikalov A, Loebel A. Effects on health-related quality of life in patients treated with lurasidone for bipolar depression: results from two placebo controlled bipolar depression trials. BMC Psychiatry. 2016;16:157.
124. Gonda X, Kalman J, Dome P, Rihmer Z. [Changes in quality of life and work function during phase prophylactic lamotrigine treatment in bipolar patients: 6 month, prospective, observational study]. Neuropsychopharmacol Hung. 2016;18(1):57–67.
125. Walker DJ, DelBello MP, Landry J, D'Souza DN, Detke HC. Quality of life in children and adolescents with bipolar I depression treated with olanzapine/fluoxetine combination. Child Adolesc Psychiatry Ment Health. 2017;11:34. http://www.ncbi.nlm.nih.gov/pubmed/28706563.
126. Vancampfort D, Van Damme T, Probst M, Firth J, Stubbs B, Basangwa D, et al. Physical activity is associated with the physical, psychological, social and environmental quality of life in people with mental health problems in a low resource setting. Psychiatry Res. 2017;258:250–4. http://www.ncbi.nlm.nih.gov/sites/entrez?Db=pubmed&DbFrom=pubmed&Cmd=Link&LinkName=pubmed_pubmed&LinkReadableName=RelatedArticles&IdsFromResult=28844560&ordinalpos=3&itool=EntrezSystem2.PEntrez.Pubmed.Pubmed_ResultsPanel.Pubmed_RVDocSum.
127. O'Donnell LA, Axelson DA, Kowatch RA, Schneck CD, Sugar CA, Miklowitz DJ. Enhancing quality of life among adolescents with bipolar disorder: a randomized trial of two psychosocial interventions. J Affect Disord. 2017;219:201–8. http://www.ncbi.nlm.nih.gov/pubmed/28570966.
128. Lauder S, Chester A, Castle D, Dodd S, Gliddon E, Berk L, et al. A randomized head to head trial of MoodSwings.net.au: an Internet based self-help program for bipolar disorder. J Affect Disord. 2015;171:13–21. http://www.ncbi.nlm.nih.gov/pubmed/25282145.
129. Hidalgo-Mazzei D, Reinares M, Mateu A, Nikolova VL, Bonnín CDM, Samalin L, et al. OpenSIMPLe: a real-world implementation feasibility study of a smartphone-based psychoeducation programme for bipolar disorder. J Affect Disord. 2018;241:436–45. http://www.ncbi.nlm.nih.gov/pubmed/30145515.
130. Bauer R, Glenn T, Strejilevich S, Conell J, Alda M, Ardau R, et al. Internet use by older adults with bipolar disorder: international survey results. Int J bipolar Disord. 2018;6(1):20. http://www.ncbi.nlm.nih.gov/pubmed/30178112.
131. Hidalgo-Mazzei D, Reinares M, Mateu A, Juruena MF, Young AH, Pérez-Sola V, et al. Is a SIMPLe smartphone application capable of improving biological rhythms in bipolar disorder? J Affect Disord. 2017;223:10–6. http://www.ncbi.nlm.nih.gov/pubmed/28711743.
132. Bonnín CDM, Solé B, Reinares M, García-Estela A, Samalin L, Martínez-Arán A, et al. Does cognitive impairment in bipolar disorder impact on a SIMPLe app use? J Affect Disord. 2021;282:488–94. http://www.ncbi.nlm.nih.gov/pubmed/33422826.
133. IsHak WW, Brown K, Aye SS, Kahloon M, Mobaraki S, Hanna R. Health-related quality of life in bipolar disorder. Bipolar Disord. 2012;14(1):6–18. http://www.ncbi.nlm.nih.gov/pubmed/22329468.
134. Sylvia LG, Montana RE, Deckersbach T, Thase ME, Tohen M, Reilly-Harrington N, et al. Poor quality of life and functioning in bipolar disorder. Int J bipolar Disord. 2017;5(1):10. http://www.ncbi.nlm.nih gov/sites/entrez?Db=pubmed&DbFrom=pubmed&Cmd=Link&LinkName=pubmed_pubmed&LinkReadableName=RelatedArticles&IdsFromResult=28188565&ordinalpos=3&itool=EntrezSystem2.PEntrez.Pubmed.Pubmed_ResultsPanel.Pubmed_RVDocSum.

135. Marwaha S, Durrani A, Singh S. Employment outcomes in people with bipolar disorder: a systematic review. Acta Psychiatr Scand. 2013;128(3):179–93. http://www.ncbi.nlm.nih.gov/pubmed/23379960.

136. Träger C, Decker L, Wæhrens EE, Knorr U, Miskowiak K, Vinberg M. Influences of patient informed cognitive complaints on activities of daily living in patients with bipolar disorder. An exploratory cross-sectional study. Psychiatry Res. 2017;249:268–74. http://www.ncbi.nlm.nih.gov/sites/entrez?Db=pubmed&DbFrom=pubmed&Cmd=Link&LinkName=pubmed_pubmed&LinkReadableName=RelatedArticles&IdsFromResult=28135597&ordinalpos=3&itool=EntrezSystem2.PEntrez.Pubmed.Pubmed_ResultsPanel.Pubmed_RVDocSum.

137. Ehrminger M, Brunet-Gouet E, Cannavo A-S, Aouizerate B, Cussac I, Azorin J-M, et al. Longitudinal relationships between cognition and functioning over 2 years in euthymic patients with bipolar disorder: a cross-lagged panel model approach with the FACE-BD cohort. Br J Psychiatry. 2021;218(2):80–7. http://www.ncbi.nlm.nih.gov/pubmed/31407639.

138. Salagre E, Dodd S, Aedo A, Rosa A, Amoretti S, Pinzon J, et al. Toward precision psychiatry in bipolar disorder: staging 2.0. Front Psych. 2018;9:641. http://www.ncbi.nlm.nih.gov/sites/entrez?Db=pubmed&DbFrom=pubmed&Cmd=Link&LinkName=pubmed_pubmed&LinkReadableName=RelatedArticles&IdsFromResult=30555363&ordinalpos=3&itool=EntrezSystem2.PEntrez.Pubmed.Pubmed_ResultsPanel.Pubmed_RVDocSum.

Psychopharmacological Recovery-Oriented Treatments in Bipolar Disorders

12

Alessandro Cuomo, Alessandro Spiti, Marco Chioccioli, Despoina Koukouna, Arianna Goracci, Simone Bolognesi, and Andrea Fagiolini

12.1 Introduction

Most people with a mental health disease can recover from their acute symptoms and live a fulfilling life. Ideally, all patients with a mental disease would become and remain symptom free, discontinue all treatments, and be able to function at the highest levels, for the rest of their life. For most patients, this is a reasonable hope for the future, as new treatment will optimistically be discovered. The bad news is that, at present, this goal is unrealistic for the majority of patients with severe mental illnesses. The good news is that, if recovery means achieving a good quality of life, functioning at the best, being socially included, reaching and maintaining remission, the goal is realizable and we can succeed. Indeed, assisting the personal recovery of people with mental illness has become a high-value target for mental health services, and this process has been integrated into all the mental health policies [1–3]. Mental health systems based on recovery orientation encourage cooperation between patients and their caregivers for the accomplishment of patients' personal goals, purposes, and ambitions so that they can realize their abilities and disabilities, facilitate their social inclusion, and achieve independence and autonomy. A recovery-oriented approach aims to reduce the incidence, prevalence, and recurrence of mental health disorders and their associated disabilities *(prevention)*, thereby restraining the risk exposure before the onset of symptoms and intensifying the coping and social support mechanisms of the individual [4]. Finally, the

---

A. Cuomo · A. Spiti · M. Chioccioli · D. Koukouna · A. Goracci · S. Bolognesi · A. Fagiolini (✉)
Department of Molecular Medicine, University of Siena School of Medicine,
Siena, Tuscany, Italy
e-mail: alessandrocuomo86@gmail.com; alessandrospiti93@gmail.com;
m.chioccioli22@gmail.com; despinakoukouna@hotmail.com; a.goracci@gmail.com;
simbolognesi@gmail.com; andrea.fagiolini@unisi.it

© The Author(s), under exclusive license to Springer Nature
Switzerland AG 2022
B. Carpiniello et al. (eds.), *Recovery and Major Mental Disorders*,
Comprehensive Approach to Psychiatry 2,
https://doi.org/10.1007/978-3-030-98301-7_12

recovery-oriented health care model emphasizes the early detection of mental illnesses and their treatment systems based on shared decision-making for the stabilization and remission of symptoms while aiming to improve the general functioning of patients [5, 6].

Recovery in the mental health research literature can be differentiated according to the following three types:

- Clinical or symptomatic recovery: defined as a decrease or remission of symptoms and revitalization of the social functioning.
- Functional or objective recovery: described as the degree of social and occupational functioning, independence, and autonomy.
- Personal or subjective recovery: conceptualized as attaining hope and self-esteem while prevailing over stigma and discrimination via the activation of all accessible resources [7–9].

Even over the past decades, mental disease was considered chronic and degenerative condition with a poor prospect of improvement. However, studies have reported that 20–25% patients experiencing mental illness recovered completely to a premorbid state, and 50–60% patients recovered to a state of substantial decrease in symptoms and achieved high functioning levels. Considering that the medication's efficacy, tolerability, safety, and acceptability; the symptom management strategies; and the access to mental health services play a key role in patient's recovery, the mental health care team has a huge responsibility to recognize the decisive impact of social inclusion, personal relationships, lifestyle, job, education, economic conditions, and the key role of local community [10–15]. Currently, one of the most pivotal problems in the public mental health system is the chasm between the availability of evidence-based, person-centered, and recovery-oriented rehabilitative procedures and the real capacity of mental health professionals to provide them to the patients. Actually, there is a plethora of quality improvement strategies for the optimization of the mental health care system, but the most effective ones are the remodeling services supported by the concept of recovery (personal orientation, involvement, choice, and development along with self-determination) [16] and organizing services that facilitate strategies and interventions based on scientific evidence [17]. Furthermore, it is very crucial to expand our knowledge on the distinct forms of strategies, their distribution methods, evaluation instruments, assessment impact of endpoints, predictors of therapy's reactions, and the combination of psychopharmacological treatments and other psychosocial rehabilitation processes [18].

12.2 Psychopharmacological Treatment of Bipolar Phases

The past half-century has witnessed breakthrough innovation in the mental health methods and pharmacological treatments. Nevertheless, an approach that focuses on the complexity of the individual patient is always essential, wherein psychotropic drugs positively affect cognition, mood, and behavior, but do not change the underlying illness process. Favorable results can be achieved by lessening the symptoms and encouraging the patients' ability to adapt to the requirements of their lives [19].

In this extremely heterogeneous scenario in which each patient is a changing and independent entity, the main objective of treatment must be a complete remission of the symptoms that allows the patient to return to full functionality. Therefore, the mission of psychiatry is to eliminate symptoms, alleviate suffering, and restore patients to their maximum functioning levels. The success of drug therapy in the field of mental health is based on understanding exactly where, how, and when to use the most appropriate drugs for each patient. Although there is no certainty in medicine, it is well known that a more long-term treatment is required with the progression and persistence of a disease. For this reason, the psychiatrist has the intense task of educating the patient on the symptoms of relapse or recurrence and explaining that the symptoms are the results of biopsychosocial factors.

The drugs belonging to the class of so-called "*mood stabilizers*" are characterized by the presence of antimanic and antidepressant actions, which establishes their ability to act on both polarities [20, 21] and in all the phases of the disease including the maintenance phase and prophylaxis [22, 23].

Cognitive behavioral therapy (CBT) is frequently considered as an adjuvant to pharmacotherapy in the treatment of bipolar disorder (BD). CBT focuses on identifying, challenging, and correcting the automatic, negative, distorted, and dysfunctional thinking. Interpersonal and social rhythm therapy are also useful for the patients to help them understand the importance of stabilizing the disruptions in the circadian rhythm and maintaining a proper routine for performing their daily activities.

12.2.1 Acute Mania in Bipolar Disorder

Pharmacotherapy is the cornerstone of the treatment of manic and mixed acute episodes in BD. The mainstay of treatment for manic states is the rapid reduction of symptoms, followed by a complete remission of symptoms and restoration of psychosocial functioning [24]. First-line medications for manic episodes include lithium (it is necessary to ensure that the dosage is adequate, and its blood concentrations are in the upper therapeutic range of 1.0–1.4 mmol/L), valproate, or a second-generation antipsychotic (SGA) [25].

The common side effects associated with acute *lithium* treatment are nausea, diarrhea, vomiting, tremor, drowsiness, weight gain, and cognitive decline. Lithium can also interfere with thyroid and parathyroid functions and exacerbate renal impairment; therefore, the assessment of both thyroid and kidney functions can ensure the efficacy of treatment and patient's safety. A careful monitoring of lithium blood concentrations is recommended at the beginning of treatment and whenever there is a change in its dosage to avoid its excessive concentrations that can cause even severe toxicity with the manifestations of encephalopathy and potentially fatal cardiac arrhythmias [26].

Antiepileptics. Various guidelines have indicated valproate as a first-line agent for the treatment of manic episodes. Carbamazepine is considered as a second-line agent, whereas lamotrigine is approved for the treatment of both acute and maintenance phases. For the treatment of bipolar depression, the mental team considers lamotrigine as the first-line agent.

The effectiveness of *valproate* in the manic phases, as well as for lithium, is related to its concentrations in the blood (50–125 mg/L). Valproate exerts a greater response when it is administered in the upper limit [27, 28]. It does not interact directly with postsynaptic gamma aminobutyric acid (GABA) receptors. In fact, valproate increases the regional neuronal concentrations of GABA by inhibiting its metabolism and synthesis. The association of valproate with antipsychotics causes a reduction in the dosages of the latter and higher response rates as compared to placebo added with antipsychotics in the patients with acute mania. Valproate is, generally, a well-tolerated drug during the treatment of the manic phase; its commonly reported side effects, usually transient, are drowsiness, fatigue, nausea, vomiting, tremors, weight gain, cognitive decline, and dizziness. Although extremely safe, it is important to report some possible serious, rare, and adverse events such as pancreatitis, thrombocytopenia, a significant increase in liver transaminases, hyperammonemic encephalopathy in the patients with urea cycle disorders, and liver failure. *Carbamazepine*'s mechanism of action is believed to occur because of the inactivation of sodium ion channels or potentiation of GABA, which is the main inhibitory neurotransmitter in the central nervous system [29].

The most frequently encountered side effects of carbamazepine are sedation, dizziness, drowsiness, blurred vision, difficulty in motor coordination, nausea, vomiting, diarrhea, and abdominal pain (often related to dose, these side effects can be minimized by slowly increasing the dosage of the drug or taking the drug on a full stomach). Additionally, dermatological side effects (red, itchy, or hives rash) may also manifest, thus necessitating the discontinuation of treatment [30]. Carbamazepine must be used with caution in the patients with hepatic or renal impairment and cardiac abnormalities. Moreover, it may induce blood dyscrasias such as agranulocytosis and thrombocytopenia necessitating hematological monitoring in the first month of therapy. A periodic monitoring of serum carbamazepine concentrations may be useful in dose selection and avoiding toxicity.

The molecular structure of *oxcarbazepine* is the foundation of its peculiar pharmacokinetic and pharmacodynamic properties, which ensure a better tolerability profile, thereby leading to a fewer adverse reactions (less frequency of blood dyscrasias) and drug interactions [24].

Lamotrigine inhibits the action of glutamate, which is an excitatory neurotransmitter, establishing its effectiveness in the treatment of BD. Although the US Food and Drug Administration (FDA) has not authorized the use of lamotrigine for the acute treatment of bipolar depression, it is indicated as maintenance therapy in the prevention of depressive, manic, and hypomanic episodes. Lamotrigine can help prevent manic phases; however, the results are not as strong as those of lithium [31]. Other studies have suggested the possibility of combining lamotrigine with lithium to achieve synergistic results in the prevention of relapse [32].

Lamotrigine is generally a well-tolerated drug; its most common side effects were influencing the central nervous system (dizziness, headache, ataxia, drowsiness, and tremors) and the gastrointestinal apparatus (nausea and vomiting), along with dermatological conditions (Stevens-Johnson syndrome). Stevens-Johnson syndrome is more likely to affect high-risk groups such as slow acetylators, immunosuppressed population, patients with human leukocyte antigen associations, and people in therapy with valproate [33]. In the latter case, we know that valproate, by inhibiting UDP-glucuronosyltransferase (UGT) which metabolizes lamotrigine, increases the blood levels of this drug, raising the risk for serious adverse skin events: we must therefore be very careful using initial, titration and maintenance dosages of lamotrigine at half of the usual ones.

There is scientific evidence that a rapid increase of lamotrigine levels may increase the occurrence of lamotrigine-related skin lesions and rashes [34]; therefore, the lower starting dose of lamotrigine and slower dose escalations are recommended. Titration of the drug usually takes place according to the following scheme: 25 mg for 2 weeks, then 50 mg for 2 weeks, before increasing to 100 mg and, if necessary, 1 week later to 200 mg. In addition, lamotrigine is also potentially able to bind with the ocular tissue containing melanin.

Gabapentin was one of the first third-generation antiepileptic drugs to be studied for BD, particularly for the treatment of mania. Although gabapentin does not have an important stabilizing power in monotherapy, it can be used in combination with other mood stabilizers to enhance its effectiveness and in patients with a high anxiety component [35, 36].

Atypical (Second-Generation) Antipsychotics. The class of atypical antipsychotic drugs called SGAs has demonstrated efficacy in the treatment of the acute manic phase. These drugs are considered as primary agents in the treatment of the manic phase or mixed states [37]. This category of drugs has a huge advantage of generating fewer extrapyramidal side effects such as tardive dyskinesia and depression [38]; however, the possibility of other side effects such as seizures, cardiac arrhythmias, hypertension, and metabolic syndrome (weight gain, Type 2 diabetes mellitus, and hyperlipidemia) should also be considered.

Olanzapine was the first FDA-approved SGA for treating the manic episodes in BD in 2000 [39, 40], that today is licensed also for prophylaxis. Various studies have shown that the add-on treatment with olanzapine is superior to placebo in patients whose symptoms were inadequately responsive to lithium or valproate monotherapy [41–43]. Further data suggest that olanzapine may offer long-term treatment benefits [44, 45] and can be more effective than lithium [46–48]. Olanzapine has demonstrated its effectiveness to be, at least, on a par with valproate [49, 50] and risperidone [51]. The most common side effects associated with olanzapine in the short-term studies were somnolence, constipation, dry mouth, increased appetite, weight gain, and orthostatic hypotension.

Several studies lasting 3–4 weeks on an average have demonstrated that *risperidone* is superior to placebo [52, 53] and comparable to olanzapine [54], haloperidol [55], and lithium [33] in the reduction of manic and mixed symptoms in monotherapy. The rates of side effects, predominantly extrapyramidal symptoms

(EPS), associated with risperidone were low when the drug was administered at the medium doses of up to 4 mg/day [22, 52, 56], but not when administered at the average doses of 6 mg/day or higher [33, 53]. Other commonly occurring side effects reported in the short-term studies were high prolactin levels, akathisia, drowsiness, dyspepsia, and nausea.

The use of *quetiapine* for 12 weeks in monotherapy was superior to placebo [57, 58] and comparable to the use of lithium in the treatment at 4 weeks of adult age [59]. Most studies suggest approximately 600 mg/day as an antimanic dose of quetiapine [60]. Headache, xerostomia, weight gain, sedation, dizziness, and constipation are some of the commonly reported side effects of quetiapine.

Ziprasidone was superior to placebo (average dosage = 120–130 mg/day) in two 3-week monotherapy studies in the adult patients and comparable to haloperidol in a 12-week study. The recorded side effects of ziprasidone were headache, drowsiness, EPS, akathisia, and dizziness [61, 62].

Aripiprazole had a significantly greater efficacy in the reduction of manic symptoms as compared to placebo in three different 3-week trials [63, 64]. It showed equivalent efficacy as compared with haloperidol and lithium in the adequately powered 12-week comparison trials [63]. Aripiprazole is initiated at the doses of 15 or 30 mg/day and its most frequently encountered adverse reactions are headache, nausea, vomiting, constipation, insomnia, and akathisia.

Asenapine was superior to placebo in the mean reduction of the manic symptoms in two different 3-week studies [65, 66]. It is a sublingually administered drug, which is effective in mania. Asenapine has a less sedative effect than olanzapine with a similar propensity, albeit low, to the possible development of akathisia and other movement disorders [67]; however, it has a less likely sedative and antihistaminic effect than olanzapine that generates the metabolic syndrome. The efficacy of this drug appears to be maintained even in the long term [68].

Cariprazine is a partial agonist of dopamine D3 and D2 receptors, which was approved for the treatment of mania [69–71]. The most common side effects associated with cariprazine (occurring in about 10% of subjects and twice as frequently as placebo) were akathisia, extrapyramidal symptoms (EPS), tremors, dyspepsia, and vomiting, but it has the advantage of having a low propensity to deteriorate the weight gain and metabolic profile of the patients.

Overall, the response rate for mood stabilizers and SGAs is around 50%, where the response to treatment is defined as a reduction of 50% in manic symptoms as compared to a response rate of around 25% in the placebo group. A patient who does not respond or tolerate the first prescribed drug must switch to another agent, which can be another mood stabilizer or a SGA. The association of lithium or valproate with a SGA has proven to be the most used combination in clinical practice as well as the most effective one in all the stages of BD. These are the reasons why FDA approved so many SGAs as an adjunct treatment to mood stabilizers in the treatment of manic phases or in the mixed states. In an aggregate analysis of five of the largest controlled trials of SGAs used in association with lithium or valproate in patients with mania, Ketter and colleagues concluded that there was an approximate 20% advantage of combination treatment as compared to the use of a single mood stabilizer. This is roughly equivalent to the advantage of using a single mood stabilizer or SGAs over placebo in the treatment of acute mania. Therefore, the authors concluded the combination of SGA and lithium or valproate appears to have a distinct advantage in acute mania [69]. Similarly, an added antipsychotic is more effective than a single use of mood stabilizer in the acute manic episodes that present significant psychomotor agitation and delusions or hallucinations.

Combining antipsychotics could be a treatment choice when the benefits outweigh the risks of ineffective therapy by considering the eventual development of neuroleptic malignant syndrome (NMS), which is a life-threatening reaction in response to an antipsychotic drug. In fact, it paints a very serious clinical picture, rare but potentially fatal, characterized by muscle stiffness, fever, altered mental state, irregular pulse or blood pressure, high pulse rate, sweating, and arrhythmia, which are associated with the laboratory abnormalities that indicate muscle, kidney, and heart problems, including increased creatine phosphokinase, myoglobinuria, and acute renal failure, requiring urgent and intensive medical treatment.

12.2.2 Rapid Cycling Bipolar Disorder

The fundamental aspects of this disorder are the lower responsiveness to drug treatment as compared to the non-rapid-cycling BD [72, 73] and the considerable depressive morbidity as well as a high risk of suicide [74]. Table 12.1 outlines the steps for the treatment of rapid cycling BD.

Anti-kindling agents are the drugs of choice for treatment, whereas it has been suggested that valproate is more effective than lithium for this disorder; however, controlled studies have not necessarily supported this idea [75]. The addition of valproate to lithium may not be better than the single administration of lithium in the management of rapid cycling in BD [76]. There is also evidence that the combination of lithium and carbamazepine can be particularly useful. Lamotrigine is considered as a second-line agent, but it has demonstrated superiority over placebo in improving the depressive symptoms in patients with bipolar I or II rapid-cycle refractory treatment [77, 78].

Table 12.1 Possible therapeutic intervention strategies for increasing degrees of intervention in rapid cycling bipolar disorder

Treatment strategies for rapid cycling bipolar disorder	
First step	Stop treatment with antidepressants
Second step	Consider the possible precipitating factors
Third step	Optimize treatment with mood stabilizer drugs
	Evaluate possible associations: lithium + valproate/lamotrigine
Fourth step	Consider using the combination of olanzapine, quetiapine, aripiprazole, risperidone, lamotrigine, and topiramate

Furthermore, the addition of high doses of T4, T3, or the combination of these two would be a second- or third-level option in the patients with bipolar or rapid cycling depression.

12.2.3 Bipolar Depression

In the treatment of an acute depressive episode, lithium and/or lamotrigine are widely considered as first-line treatments. The FDA had also approved the use of some SGAs in BD. If the antidepressant therapy needs to be initiated, then a recommended selective serotonin reuptake inhibitor (SSRI) or bupropion would be preferred over a tricyclic antidepressant (TCA) or serotonin–norepinephrine reuptake inhibitor (SNRI) by focusing on the signs of dysphoria, mixed symptoms, hypomania, mania, and rapid cycles.

Young et al. conducted a short trial in 2000, wherein they assigned 27 patients with bipolar depression to either paroxetine or an additional mood stabilizer (either lithium or valproate). Over the 6-week trial, both the strategies improved depression, but the patients were more likely to benefit from the paroxetine than they were from the mood stabilizer [79].

It has been observed that most cases of rapid cycling in BD induction can occur with the use of TCA and SNRI, but it can also occur with monoamine oxidase inhibitor (MAOI), SSRI, and other classes of drugs. Bupropion was initially believed to less likely induce rapid cycles or mixed states, but some cases of the same have been reported in literature. Researchers have concluded that it is preferable for patients with depression in the context of a BD to try bupropion or SSRI before a noradrenergic antidepressant, including a TCA or SNRI. This observation was confirmed when the conversion rates associated with new antidepressants in the short-term studies generally appear to be lower than those associated with TCAs [80]. The greatest efficacy has been observed with tranylcypromine (MAOI) [81], but the safety problems associated with it do not make it a first-line treatment [82]. Bupropion and SSRIs are the common first-line agents administered in combination with mood stabilizers [83, 84].

The Systematic Treatment Enhancement Program for Bipolar Disorder study examined how the duration of treatment with an antidepressant affects the possibility to develop further depressive, manic, or hypomanic episodes. The collected data revealed that 23% of patients with bipolar depression treated with an antidepressant in combination with a mood stabilizer reached euthymia in at least 8 consecutive weeks as compared to the 27% of patients who received placebo added to a mood stabilizer [85]. Likewise, Nemeroff and colleagues (2001) did not find any advantage for adding imipramine or paroxetine to lithium over adding placebo for the patients with bipolar depression [84]. However, patients with lower serum lithium levels (<0.8 mEq/L) performed better with the addition of an antidepressant than those with the addition of placebo. This observation suggests that patients with bipolar depression who cannot tolerate a higher lithium level could benefit from the addition of an antidepressant.

The first SGA to obtain approval from the FDA for the treatment of bipolar depression in monotherapy was *quetiapine* in 2008. At the doses of 300 mg/day and 600 mg/day, quetiapine proved to be superior to placebo in reducing the depressive symptoms in four large multi-center and 8-week-long studies of outpatients with bipolar I and II depression [86–88]. From a pharmacological point of view, norquetiapine, which is an active metabolite of quetiapine, helps in serotonergic transmission by acting as a partial agonist of 5-HT1A receptors and a powerful inhibitor of the norepinephrine transporter that consequently increases the noradrenergic function [89, 90].

Lurasidone is effective in the treatment of type I bipolar depressive episodes and approved for monotherapy and for the additional use with lithium or valproate in bipolar depression [61]. Various clinical trials found that it has a significant lower probability than other atypical agents for producing metabolic side effects. The recording study of adding lurasidone to valproate or lithium at the therapeutic levels found that the combination of lurasidone and a mood stabilizer at the dosages of 20–120 mg/day was significantly more effective than one of the mood stabilizers in the acute treatment of bipolar depression [91]. Lurasidone is one of the first SGAs whose efficacy in BD has been studied exclusively in the treatment of depressive phase. The decision to conduct the clinical pharmacological trials of lurasidone in the patients with depressive episodes in BD was affected by three relevant factors [92]: the peculiar pharmacological profile of receptor affinity (mainly as a 5-HT1A receptor agonist and a 5-HT7 receptor) [93], efficacy in the animal models of acute and chronic depression [94], and a favorable improvement in the depressive mood in the previous efficacy studies of schizophrenia [95].

The *olanzapine-fluoxetine combination* (OFC) was approved in 2003 by the FDA for the acute treatment of depressive episodes associated with bipolar I disorder. The effectiveness of this original drug combination was demonstrated in a double-blind, 8-week, randomized controlled trial that compared the efficacy of OFC in the treatment of bipolar depressive phases versus olanzapine alone and placebo. The results showed that OFC was superior in terms of depressive symptomatology reduction compared to the olanzapine and placebo groups without increased risk of developing manic symptoms. In particular, remission criteria were met by 24.5% of the placebo group, 32.8% of the olanzapine group, and 48.8% of the olanzapine-fluoxetine group [96].

A later study evaluated the risk of manic switch in bipolar patients from using OFC versus using olanzapine alone and placebo in the treatment of bipolar depression. Incidence of treatment-emergent mania (defined as a YMRS score < 15 at baseline and > or = 15 at any subsequent visit) did not differ significantly among the groups (olanzapine 5.7%, placebo 6.7%, olanzapine/fluoxetine combination 6.4%; $p = 0.861$). The results indicate that olanzapine/fluoxetine combination does not present a greater risk of treatment-emergent mania compared to olanzapine or placebo over 8 weeks of acute treatment for bipolar I depression [97].

Lamotrigine is effective in preventing the depressive episodes in the patients with BD. Its combination with other mood stabilizers can be even more effective in preventing bipolar depression. In a controlled study, Bowden and colleagues found that the combination of lamotrigine and valproate was significantly more effective than the single administration of lamotrigine in preventing the bipolar depressive episodes [98]. The use of lamotrigine in combination with lithium in the treatment of bipolar depression has proven effective at the dosages between 50 and 200 mg/day. Lamotrigine proved to be superior to placebo in the treatment of patients with type I bipolar depression in a large randomized controlled trial (RCT) [99]. A double-blind crossover study found lamotrigine to be superior to placebo when it was added to lithium treatment in an 8-week study in the patients with recurrent depressive episodes [100].

12.2.4 Mixed States in Bipolar Disorder

The concept of mixed states has widened with the Diagnostic and Statistical Manual of Mental Disorders' mixed specifier, but there are yet very few studies that have used this concept. Mixed states are also common and present an increased risk of suicide [101]. Iloperidone may be effective in the mixed episodes, but there are scarce data on its efficacy [102]. For mixed episodes, valproate is recommended as one of the first-line agents, whereas carbamazepine is generally considered a first- or second-line agent for mixed episodes.

12.3 Treatment-Resistant Bipolar Disorder (Augmentation Strategies)

Despite the progress made over the years in the field of BD treatment, there are still four main shortcomings: many patients are resistant to the conventional treatments; a significant proportion of patients has tolerability problems; the used drugs determine significant adverse effects; and the depressive phase constitutes a clinical problem that relates to the frequency, duration, and intensity of the phases [103–105].

For these reasons, many patients require polypharmacological therapy with the different classes of drugs to obtain an adequate response. There are various motivations that push the clinician to combine several medications, such as increasing the effect of an agent with a synergistic mechanism, treating a particular aspect of the disease (e.g., adding a hypnotic to an antidepressant to help with sleep or a stimulant is added to combat residual fatigue), and reducing the side effects that could be created by the treatment.

Lithium can be used in combination with anticonvulsants in the treatment of patients with refractory mania. A few number of reports have indicated that the combined administration of carbamazepine and lithium is more effective in patients who have not responded to the separate single administration of these two agents. Retrospective reviews have generally evidenced that the combination of lithium and *carbamazepine* is useful and synergistic [106, 107], and this association appears to be well tolerated by patients. However, among the adverse reactions, an increased risk of sinus node dysfunction with this combination should be noted, but this effect

12 Psychopharmacological Recovery-Oriented Treatments in Bipolar Disorders

appears to be rare [108]. Furthermore, the combination of lithium and carbamazepine may have a cumulative antithyroid effect, but there is no evidence of increased neurotoxicity or blood dyscrasias with respect to this combination. This action indicates that the combination of lithium and carbamazepine appears to be well tolerated [109]. A prospective randomized study showed the effectiveness of both carbamazepine and oxcarbazepine in treating the residual BD symptoms that had not responded to the single administration of lithium [110].

Lithium is usually combined with *valproate* in the treatment of BD; however, valproate and carbamazepine compete for liver metabolism, which can increase the risk of carbamazepine toxicity. For this reason, some researchers have suggested that the combination of valproate and carbamazepine is contraindicated. Our experience suggests that the combination can be safely used if the serum levels of both drugs are carefully monitored and are administered with adequate doses. Other anticonvulsants that have sometimes been associated with lithium and valproate in the patients with treatment-resistant DB are gabapentin, topiramate, and lamotrigine.

The only double-blind augmentation study to date has found that *gabapentin* added to a conventional mood stabilizer may have a modest role in the prevention of relapse [111]. This combination appears to be well tolerated and seems to be useful with the symptoms of anxiety and agitation in the patients with BD even if it does not seem to be very effective in the treatment of mania or depression. We typically use 900–1200 mg/day as an adjuvant dose and do not recommend gabapentin as monotherapy for BD.

Topiramate may be more useful as an adjuvant drug than as an augmenting agent. Adding 50–200 mg of topiramate to a standard mood stabilizer regimen can play an important role in mitigating weight gain.

The prototypical atypical agent *clozapine* was reported to have substantial efficacy in several large case series of patients with treatment refractory mania but has not been studied in placebo-controlled trials in mania [112, 113]. Clozapine tends to underlie the treatment algorithm for treatment-resistant DB because of its complex use and possible side effects. The combination of lithium and clozapine can be synergistic: additionally, lithium can mitigate leukopenia associated with clozapine [114]. In contrast, most of the known cases of clozapine-associated NMS have been associated with the concomitant use of lithium. However, for the patient with treatment-resistant BD, adding or replacing clozapine in the regimen remains an important option if other mood stabilizers and antipsychotics have failed.

12.4 Special Populations

12.4.1 Pregnancy

Depression has been shown to adversely affect fetal development (low weight infants, small for gestational age infants, preterm birth, and lower APGAR scores). Although the direct effect of mania on fetal development is unknown, we know that it is associated with poor self-care, an increased risk of suicide, poor nutrition, impaired sleep, and a tendency to use drugs, alcohol, and tobacco.

Valproate should not be used to treat a woman during pregnancy because it is associated with a significant risk of birth defects, such as heart defects and neural tube defects, and combined with the development of polycystic ovary syndrome.

Another anticonvulsant that should not be used during pregnancy is topiramate that has recently been placed in category D because of an increased risk of cleft lip and/or cleft palate. Lithium is correlated with the development of Ebstein's anomaly of the cardiac tricuspid valve. The preferred mood stabilizer during pregnancy is lamotrigine, which does not appear to have an increased risk of serious birth defects. All SGAs belong to pregnancy category C except for lurasidone and Clozapine which belong to category B.

12.4.2 Breastfeeding

All psychotropic drugs are fat-soluble and dissolve easily in the adipose tissues, which is why they pass easily into the breast milk through passive diffusion in the cell membranes. The American Academy of Pediatrics (AAP) Drug Safety Committee has expressed concerns about the use of lithium during breastfeeding because it is passed in the breast milk at a rate of 50% of maternal serum levels. Some clinical cases have indicated adverse outcomes in children who have been exposed to lithium during breastfeeding. Carbamazepine levels were around 25–50% of maternal serum levels, and lamotrigine levels were around 30% of maternal serum levels, but the AAP Drug Safety Committee classified lamotrigine as "unknown but could be a concern." To date, however, there have been no cases of significant adverse events in newborns, including cases of Stevens-Johnson syndrome in infants. Valproate levels in infants were approximately 5% of maternal serum concentration; however, a case of anemia was reported in a child exposed to valproate while breastfeeding.

12.5 Maintenance of Bipolar Disorder

There are many reasons why patients abandon treatment along with some following risk factors for non-adherence:

- Age, with a higher frequency among the young and the elderly.
- Substance abuse and other associated psychiatric and medical conditions.
- Socio-economic barriers including lower income and lower education.

There have been two most effective strategies: evaluating the patient on the nature of his/her disorders and the benefits of treatment and motivational interview strategies. Successful treatment recognizes the importance of basing the clinical decisions on the available research and evidence-based medicine in this activity.

12 Psychopharmacological Recovery-Oriented Treatments in Bipolar Disorders

Therapeutic decisions must be based on a combination of available research, clinical judgment, and the therapist's acumen.

Unfortunately, patients with BD are at a very high risk of therapeutic non-compliance; in fact, almost two-thirds of patients do not respect drug treatment in the entire first year of treatment. Effective BD treatment requires patients' participation in agreeing to treatment goals, monitoring of response and possible side effects, evaluating their functioning levels, and recognizing and managing stressors in their lives. Effective treatment BD requires flexibility for all these reasons.

BD is a chronic disease with a high morbidity that tends to recur in the subject's life with a high frequency (about 90%) [115]. For this reason, maintenance therapy is indicated and recommended only after a single manic episode [24]. Further objectives of maintenance therapy include the prevention of recurrence, the optimization of biopsychosocial functioning for obtaining a complete recovery and mostly the prevention of suicide. It is a fact that the best way to treat an acute episode is to prevent it. Numerous medications have received the FDA's approval for monotherapy maintenance treatment, including lithium, lamotrigine, aripiprazole, olanzapine, and risperidone. The FDA has also approved quetiapine, ziprasidone, and asenapine for maintenance as an additional treatment with lithium or valproate. Some patients responded very well with monotherapy, but combination treatment is required in most cases. Patients should generally start monotherapy with a mood stabilizer. Those who do not undergo a complete remission of symptoms but only a partial response with monotherapy at the maximum tolerated dosage, or in the case of lithium or valproate, at the doses that guarantee a level within the therapeutic range, must receive combined treatment to keep the possible side effects under control.

Patients who experience breakthrough manic or hypomanic episodes while on maintenance treatment should receive effective medications, which should essentially contain all the antipsychotics and/or effective mood stabilizers. The breakthrough episodes of depression should be treated with medications that have demonstrated a higher efficiency for BD.

Quetiapine, approved in 2008 in combination with valproate or lithium for the maintenance treatment of BD-I, can be also associated with valproate or carbamazepine but poses greater risks of interaction [32]. The most common pharmacological association is of a mood stabilizer and an antipsychotic. There are few reasons to combine two antipsychotics: this solution can be considered only in the cases of patients who are ultra-resistant to treatment while paying close attention on monitoring the side effects that could also be serious, especially at the cardiovascular level. In the latter case, the risk-benefit ratio must be carefully considered along with the assessment of all the possible advantages and disadvantages.

Lithium is certainly the most widely studied drug in the maintenance treatment of BD. Serum lithium concentrations in the maintenance therapy are generally lower than those needed to produce efficacy in an acute manic episode. The optimal level of lithium for many patients will be considered as the level that balances the prevention of relapses and suppresses the subsyndromal symptoms as compared to the minimization of annoying everyday side effects. The lithium dose in maintenance treatment is controversial. Studies have shown that low levels such as

0.4–0.6 mEq/L are effective for maintenance; instead a controlled study found that patients who presented low lithium level (0.4–0.6 mEq/L) experienced more illness episodes than patients who presented standard lithium level (0.8–1 mEq/L), showing a higher rate of relapse (38% vs. 13%)" [116].

Two large 18-month placebo-controlled maintenance trials comparing *lamotrigine* (200–400 mg/day) and lithium (0.8–1.1 mEq/L) found lamotrigine, but not lithium, superior to placebo in preventing the depressive episodes [31, 32]. In contrast, lithium, but not lamotrigine, was superior to placebo in preventing the manic episodes.

The only randomized, placebo-controlled maintenance study of *valproate* in BD-I found no significant difference in time for the development of any mood episode among the patients receiving valproate, lithium, or placebo [117]. Calabrese et al. compared valproate and lithium in a 20-month study of patients with rapid cycling in BD and found comparable relapse rates in both the treatment groups [86]. To date, there are no clear data regarding the optimal concentration of valproic acid in maintenance therapy in BD. Usually, the current practice consists of titrating the therapeutic serum concentrations (50–125 µg/mL) and, as in lithium, balancing relapse and preventing subsyndromal symptoms against the minimization of side effects [24].

Among the BD maintenance treatments, the use of *olanzapine* is indicated to be superior to placebo in the prevention of manic and depressive episodes [118]. The combination of olanzapine with lithium or valproate has also shown to be more effective in preventing relapses than placebo, lithium, or valproate [41, 42].

Aripiprazole was superior to placebo in preventing the manic relapse over a 6-month follow-up period in the patients with BD who were initially stabilized on the aripiprazole monotherapy for an acute manic or mixed episode [33, 119]. In contrast, there was no significant difference between aripiprazole and placebo for the rates of depressive relapse.

A 6-month maintenance study found *ziprasidone* to be superior in prolonging the intervention time for a mood episode than placebo when it was used in combination with lithium or valproate and also in the proportion of patients who needed intervention during the study's duration [120].

Risperidone (long-acting injectable formulation) was encountered to be superior to placebo in the prevention of relapse, both as monotherapy and as adjunctive therapy [121, 122].

The extended release of *paliperidone* may be efficacious as a maintenance treatment in the patients with BD [123].

12.6 Prophylaxis of Bipolar Disorder

Although the use of antidepressants and antipsychotics is limited to the specific disease stages, the use of a mood stabilizer is considered as a standard maintenance therapy for most patients. Table 12.2 outlines the stepwise recommendations. Recent studies propose the combination of antidepressants and mood stabilizers as a

12 Psychopharmacological Recovery-Oriented Treatments in Bipolar Disorders 213

Table 12.2 Description of the main recommendations for the prophylaxis of patients with bipolar disorder both in pharmacological and psychoeducational terms

Recommendation for the prophylaxis of Bipolar Disorder
• In long-term treatment, it is necessary to use antimanic and antidepressant drugs to prevent the repetition of the disease phase. Lithium is considered as the gold standard drug.
• If lithium is not effective, then evaluate the association with valproate.
• If lithium is not tolerated, then evaluate valproate or olanzapine. Quetiapine should also be evaluated if it was effective during an episode of mania or bipolar depression.
• Avoid the use of valproate in the women of childbearing age.
• The efficacy and tolerability of antipsychotic drugs must be assessed until the clinical picture stabilizes.
• Perform psychoeducation on the importance of continuing treatment and self-monitoring on the possible prodromal symptoms of a relapse.
• Never stop a drug suddenly but only gradually and under medical supervision.
• Monitor symptoms for at least 2 years after stopping treatment.

maintenance strategy, and it may be important to prevent depressive relapse in some patients. The median duration of mood episodes in people with BD has reported to be 13 weeks, with a quarter of patients remaining ill for 1 year [124]. Residual symptoms after an acute episode are a strong predictor of recurrence [125].

Most of the evidence supports the application of lithium in the prevention of episodes of mania and depression [126–130]. Although lithium has the disadvantage of producing worsening results after its sudden interruption compared to other mood stabilizers [131–134], it has the advantage of a proven anti-suicide effect [135–138]. Among antiepileptics, carbamazepine is considered as the third-line approach and appears to be the least effective [139].

The long-term use of valproate appears uncertain [140]. The BALANCE study found that the individual use of valproate was less effective than lithium or the combination of lithium and valproate [141]. A large observational study, in fact, has shown that lithium is much more effective than valproate in preventing relapse in any condition and in preventing re-hospitalization [142]. Some SGAs such as olanzapine [129], quetiapine [143], aripiprazole [144, 145], and risperidone [146] have also proven to be more effective than valproate. It is no coincidence, in fact, that among these SGAs, the first three have received approval for the prophylaxis of BD. The use of long-acting injection (LAI) of FGAs and SGAs probably plays an important role in the prevention of mania, especially in the subjects who are not compliant with drug therapy but can have a negative effect on depressive symptoms [147].

The use of polypharmacy must always be calibrated with the possible increase in adverse effects. The National Institute for Health and Care Excellence and the most recent British Association for Psychopharmacology guidelines recommend the combinations of olanzapine, risperidone, quetiapine, or haloperidol with lithium or valproate. Antipsychotics such as aripiprazole are also viable options when combined with lithium or valproate, particularly if they have been proven effective during the treatment of an acute episode of mania or depression [31, 131]. Lurasidone may have a substantially similar long-term efficacy, both in monotherapy and in combination with a mood stabilizer [148] (Table 12.3).

Table 12.3 First-, second-, and third-line treatments in the prevention of relapses in the patient with bipolar disorder

Prophylaxis in bipolar disorder	First line	Lithium
	Second line	Valproate (not in women of childbearing potential), olanzapine, aripiprazole, risperidone, or quetiapine
	Third line	Alternative antipsychotics that have been effective during an acute episode: carbamazepine, lurasidone, and lamotrigine
	• Always maintain successful acute treatment regimens (e.g., mood stabilizer + antipsychotic) as prophylaxis • Avoid long-term antidepressants if possible	

12.6.1 Antipsychotic Long-Acting Injections in Bipolar Disorder

LAIs are widely used in BD; however, none of them are formally authorized for this indication. LAIs of risperidone and aripiprazole are strongly associated with a reduced risk of high mood recurrence as compared to placebo but have a little effect on the risk of depressive recurrence; however, risperidone may be less effective than the oral administration of olanzapine [149]. It can be effective as a single treatment or as an adjuvant, but it only provides protection against manic, hypomanic, and mixed episodes, and does not decrease or increase the risk of depressive recurrence.

The LAI of aripiprazole has proven effective in reducing the frequency and recurrence of manic episodes, but it is also extremely useful for BD-I prophylaxis with an effect mainly on the prevention of manic episodes [150]. Moreover, it is generally safe and well tolerated, and does not adversely affect the risk of depression.

The support for using FGA-LAIs in BD is currently weak, and very limited evidence suggests that FGA-LAIs may be effective in reducing the recurrence of high mood but do not prevent the recurrence of depression and may indeed increase the risk. The largest (open) study ($n = 85$) suggested that flupentixol decanoate (20 mg every 2–3 weeks) reduces the risk of recurrence of manic episodes and there are also other reports that describe similar effects for other LAIs of FGA. However, the only RCT conducted with the LAI form of flupentixol showed no effect and superiority over lithium [151].

Oral paliperidone is useful in the prevention of manic phases as well as its LAI formulation. It could be assumed that the LAI of paliperidone has similar effects as the LAI of risperidone [152, 153].

12.7 Conclusions

The introduction of the first psychotropic drugs in the 1950s had numerous direct and future consequences. Moreover, lithium salts have played a fundamental role in producing these results [154–158]. On a purely scientific level, they favored the postulate of the first biological hypotheses on the genesis of mental illnesses,

12 Psychopharmacological Recovery-Oriented Treatments in Bipolar Disorders

thus giving rise to the so-called "biological psychiatry." From the historical point of view, another important contribution of the clinical introduction of lithium and FGAs resides at the level of health care, giving rise to the progressive phenomenon of "deinstitutionalization" in psychiatry. This fact mitigated the component of the stigma that had accompanied psychiatric care. In this sense, the FGAs not only allowed patients to leave psychiatric hospitals, but also helped their socialization.

References

1. Delaney KR. Moving to a recovery framework of care: focusing attention on process. Arch Psychiatr Nurs. 2012;26(2):165–6. https://doi.org/10.1016/j.apnu.2011.12.005.
2. Glick ID, Sharfstein SS, Schwartz HI. Inpatient psychiatric care in the 21st century: the need for reform. Psychiatr Serv. 2011;62(2):206–9. https://doi.org/10.1176/ps.62.2.pss6202_0206.
3. Shepherd G, Boardman J, Slade M. Making recovery a reality. London: Sainsbury Centre for Mental Health; 2008. p. 1–3.
4. Mental Health Foundation. Prevention review: landscape paper. London; 2016. https://www.mentalhealth.org.uk/publications/prevention-review.
5. Korsbek L. How to recover? Recovery in Denmark: a work in progress. J Recovery Mental Health. 2011;1(1):25–33.
6. The Regional Council. Visions for the future of mental health service. Copenhagen; 2016. http://www.psykiatri-regionh.dk/NR/rdonlyres/97E44B23-FCC0-4C7F-A62BE9580913925D/0/Visioner_Katalog_lilla_version.pdf.
7. Roosenschoon BJ, Kamperman AM, Deen ML, van Weeghel J, Mulder CL. Determinants of clinical, functional and personal recovery for people with schizophrenia and other severe mental illnesses: a cross-sectional analysis. PLoS One. 2019;14(9):e0222378.
8. Davidson L, O'Connell M, Tondora J, Styron T, Kangas K. The top ten concerns about recovery encountered in mental health system transformation. Psychiatr Serv. 2006;57(5):640–5. https://doi.org/10.1176/ps.2006.57.5.640.
9. Spaulding WD, Montague E, Avila A, Sullivan ME. The idea of recovery. In: Singh N, Barber JW, Van Sant S, editors. Handbook of recovery in inpatient psychiatry. Cham: Springer. p. 3–38.
10. Bellack AS. Scientific and consumer models of recovery in schizophrenia: concordance, contrasts, and implications. Schizophr Bull. 2006;32(3):432–42. https://doi.org/10.1093/schbul/sbj044.
11. Liberman RP, Kopelowicz A. Recovery from schizophrenia: a challenge for the 21st century. Schizophr Bull. 2009;35(2):370–80. https://doi.org/10.1093/schbul/sbn175.
12. Silverstein SM, Bellack AS. A scientific agenda for the concept of recovery as it applies to schizophrenia. Clin Psychol Rev. 2008;28(7):1108–24. https://doi.org/10.1016/j.cpr.2008.03.004.
13. Spaniol L, Wewiorski NJ, Gagne C, Anthony WA. The process of recovery from schizophrenia. Int Rev Psychiatry. 2002;14(4):327–36.
14. Borg M, Davidson L. The nature of recovery as lived-in everyday experience. J Ment Health. 2008;17(2):129–40.
15. Schön UK, Denhov A, Topor A. Social relationships as a decisive factor in recovering from severe mental illness. Int J Soc Psychiatry. 2009;55(4):336–47. https://doi.org/10.1177/0020764008093686.
16. Farkas M, Gagne C, Anthony W, Chamberlin J. Implementing recovery-oriented evidence based programs: identifying the critical dimensions. Community Ment Health J. 2005;41(2):141–58. https://doi.org/10.1007/s10597-005-2649-6.
17. Drake RE, Essock SM. The science-to-service gap in real-world schizophrenia treatment: the 95% problem. Schizophr Bull. 2009;35(4):677–8. https://doi.org/10.1093/schbul/sbp047.

18. Vita A, Barlati S. The implementation of evidence-based psychiatric rehabilitation: challenges and opportunities for mental health services. Front Psych. 2019;10:147. https://doi.org/10.3389/fpsyt.2019.00147.
19. Schatzberg AF, Charles DeBattista DMH. Schatzberg's manual of clinical psychopharmacology. 9th ed. Washington, DC: American Psychiatric Association Publication; 2019. p. 3–8.
20. Calabrese JR, Rapport DJ. Mood stabilizers and the evolution of maintenance study designs in bipolar I disorder. J Clin Psychiatry. 1999;60(Suppl 5):5–13; discussion 14–5.
21. Ghaemi SN. New treatments for bipolar disorder: the role of atypical neuroleptic agents. J Clin Psychiatry. 2000;61(Suppl 14):33–42.
22. Sachs GS. Bipolar mood disorder: practical strategies for acute and maintenance phase treatment. J Clin Psychopharmacol. 1996;16(2 Suppl 1):32S–47S. https://doi.org/10.1097/00004714-199604001-00005.
23. Bowden CL. New concepts in mood stabilization: evidence for the effectiveness of valproate and lamotrigine. Neuropsychopharmacology. 1998;19(3):194–9.
24. Hirschfeld RM, Bowden CL, Gitlin MJ, et al. Practice guideline for the treatment of patients with bipolar disorder (revision). Am J Psychiatry. 2002;159(4 suppl):1–50.
25. Stokes PE, Kocsis JH, Arcuni OJ. Relationship of lithium chloride dose to treatment response in acute mania. Arch Gen Psychiatry. 1976;33(9):1080–4.
26. Allen MH, Hirschfeld RM, Wozniak PJ, Baker JD, Bowden CL. Linear relationship of valproate serum concentration to response and optimal serum levels for acute mania. Am J Psychiatry. 2006;163(2):272–5. https://doi.org/10.1176/appi.ajp.163.2.272.
27. Baird-Gunning J, Lea-Henry T, Hoegberg LCG, Gosselin S, Roberts DM. Lithium poisoning. J Intensive Care Med. 2017;32(4):249–63. https://doi.org/10.1177/0885066616651582.
28. Müller-Oerlinghausen B, Retzow A, Henn FA, Giedke H, Walden J, European Valproate Mania Study Group. Valproate as an adjunct to neuroleptic medication for the treatment of acute episodes of mania: a prospective, randomized, double-blind, placebo-controlled, multicenter study. J Clin Psychopharmacol. 2000;20(2):195–203.
29. Takezaki H. The use of carbamazepine (Tegretol) in the control of manic depressive psychosis and other manic depressive states. Seishin Igaku. 1971;13:1310–8.
30. Hollister LE. Stability of psychiatric diagnoses among acutely ill patients. Psychopathology. 1992;25(4):204–8.
31. Bowden CL, Calabrese JR, Sachs G, Yatham LN, Asghar SA, Hompland M, et al. A placebo-controlled 18-month trial of lamotrigine and lithium maintenance treatment in recently manic or hypomanic patients with bipolar I disorder. J Clin Psychiatry. 2003;64(9):1013–24. https://doi.org/10.4088/jcp.v64n0906.
32. Calabrese JR, Vieta E, Shelton MD. Latest maintenance data on lamotrigine in bipolar disorder. Eur Neuropsychopharmacol. 2003;13(Suppl 2):S57–66.
33. Cuomo A, Crescenzi B, Goracci A, Bolognesi S, Giordano N, et al. Drug safety evaluation of aripiprazole in bipolar disorder. Expert Opin Drug Saf. 2019;18(6):455–63. https://doi.org/10.1080/14740338.2019.1617847.
34. Cramer JA, Mintzer S, Wheless J, Mattson RH. Adverse effects of antiepileptic drugs: a brief overview of important issues. Expert Rev Neurother. 2010;10(6):885–91.
35. Vieta E. Diagnosis and classification of psychiatric disorders. In: Sussman N, editor. Anticonvulsants in psychiatry. London: The Royal Society of Medicine Press; 1999. p. 3–8.
36. Post RM, Frye MA, Leverich GS, Denicoff KD. The role of complex combination therapy in the treatment of refractory bipolar illness. CNS Spectr. 1998;3(5):66–86.
37. Perlis RH. Treatment of bipolar disorder: the evolving role of atypical antipsychotics. Am J Manag Care. 2007;13(7 Suppl):S178–88.
38. Goikolea JM, Colom F, Torres I, Capapey J, Valentí M, Undurraga J, et al. Lower rate of depressive switch following antimanic treatment with second-generation antipsychotics versus haloperidol. J Affect Disord. 2013;144(3):191–8. https://doi.org/10.1016/j.jad.2012.07.038.
39. Tohen M, Sanger TM, McElroy SL, Tollefson GD, Chengappa KR, Daniel DG, et al. Olanzapine versus placebo in the treatment of acute mania. Am J Psychiatry. 1999;156(5):702–9. https://doi.org/10.1176/ajp.156.5.702.

12 Psychopharmacological Recovery-Oriented Treatments in Bipolar Disorders

40. Tohen M, Jacobs TG, Grundy SL, McElroy SL, Banov MC, Janicak PG, et al. Efficacy of olanzapine in acute bipolar mania: a double-blind, placebo-controlled study. Arch Gen Psychiatry. 2000;57(9):841–9. https://doi.org/10.1001/archpsyc.57.9.841.
41. Tohen M, Chengappa KR, Suppes T, Zarate CA, Calabrese JR, Bowden CL, et al. Efficacy of olanzapine in combination with valproate or lithium in the treatment of mania in patients partially nonresponsive to valproate or lithium monotherapy. Arch Gen Psychiatry. 2002;59(1):62–9. https://doi.org/10.1001/archpsyc.59.1.62.
42. Tohen M, Chengappa KR, Suppes T, Baker RW, Zarate CA, Bowden CL, et al. Relapse prevention in bipolar I disorder: 18-month comparison of olanzapine plus mood stabiliser v. mood stabiliser alone. Br J Psychiatry. 2004;184:337–45. https://doi.org/10.1192/bjp.184.4.337.
43. Fagiolini A, Coluccia A, Maina G, Forgione RN, Goracci A, Cuomo A, et al. Diagnosis, epidemiology and management of mixed states in bipolar disorder. CNS Drugs. 2015;29(9):725–40. https://doi.org/10.1007/s40263-015-0275-6.
44. Sanger TM, Grundy SL, Gibson PJ, Namjoshi MA, Greaney MG, Tohen MF. Long-term olanzapine therapy in the treatment of bipolar I disorder: an open-label continuation phase study. J Clin Psychiatry. 2001;62(4):273–81. https://doi.org/10.4088/jcp.v62n0410.
45. Vieta E, Reinares M, Corbella B, Benabarre A, Gilaberte I, Colom F, et al. Olanzapine as long-term adjunctive therapy in treatment-resistant bipolar disorder. J Clin Psychopharmacol. 2001;21(5):469–73. https://doi.org/10.1097/00004714-200110000-00002.
46. Berk M, Ichim L, Brook S. Olanzapine compared to lithium in mania: a double-blind randomized controlled trial. Int Clin Psychopharmacol. 1999;14(6):339–43. https://doi.org/10.1097/00004850-199911000-00003.
47. Niufan G, Tohen M, Qiuqing A, Fude Y, Pope E, McElroy H, et al. Olanzapine versus lithium in the acute treatment of bipolar mania: a double-blind, randomized, controlled trial. J Affect Disord. 2010;122(3):273–6.
48. Tohen M, Greil W, Calabrese JR, et al. Olanzapine versus lithium in the maintenance treatment of bipolar disorder: a 12-month, randomized, double-blind, controlled clinical trial. Am J Psychiatry. 2005;162(7):1281–90. https://doi.org/10.1176/appi.ajp.162.7.1281.
49. Tohen M, Baker RW, Altshuler LL, Zarate CA, Suppes T, Ketter TA, et al. Olanzapine versus divalproex in the treatment of acute mania. Am J Psychiatry. 2002;159(6):1011–7. https://doi.org/10.1176/appi.ajp.159.6.1011.
50. Tohen M, Vieta E, Goodwin GM, Sun B, Amsterdam JD, Banov M, et al. Olanzapine versus divalproex versus placebo in the treatment of mild to moderate mania: a randomized, 12-week, double-blind study. J Clin Psychiatry. 2008;69(11):1776–89. https://doi.org/10.4088/jcp.v69n1113. Epub 2008 Oct 7.
51. Yatham LN, Beaulieu S, Schaffer A, Kauer-Sant'Anna M, Kapczinski F, Lafer B, et al. Optimal duration of risperidone or olanzapine adjunctive therapy to mood stabilizer following remission of a manic episode: a CANMAT randomized double-blind trial. Mol Psychiatry. 2016;21(8):1050–6. https://doi.org/10.1038/mp.2015.158. Epub 2015 Oct 13.
52. Hirschfeld RM, Keck PE Jr, Kramer M, Karcher K, Canuso C, et al. Rapid antimanic effect of risperidone monotherapy: a 3-week multicenter, double-blind, placebo-controlled trial. Am J Psychiatry. 2004;161(6):1057–65. https://doi.org/10.1176/appi.ajp.161.6.1057.
53. Khanna S, Vieta E, Lyons B, Grossman F, Eerdekens M, Kramer M. Risperidone in the treatment of acute mania: double-blind, placebo-controlled study. Br J Psychiatry. 2005;187:229–34. https://doi.org/10.1192/bjp.187.3.229.
54. Perlis RH, Welge JA, Vornik LA, Hirschfeld RM, Keck PE Jr. Atypical antipsychotics in the treatment of mania: a meta-analysis of randomized, placebo-controlled trials. J Clin Psychiatry. 2005;67(4):509–16.
55. Smulevich AB, Khanna S, Eerdekens M, Karcher K, Kramer M, Grossman F. Acute and continuation risperidone monotherapy in bipolar mania: a 3-week placebo-controlled trial followed by a 9-week double-blind trial of risperidone and haloperidol. Eur Neuropsychopharmacol. 2005;15(1):75–84.
56. Yatham LN, Grossman F, Augustyns I, Vieta E, Ravindran A. Mood stabilisers plus risperidone or placebo in the treatment of acute mania: international, double-blind, randomised controlled trial. Br J Psychiatry. 2003;182:141–7. https://doi.org/10.1192/bjp.182.2.141.

57. Bowden CL, Grunze H, Mullen J, Brecher M, Paulsson B, Jones M, et al. A randomized, double-blind, placebo-controlled efficacy and safety study of quetiapine or lithium as monotherapy for mania in bipolar disorder. J Clin Psychiatry. 2005;66(1):111–21. https://doi.org/10.4088/jcp.v66n0116.
58. McIntyre RS, Brecher M, Paulsson B, Huizar K, Mullen J. Quetiapine or haloperidol as monotherapy for bipolar mania—a 12-week, double-blind, randomised, parallel-group, placebo-controlled trial. Eur Neuropsychopharmacol. 2005;15(5):573–85. https://doi.org/10.1016/j.euroneuro.2005.02.006. Epub 2005 Apr 18.
59. Li H, Ma C, Wang G, Zhu X, Peng M, Gu N. Response and remission rates in Chinese patients with bipolar mania treated for 4 weeks with either quetiapine or lithium: a randomized and double-blind study. Curr Med Res Opin. 2008;24(1):1–10. https://doi.org/10.1185/030079908x253933.
60. Vieta E, Mullen J, Brecher M, Paulsson B, Jones M. Quetiapine monotherapy for mania associated with bipolar disorder: combined analysis of two international, double-blind, randomised, placebo-controlled studies. Curr Med Res Opin. 2005;21(6):923–34. https://doi.org/10.1185/030079905X46340.
61. Fagiolini A, Bolognesi S, Goracci A, Beccarini Crescenzi B, Cuomo A. Principi di farmacodinamica e farmacocinetica nello switch tra antipsicotici: focus su cariprazina. Riv Psichiatr. 2019;54(6):1–6. https://doi.org/10.1708/3340.33095.
62. Potkin SG, Keck PE Jr, Segal S, Ice K, English P. Ziprasidone in acute bipolar mania: a 21-day randomized, double-blind, placebo-controlled replication trial. J Clin Psychopharmacol. 2005;25(4):301–10. https://doi.org/10.1097/01.jcp.0000169068.34322.70.
63. Keck PE, Orsulak PJ, Cutler AJ, Sanchez R, Torbeyns A, Marcus RN, et al. Aripiprazole monotherapy in the treatment of acute bipolar I mania: a randomized, double-blind, placebo- and lithium-controlled study. J Affect Disord. 2009;112(1–3):36–49. https://doi.org/10.1016/j.jad.2008.05.014. Epub 2008 Oct 2.
64. Sachs G, Sanchez R, Marcus R, Stock E, McQuade R, Carson W, et al. Aripiprazole in the treatment of acute manic or mixed episodes in patients with bipolar I disorder: a 3-week placebo-controlled study. J Psychopharmacol. 2006;20(4):536–46. https://doi.org/10.1177/0269881106059693. Epub 2006 Jan 9.
65. McIntyre RS, Cohen M, Zhao J, Alphs L, Macek TA, Panagides J. Asenapine in the treatment of acute mania in bipolar I disorder: a randomized, double-blind, placebo-controlled trial. J Affect Disord. 2010;122:27–38.
66. McIntyre RS, Cohen M, Zhao J, Alphs L, Macek TA, Panagides J. Asenapine versus olanzapine in acute mania: a double-blind extension study. Bipolar Disord. 2009;11(1):815–26.
67. McIntyre RS, Cohen M, Zhao J, Alphs L, Macek TA, Panagides J. Asenapine for long-term treatment of bipolar disorder: a double-blind 40-week extension study. J Affect Disord. 2010;126:358–65.
68. Kemp DE, et al. Weight change and metabolic effects of asenapine in patients with schizophrenia and bipolar disorder. J Clin Psychiatry. 2014;75:238–45.
69. Lao KS, He Y, Wong ICK, Besag FMC, Chan EW. Tolerability and safety profile of cariprazine in treating psychotic disorders, bipolar disorder and major depressive disorder: a systematic review with meta-analysis of randomized controlled trials. CNS Drugs. 2016;30:1043–54.
70. Sachs GS, Greenberg WM, Starace A, Lu K, Ruth A, Laszlovszky I. Cariprazine in the treatment of acute mania in bipolar I disorder: a double-blind, placebo-controlled, phase III trial. J Affect Disord. 2015;174:296–302. https://doi.org/10.1016/j.jad.2014.11.018. Epub 2014 Nov 24.
71. Calabrese JR, Keck PE Jr, Starace A, Lu K, Ruth A, Laszlovszky I. Efficacy and safety of low- and high-dose cariprazine in acute and mixed mania associated with bipolar I disorder: a double-blind, placebo-controlled study. J Clin Psychiatry. 2015;76(3):284–92. https://doi.org/10.4088/JCP.14m09081.
72. Calabrese JR, Shelton MD, Rapport DJ, Kujawa M, Kimmel SE, Caban S. Current research on rapid cycling bipolar disorder and its treatment. J Affect Disord. 2001;67(1–3):241–55. https://doi.org/10.1016/s0165-0327(98)00161-x.

73. Kupka RW, Luckenbaugh DA, Post RM, Leverich GS, Nolen WA. Rapid and non-rapid cycling bipolar disorder: a meta-analysis of clinical studies. J Clin Psychiatry. 2003;64(12):1483–94. https://doi.org/10.4088/jcp.v64n1213.
74. Coryell W, Solomon D, Turvey C, Keller M, Leon AC, Endicott J, et al. The long-term course of rapid-cycling bipolar disorder. Arch Gen Psychiatry. 2003;60(9):914–20. https://doi.org/10.1001/archpsyc.60.9.914.
75. Calabrese JR, Rapport DJ, Youngstrom EA, Jackson K, Bilali S, Findling RL. New data on the use of lithium, divalproate, and lamotrigine in rapid cycling bipolar disorder. Eur Psychiatry. 2005;20(2):92–5. https://doi.org/10.1016/j.eurpsy.2004.12.003.
76. Kemp DE, Gao K, Ganocy SJ, Rapport DJ, Elhaj O, Bilali S, et al. A 6-month, double-blind, maintenance trial of lithium monotherapy versus the combination of lithium and divalproex for rapid-cycling bipolar disorder and co-occurring substance abuse or dependence. J Clin Psychiatry. 2009;70(1):113–21. https://doi.org/10.4088/jcp.07m04022. Epub 2008 Dec 30.
77. Post RM, Frye MA, Denicoff KD, Leverich GS, Dunn RT, Osuch EA, et al. Emerging trends in the treatment of rapid cycling bipolar disorder: a selected review. Bipolar Disord. 2000;2(4):305–15. https://doi.org/10.1034/j.1399-5618.2000.020403.x.
78. Calabrese JR, Suppes T, Bowden CL, Sachs GS, Swann AC, McElroy SL, et al. A double-blind, placebo-controlled, prophylaxis study of lamotrigine in rapid-cycling bipolar disorder. J Clin Psychiatry. 2000;61(11):841–50. https://doi.org/10.4088/jcp.v61n1106.
79. Young LT, Joffe RT, Robb JC, MacQueen GM, Marriott M, Patelis-Siotis I. Double-blind comparison of addition of a second mood stabilizer versus an antidepressant to an initial mood stabilizer for treatment of patients with bipolar depression. Am J Psychiatry. 2000;157(1):124–6. https://doi.org/10.1176/ajp.157.1.124.
80. Thase ME, Sachs GS. Bipolar depression: pharmacotherapy and related therapeutic strategies. Biol Psychiatry. 2000;48(6):558–72. https://doi.org/10.1016/s0006-3223(00)00980-x.
81. Barbato A, Bossini L, Calugi S, D'Avanzo B, Fagiolini A, Koukouna D, et al. Validation of the Italian version of the Functioning Assessment Short Test (FAST) for bipolar disorder. Epidemiol Psychiatr Sci 2013;22(2):187–194. DOI: https://doi.org/10.1017/S2045796012000522. Epub 2012 Sep 19..
82. Hirschfeld R, Montgomery SA, Aguglia E, Amore M, Delgado PL, Gastpar M, et al. Partial response and nonresponse to antidepressant therapy: current approaches and treatment options. J Clin Psychiatry. 2002;63(9):826–37. https://doi.org/10.4088/jcp.v63n0913.
83. Sachs GS, Lafer B, Stoll AL, Banov M, Thibault AB, Tohen M, et al. A double-blind trial of bupropion versus desipramine for bipolar depression. J Clin Psychiatry. 1994;55(9):391–3.
84. Nemeroff CB, Evans DL, Gyulai L, Sachs GS, Bowden CL, Gergel IP, et al. Double-blind, placebo-controlled comparison of imipramine and paroxetine in the treatment of bipolar depression. Am J Psychiatry. 2001;158(6):906–12. https://doi.org/10.1176/appi.ajp.158.6.906.
85. Sachs GS, Nierenberg AA, Calabrese JR, Marangell LB, Wisniewski SR, Gyulai L, et al. Effectiveness of adjunctive antidepressant treatment for bipolar depression. N Engl J Med. 2007;356(17):1711–22.
86. Calabrese JR, Keck PE Jr, MacFadden W, Minkwitz M, Ketter TA, Weisler RH, et al. A randomized, double-blind, placebo-controlled trial of quetiapine in the treatment of bipolar I or II depression. Am J Psychiatry. 2005;162(7):1351–60. https://doi.org/10.1176/appi.ajp.162.7.1351.
87. McElroy SL, Weisler RH, Chang W, Olausson B, Paulsson B, Brecher M, et al. A double-blind, placebo-controlled study of quetiapine and paroxetine as monotherapy in adults with bipolar depression (EMBOLDEN II). J Clin Psychiatry. 2010;71(2):163–74. https://doi.org/10.4088/JCP.08m04942gre. Epub 2010 Jan 26.
88. Rush AJ, Trivedi MH, Wisniewski SR, Nierenberg AA, Stewart JW, Warden D, et al. Acute and longer-term outcomes in depressed outpatients requiring one or several treatment steps: a STAR*D report. Am J Psychiatry. 2006;163(11):1905–17. https://doi.org/10.1176/ajp.2006.163.11.1905.

89. López-Muñoz F, Álamo C. Active metabolites as antidepressant drugs: the role of norquetiapine in the mechanism of action of quetiapine in the treatment of mood disorders. Front Psych. 2013;4:102. https://doi.org/10.3389/fpsyt.2013.00102.

90. Miranda ASD, Moreira FA, Teixeira AL. The preclinical discovery and development of quetiapine for the treatment of mania and depression. Expert Opin Drug Discov. 2017;12(5):525–35. https://doi.org/10.1080/17460441.2017.1304378. Epub 2017 Mar 14.

91. Loebel A, Cucchiaro J, Silva R, Kroger H, Sarma K, Xu J, Calabrese JR. Lurasidone as adjunctive therapy with lithium or valproate for the treatment of bipolar I depression: a randomized, double-blind, placebo-controlled study. Am J Psychiatry. 2014;171(2):169–77. https://doi.org/10.1176/appi.ajp.2013.13070985.

92. Loebel A, Xu J, Hsu J, Cucchiaro J, Pikalov A. The development of lurasidone for bipolar depression. Ann N Y Acad Sci. 2015;1358:95–104. https://doi.org/10.1111/nyas.12965.

93. Ishibashi T, Horisawa T, Tokuda K, Ishiyama T, Ogasa M, Tagashira R, et al. Pharmacological profile of lurasidone, a novel antipsychotic agent with potent 5-hydroxytryptamine 7 (5-HT7) and 5-HT1A receptor activity. J Pharmacol Exp Ther. 2010;334(1):171–81. https://doi.org/10.1124/jpet.110.167346. Epub 2010 Apr 19.

94. Cates LN, Roberts AJ, Huitron-Resendiz S, Hedlund PB. Effects of lurasidone in behavioral models of depression. Role of the 5-HT7 receptor subtype. Neuropharmacology. 2013;70:211–7. https://doi.org/10.1016/j.neuropharm.2013.01.023. Epub 2013 Feb 13.

95. Nasrallah HA, Cucchiaro J, Mao Y, Pikalov AA, Loebel AD. Lurasidone for the treatment of depressive symptoms in schizophrenia: analysis of 4 pooled, 6-week, placebo-controlled studies. CNS Spectr. 2015;20(2):140–7. https://doi.org/10.1017/S1092852914000285. Epub 2014 Jun 23.

96. Tohen M, Vieta E, Calabrese J, et al. Efficacy of olanzapine and olanzapine-fluoxetine combination in the treatment of bipolar I depression. Arch Gen Psychiatry. 2003;60:1079–88. https://doi.org/10.1001/archpsyc.60.11.1079.

97. Keck PE Jr, Corya SA, Altshuler LL, et al. Analyses of treatment-emergent mania with olanzapine/fluoxetine combination in the treatment of bipolar depression. J Clin Psychiatry. 2005;66:611–6. https://doi.org/10.4088/jcp.v66n0511.

98. Bowden CL, Singh V, Weisler R, Thompson P, Chang X, Quinones M, et al. Lamotrigine vs. lamotrigine plus divalproex in randomized, placebo-controlled maintenance treatment for bipolar depression. Acta Psychiatr Scand. 2012;126(5):342–50. https://doi.org/10.1111/j.1600-0447.2012.01890.x. Epub 2012 Jun 18.

99. Calabrese JR, Bowden CL, Sachs GS, Ascher JA, Monaghan E, Rudd GD. A double-blind placebo-controlled study of lamotrigine monotherapy in outpatients with bipolar I depression. J Clin Psychiatry. 1999;60(2):79–88. https://doi.org/10.4088/jcp.v60n0203.

100. van der Loos ML, Mulder PG, Hartong EGTM, Blom MB, Vergouwen AC, de Keyzer HJ, et al. Efficacy and safety of lamotrigine as add-on treatment to lithium in bipolar depression: a multicenter, double-blind, placebo-controlled trial. J Clin Psychiatry. 2009;70(2):223–31. https://doi.org/10.4088/jcp.08m04152. Epub 2008 Dec 30.

101. Singh V, Arnold JG, Prihoda TJ, Martinez M, Bowden CL. An open trial of iloperidone for mixed episodes in bipolar disorder. J Clin Psychopharmacol. 2017;37(5):615–9.

102. Houston JP, Ahl J, Meyers AL, Kaiser CJ, Tohen M, Baldessarini RJ. Reduced suicidal ideation in bipolar I disorder mixed-episode patients in a placebo-controlled trial of olanzapine combined with lithium or divalproex. J Clin Psychiatry. 2006;67(8):1246–52. https://doi.org/10.4088/jcp.v67n0811.

103. Dardennes R, Even C, Bange F, Heim A. Comparison of carbamazepine and lithium in the prophylaxis of bipolar disorders: a meta-analysis. Br J Psychiatry. 1995;166(3):378–81. https://doi.org/10.1192/bjp.166.3.378.

104. Keck PE Jr, McElroy SL. Outcome in the pharmacologic treatment of bipolar disorder. J Clin Psychopharmacol. 1996;16(2 Suppl 1):15S–23S. https://doi.org/10.1097/00004714-199604001-00003.

105. Macritchie KAN, Geddes JR, Scott J, Haslam DR, Goodwin GM. Valproic acid, valproate and divalproex in the maintenance treatment of bipolar disorder. Cochrane Database Syst Rev. 2013;2013(10):CD003196. https://doi.org/10.1002/14651858.CD003196.pub2.
106. Peselow ED, Fieve RR, Difiglia C, Sanfilipo MP. Lithium prophylaxis of bipolar illness: the value of combination treatment. Br J Psychiatry. 1994;164(2):208–14. https://doi.org/10.1192/bjp.164.2.208.
107. Steckler TL. Lithium- and carbamazepine-associated sinus node dysfunction: nine-year experience in a psychiatric hospital. J Clin Psychopharmacol. 1994;14(5):336–9.
108. Juruena MF, Ottoni GL, Machado-Vieira R, Carneiro RM, Weingarthner N, Marquardt AR, et al. Bipolar I and II disorder residual symptoms: oxcarbazepine and carbamazepine as add-on treatment to lithium in a double-blind, randomized trial. Prog Neuro-Psychopharmacol Biol Psychiatry. 2009;33(1):94–9. https://doi.org/10.1016/j.pnpbp.2008.10.012. Epub 2008 Oct 31.
109. Kramlinger KG, Post RM. Addition of lithium carbonate to carbamazepine: hematological and thyroid effects. Am J Psychiatry. 1990;147(5):615–20. https://doi.org/10.1176/ajp.147.5.615.
110. Lipinski JF, Pope HG. Possible synergistic action between carbamazepine and lithium carbonate in the treatment of three acutely manic patients. Am J Psychiatry. 1982;139(7):948–9. https://doi.org/10.1176/ajp.139.7.948.
111. Vieta E, Manuel JG, Martínez-Arán A, Comes M, Verger K, Masramon X, et al. A double-blind, randomized, placebo-controlled, prophylaxis study of adjunctive gabapentin for bipolar disorder. J Clin Psychiatry. 2006;67(3):473–7. https://doi.org/10.4088/jcp.v67n0320.
112. Calabrese JR, Kimmel SE, Woyshville MJ, Rapport DJ, Faust CJ. Clozapine in treatment-refractory mania. Am J Psychiatry. 1996;153(6):759–64. https://doi.org/10.1176/ajp.153.6.759.
113. Drake RE, Xie H, McHugo GJ, Green AI. The effects of clozapine on alcohol and drug use disorders among patients with schizophrenia. Schizophr Bull. 2000;26(2):441–9. https://doi.org/10.1093/oxfordjournals.schbul.a033464.
114. Adityanjee. Modification of clozapine-induced leukopenia and neutropenia with lithium carbonate (letter). Am J Psychiatry. 1995;152(4):648–9. https://doi.org/10.1176/ajp.152.4.648.
115. Goodwin FK, Jamison KR. Manic-depressive illness. Bipolar disorders and recurrent depression. Oxford: Oxford University Press; 2007.
116. Gelenberg AJ, Kane JM, Keller MB, Lavori P, Rosenbaum JF, Cole K, Lavelle J. Comparison of standard and low serum levels of lithium for maintenance treatment of bipolar disorder. N Engl J Med. 1989;321:1489–93. https://doi.org/10.1056/NEJM198911303212201.
117. Malhi GS, Mitchell PB, Salim S. Bipolar depression. CNS Drugs. 2000;17(1):9–25.
118. Tohen M, Calabrese JR, Sachs GS, Banov MD, Detke HC, Risser R, et al. Randomized, placebo-controlled trial of olanzapine as maintenance therapy in patients with bipolar I disorder responding to acute treatment with olanzapine. Am J Psychiatry. 2006;163(2):247–56.
119. McElroy SL, Suppes T, Frye MA, Altshuler LL, Stanford K, Martens B, et al. Open-label aripiprazole in the treatment of acute bipolar depression: a prospective pilot trial. J Affect Disord. 2007;101(1–3):275–81. https://doi.org/10.1016/j.jad.2006.11.025. Epub 2007 Jan 16.
120. Bowden CL. The role of ziprasidone in adjunctive use with lithium or valproate in maintenance treatment of bipolar disorder. Neuropsychiatr Dis Treat. 2011;7:87–92. https://doi.org/10.2147/NDT.S9932. Epub 2011 Mar 7.
121. Quiroz JA, Yatham LN, Palumbo JM, Karcher K, Kushner S, Kusumakar V. Risperidone long-acting injectable monotherapy in the maintenance treatment of bipolar I disorder. Biol Psychiatry. 2010;68(2):156–62. https://doi.org/10.1016/j.biopsych.2010.01.015. Epub 2010 Mar 15.
122. Popovic D, Reinares M, Goikolea JM, Bonnin CM, Gonzalez-Pinto A, Vieta E. Polarity index of pharmacological agents used for maintenance treatment of bipolar disorder. Eur Neuropsychopharmacol. 2012;22(5):339–46. https://doi.org/10.1016/j.euroneuro.2011.09.008. Epub 2011 Oct 15.

123. Berwaerts J, Melkote R, Nuamah I, Lim P. A randomized, placebo- and active-controlled study of paliperidone extended-release as maintenance treatment in patients with bipolar I disorder after an acute manic or mixed episode. J Affect Disord. 2012;138(3):247–58. https://doi.org/10.1016/j.jad.2012.01.047. Epub 2012 Feb 27.
124. Taylor DM, Cornelius V, Smith L, Young AH. Comparative efficacy and acceptability of drug treatments for bipolar depression: a multiple-treatments meta-analysis. Acta Psychiatr Scand. 2014;130(6):452–69. https://doi.org/10.1111/acps.12343. Epub 2014 Oct 6.
125. Perlis RH, Ostacher MJ, Patel JK, Marangell LB, Zhang H, Wisniewski SR, et al. Predictors of recurrence in bipolar disorder: primary outcomes from the Systematic Treatment Enhancement Program for Bipolar Disorder (STEP-BD). Am J Psychiatry. 2006;163(2):217–24. https://doi.org/10.1176/appi.ajp.163.2.217.
126. Young AH, Hammond JM. Lithium in mood disorders: increasing evidence base, declining use? Br J Psychiatry. 2007;191:474–6. https://doi.org/10.1192/bjp.bp.107.043133.
127. Biel MG, Peselow E, Mulcare L, Case BG, Fieve R. Continuation versus discontinuation of lithium in recurrent bipolar illness: a naturalistic study. Bipolar Disord. 2007;9(5):435–42. https://doi.org/10.1111/j.1399-5618.2007.00389.x.
128. Bowden CL, Calabrese JR, McElroy SL, Gyulai L, Wassef A, Petty F, et al. A randomized, placebo-controlled 12-month trial of divalproex and lithium in treatment of outpatients with bipolar I disorder. Arch Gen Psychiatry. 2000;57(5):481–9. https://doi.org/10.1001/archpsyc.57.5.481.
129. Tohen M, Ketter TA, Zarate CA, Suppes T, Frye M, Altshuler L, et al. Olanzapine versus divalproex sodium for the treatment of acute mania and maintenance of remission: a 47-week study. Am J Psychiatry. 2003;160(7):1263–71. https://doi.org/10.1176/appi.ajp.160.7.1263.
130. Sani G, Perugi G, Tondo L. Treatment of bipolar disorder in a lifetime perspective: is lithium still the best choice? Clin Drug Investig. 2017;37(8):713–27. https://doi.org/10.1007/s40261-017-0531-2.
131. Mander AJ, Loudon JB. Rapid recurrence of mania following abrupt discontinuation of lithium. Lancet. 1988;2(8601):15–7. https://doi.org/10.1016/s0140-6736(88)92947-9.
132. Faedda GL, Tondo L, Baldessarini RJ, Suppes T, Tohen M. Outcome after rapid vs gradual discontinuation of lithium treatment in bipolar disorders. Arch Gen Psychiatry. 1993;50(6):448–55.
133. Macritchie KA, Hunt NJ. Does 'rebound mania' occur after stopping carbamazepine? A pilot study. J Psychopharmacol. 2000;14(3):266–8.
134. Franks MA, Macritchie KAN, Mahmood T, Young AH. Bouncing back: is the bipolar rebound phenomenon peculiar to lithium? A retrospective naturalistic study. J Psychopharmacol. 2008;22(4):452–6.
135. Cipriani A, Pretty H, Hawton K, Geddes JR. Lithium in the prevention of suicidal behavior and all-cause mortality in patients with mood disorders: a systematic review of randomized trials. Am J Psychiatry. 2005;162(10):1805–19. https://doi.org/10.1176/appi.ajp.162.10.1805.
136. Kessing LV, Søndergård L, Kvist K, Andersen PK. Suicide risk in patients treated with lithium. Arch Gen Psychiatry. 2005;62(8):860–6. https://doi.org/10.1001/archpsyc.62.8.860.
137. Fagiolini A, Forgione R, Maccari M, Cuomo A, Morana B, Dell'Osso MC, et al. Prevalence, chronicity, burden and borders of bipolar disorder. J Affect Disord. 2013;148(2–3):161–9. https://doi.org/10.1016/j.jad.2013.02.001.
138. Song J, Sjölander A, Joas E, Bergen SE, Runeson B, Larsson H, et al. Suicidal behavior during lithium and valproate treatment: a within-individual 8-year prospective study of 50,000 patients with bipolar disorder. Am J Psychiatry. 2017;174(8):795–802. https://doi.org/10.1176/appi.ajp.2017.16050542. Epub 2017 Jun 9.
139. Hartong EG, Moleman P, Hoogduin CA, Broekman TG, Nolen WA. Prophylactic efficacy of lithium versus carbamazepine in treatment-naive bipolar patients. J Clin Psychiatry. 2003;64(2):144–51. https://doi.org/10.4088/jcp.v64n0206.
140. Cipriani A, Reid K, Young AH, Macritchie K, Geddes J. Valproic acid, valproate and divalproex in the maintenance treatment of bipolar disorder. Cochrane Database Syst Rev. 2013;2013(10):CD003196. https://doi.org/10.1002/14651858.CD003196.pub2.

141. BALANCE investigators and collaborators, Geddes JR, Goodwin GM, Rendell J, Azorin JM, Cipriani A, et al. Lithium plus valproate combination therapy versus monotherapy for relapse prevention in bipolar I disorder (BALANCE): a randomised open-label trial. Lancet. 2010;375(9712):385–95. https://doi.org/10.1016/S0140-6736(09)61828-6. Epub 2010 Jan 19.
142. Kessing LV, Hellmund G, Geddes JR, Goodwin GM, Andersen PK. Valproate vs lithium in the treatment of bipolar disorder in clinical practice: observational nationwide register-based cohort study. Br J Psychiatry. 2011;199(1):57–63. https://doi.org/10.1192/bjp.bp.110.084822. Epub 2011 May 18.
143. Vieta E, Suppes T, Eggens I, Persson I, Paulsson B, Brecher M, et al. Efficacy and safety of quetiapine in combination with lithium or divalproex for maintenance of patients with bipolar I disorder (International Trial 126). J Affect Disord. 2008;109(3):251–63. https://doi.org/10.1016/j.jad.2008.06.001. Epub 2008 Jun 24.
144. McIntyre RS. Aripiprazole for the maintenance treatment of bipolar I disorder: a review. Clin Ther. 2010;32(Suppl 1):S32–8. https://doi.org/10.1016/j.clinthera.2010.01.022.
145. Marcus R, Khan A, Rollin L, Morris B, Timko K, Carson W, et al. Efficacy of aripiprazole adjunctive to lithium or valproate in the long-term treatment of patients with bipolar I disorder with an inadequate response to lithium or valproate monotherapy: a multicenter, double-blind, randomized study. Bipolar Disord. 2011;13(2):133–44. https://doi.org/10.1111/j.1399-5618.2011.00898.x.
146. Ghaemi SN, Sachs GS. Long-term risperidone treatment in bipolar disorder: 6-month follow up. Int Clin Psychopharmacol. 1997;12(6):333–8. https://doi.org/10.1097/00004850-199711000-00006.
147. Gigante AD, Lafer B, Yatham LN. Long-acting injectable antipsychotics for the maintenance treatment of bipolar disorder. Bipolar Disord. 2018;20(Suppl 2):25–36. https://doi.org/10.1111/bdi.12698.
148. Calabrese JR, Pikalov A, Streicher C, Cucchiaro J, Mao Y, Loebel A. Lurasidone in combination with lithium or valproate for the maintenance treatment of bipolar I disorder. Eur Neuropsychopharmacol. 2017;27(9):865–76. https://doi.org/10.1016/j.euroneuro.2017.06.013. Epub 2017 Jul 6.
149. Kishi T, Oya K, Iwata N. Long-acting injectable antipsychotics for prevention of relapse in bipolar disorder: a systematic review and meta-analyses of randomized controlled trials. Int J Neuropsychopharmacol. 2016;19(9) https://doi.org/10.1093/ijnp/pyw038.
150. Calabrese JR, Sanchez R, Jin N, Amatniek J, Cox K, Johnson B, et al. Efficacy and safety of aripiprazole once-monthly in the maintenance treatment of bipolar I disorder: a double-blind, placebo-controlled, 52-week randomized withdrawal study. J Clin Psychiatry. 2017;78(3):324–31. https://doi.org/10.4088/JCP.16m11201.
151. Ahlfors UG, Baastrup PC, Dencker SJ, Elgen K, Lingjaerde O, Pedersen V, et al. Flupenthixol decanoate in recurrent manic-depressive illness: a comparison with lithium. Acta Psychiatr Scand. 1981;64(3):226–37. https://doi.org/10.1111/j.1600-0447.1981.tb00778.x.
152. Vieta E, Nuamah IF, Lim P, Yuen EC, Palumbo JM, Hough DW, et al. A randomized, placebo- and active-controlled study of paliperidone extended release for the treatment of acute manic and mixed episodes of bipolar I disorder. Bipolar Disord. 2010;12(3):230–43. https://doi.org/10.1111/j.1399-5618.2010.00815.x.
153. Buoli M, Ciappolino V, Altamura AC. Paliperidone palmitate depot in the long-term treatment of psychotic bipolar disorder: a case series. Clin Neuropharmacol. 2015;38(5):209–11. https://doi.org/10.1097/WNF.0000000000000103.
154. López-Muñoz F, González CÁ, editors. Historia de la Psicofarmacología, vol. 3. Médica Panamericana; 2007.
155. López-Muñoz F, Alamo C, Cuenca EL. Década de Oro" de la Psicofarmacología (1950–1960): Trascendencia histórica de la introducción clínica de los psicofármacos clásicos. Psiquiatria. COM (electronic journal). 2000;4(3).
156. López-Muñoz F, Alamo C, Cuenca E, Shen WW, Clervoy P, Rubio G. History of the discovery and clinical introduction of chlorpromazine. Ann Clin Psychiatry. 2005;17(3):113–35. https://doi.org/10.1080/10401230591002002.

157. López-Muñoz F, Alamo C. Psicofarmacología: El nacimiento de una nueva disciplina. In: López-Muñoz F, Alamo C, editors. Historia de la Neuropsicofarmacología. Una Nueva Aportación a la Terapéutica Farmacológica de los Trastornos del Sistema Nervioso Central. Madrid, Spain: Ediciones Eurobook SL; 1998. p. 191–206, 219.

158. Kirkby KC. Social and health consequences of the clinical introduction of psychotropic drugs. In: López-Muñoz F, Alamo C, Domino EF, editors. History of psychopharmacology (Volume 3). The consolidation of psychopharmacology as a scientific discipline: ethical-legal aspects and future prospects. Arlington, TX: NPP Books; 2014. p. 251–62.

Dimensions and Predictors of Personal Recovery in Major Depression

13

Mario Luciano, Claudia Carmassi, and Umberto Albert

13.1 Introduction

Symptomatic remission has long been the only treatment goal of severe mental disorders (SMD) [1]. It can be defined as "a period during which an improvement of sufficient magnitude is observed that the individual is asymptomatic (i.e. no longer meets syndrome criteria for the disorder and has no more than minimal symptoms)" [2]. However, current treatment guidelines suggest that symptomatic remission cannot be considered any longer the only goal of treatment, but rather the first step towards the more challenging goal of recovery. In fact, in the last decades treatment outcome in SMD has evolved from the symptomatic remission to the broader concept of recovery [3].

Recovery has been defined as "a deeply personal, unique process of changing one's attitudes, values, feelings, goals, skills, and/or roles" and "a way of living a satisfying, hopeful, and contributing life even within the limitations caused by illness" [4]. The first definition of recovery was used in the thirteenth century and referred to the act of "regaining consciousness" [5]. In the early fourteenth

---

M. Luciano
Department of Psychiatry, University of Campania "L. Vanvitelli", Naples, Italy
e-mail: mario.luciano@unicampania.it

C. Carmassi
Dipartimento di Medicina Clinica e Sperimentale, University of Pisa, Pisa, Italy
e-mail: claudia.carmassi@unipi.it

U. Albert (✉)
Department of Medicine, Surgery and Health Sciences, University of Trieste, Trieste, Italy

UCO Clinica Psichiatrica, Azienda Sanitaria Universitaria Giuliano-Isontina (ASUGI), Trieste, Italy
e-mail: ualbert@units.it

© The Author(s), under exclusive license to Springer Nature Switzerland AG 2022
B. Carpiniello et al. (eds.), *Recovery and Major Mental Disorders*, Comprehensive Approach to Psychiatry 2, https://doi.org/10.1007/978-3-030-98301-7_13

century, the term recovery was used with the meaning of "regaining health or strength", and more recently of "returning to a normal or healthy status", referring mainly to physical illnesses rather than to mental disorders. In the past, recovery was traditionally understood as a sustained remission, or as the absence of symptoms and signs, accompanied by functional improvement (e.g. cognitive, social, and vocational functioning); this concept underlined the idea that recovery could be considered as the return to a former state of health [6]. This definition refers to "clinical recovery", usually defined by a set of criteria to be met and mainly assessed by mental health professionals. Various definitions of clinical recovery have been provided. One of the most adopted and recognized definitions of clinical recovery includes full remission of symptoms, full or part-time engagement in work activities or education, independent living and the presence of friends with whom sharing pleasant activities, all sustained for a period of 2 years [7]. Clinical recovery is conceptualized as a dichotomous objective outcome (in recovery versus not in recovery) that can be rated by an expert clinician with standardized assessment instruments. The definition of clinical recovery does not vary among individuals with a given diagnosis, as the concept emerged from professional-led research and practice [8].

Despite clinical recovery can be defined as an initial attempt to assess the outcome of mental disorders beyond treatment response and remission from psychopathological symptoms, it has to be considered only a part of the process of recovery. In fact, also based on suggestions coming from individuals who have had personal experience of a severe mental illness, the term "personal recovery" came up. This definition implies that recovery can be achieved despite the presence of symptoms of a given mental disorder. The concept of personal recovery is of particular importance since it involves the process by which a person attempts to develop new goals and meaning in life, beyond the catastrophic event of having a mental illness [9]. Individuals' skills to cope with symptoms are one of the most important elements of personal recovery. They refer to the ability of an individual to overcome the negative personal and social consequences of mental disorder and regain a self-determined and meaningful life. Thus, personal recovery is not simply the acquisition of a healthy status as it was before the onset of the mental disorder, but rather the growth beyond the premorbid status [10].

Contrary to the concept of "clinical recovery", then, personal recovery is considered as a process or a continuum, and not as an outcome, founded on the concept of an individual's journey of growth and personal development [11]. It is subjectively defined by the persons with a mental disorder, and individually rated by themselves [12]. Moreover, personal recovery is a heterogeneous concept, which assumes different meanings for different people, although many aspects are shared among individuals [8, 13].

However, a widely accepted definition of personal recovery has not been achieved yet. Law et al. [14] carried out a study involving 381 patients with psychosis, in order to find a common definition of personal recovery. The highest number of participants agreed that "recovery is the achievement of a personally acceptable quality of life" and that "recovery is feeling better about yourself".

Patients' clinical and personal recovery has been extensively assessed in people with lived experience of severe mental illnesses such as schizophrenia spectrum disorders or bipolar disorders, while little is known about the process of personal recovery in patients with other severe mental disorders, including major depressive disorders (MDD) [3, 15].

The focus on recovery from depression comes from recent studies on the efficacy of antidepressants, when it became apparent that standard treatments were not sufficient for achieving clinical recovery in many patients with MDD [10]. Indeed, several clinical features associated with the naturalistic course of MDD, such as its chronicity, the associated high relapse rates, the increasing probability of recurrences with every new episode [16–18], the frequent persistence and deleterious impact of residual symptoms [19–21], and the high comorbidity with physical illnesses, with long-term damaging effects on health and well-being greater than those associated with angina, arthritis, asthma or diabetes [22], justify the recent interest in applying the concept of personal recovery to MDD. Moreover, the lack of synchronicity between symptomatic and functional improvement often seen in recovering from MDD adds interest to the study of personal recovery in mood disorders [23]. Another clinical issue that stresses the importance of considering personal recovery in MDD is the evidence that the quality of remission is different according to the number of previous episodes; past depressive episodes seem to have a negative cumulative impact on psychomotor retardation, for example [24], or on other dimensions of cognitive functioning (e.g. memory) [25], supporting the scar effect hypothesis. Living well despite the illness or the long-term negative and persistent consequences of the disorder becomes an essential goal of the treatment of MDD.

The aim of the present overview is to provide readers with a description of the components of personal recovery and report available data on personal recovery in MDD.

13.2   From *Response* to *Full Functional Recovery* in MDD: History of Outcome Definitions in the Treatment for MDD

MDD is a common mental condition ranked by the World Health Organization among one of the leading causes of health-related disability worldwide. Globally, MDD affects more than 300 million people of all ages representing one of the major contributors to the overall global burden of disease. Moreover, depression causes not only relevant economic costs due to disability, healthcare system utilization and absenteeism, but is also associated with premature loss of life, especially by suicide [26]. MDD has a high lifetime prevalence (16.2%), and two thirds of cases have an episodic recurrent course [27, 28]. More than 50% of MDD patients report not satisfying outcomes from available treatments, with a high relapse rate after 2 years from the onset of the disorder [29–31].

The magnitude of this public health problem has led researchers and clinicians on one hand to look for better treatments for this condition and, on the other, to define more specific treatment goals such as *response*, *remission* and *recovery*. These terms, in fact, have evolved as the study of novel therapeutic treatment strategies [32]. Lacking a reliable physical marker of depression, clinicians must judge wellness based on levels of symptoms and functional impairment, with the outcomes of such assessment driving the choice of therapeutic interventions [33]. Since the 1950s, after the introduction of antidepressant pharmacotherapy, the most common outcome criterion used for evaluating MDD treatment was simply symptoms improvement, and until the early 1990s, outcome terms, definitions and criteria showed inconsistencies in the literature. The introduction of standardized rating scales such as the Hamilton Rating Scale for Depression (HAM-D) or the Montgomery-Asberg Depression Rating Scale (MADRS) for evaluating treatment outcomes in the early 1980s led to some consistency in the definition of response (i.e. percentage change from baseline or reduction to a predefined cut-off score) [33]. In 1991, Frank and colleagues [2] proposed a uniform terminology for treatment outcomes aiming at allowing consistent comparisons of different clinical trials.

Response was defined as a ≥50% decrease from baseline in the total score on a standardized symptom scale (e.g. HAM-D, MADRS) and maybe represents the most consistently defined term, widely used as the acute treatment goal. How a ≥50%, instead of 40 or 60%, decrease from baseline measurements became the standard definition of symptoms improvement remains unclear [34]. In the Sequential Treatment Alternative to Relieve Depression (STAR-D), *response* rates were reported to range between 39 and 56.6% [35]. *Response* has proven useful in research settings but it is of less utility to the clinical practice. This definition does not consider symptoms severity at the end of the treatment period so that subjects in the *response* group might still have clinically significant depression at the end of the protocol. Treatment responders might, in fact, still meet MDD diagnostic criteria and paradoxically even meet inclusion criteria for the clinical trial in which they had just participated. Moreover, in clinical practice, responding to antidepressant therapy but failing to achieve symptomatic *remission* implies a negative prognosis. Residual depressive symptoms, in fact, predispose to relapse/recurrence, chronicity, and suicidality in depressed patients [19–21, 36].

Remission is considered a more rigorous definition of a positive endpoint, identified since the end of the 1990s as the treatment goal for MDD [37–39]. In clinical trials, a score reduction under a specific cut-off score on rating scales represents *remission* and operationalized criteria have been proposed depending on the specific rating scales adopted (e.g. HAM-D score ≤7; MADRS score ≤10). As compared to *response*, achieving *remission* provides a greater opportunity for improving long-term prognosis and preventing relapses and recurrences. Unfortunately, only 30–40% of individuals with MDD reach symptomatic *remission* after an adequate treatment with first-line antidepressants. Furthermore, since the definition published by Frank et al. [2], alternative thresholds continue to be utilized determining difficulties in comparing different results [40–42]. This definition of *remission* is, in fact, theoretical vague and directly depends on the psychometric characteristics of the instrument used [43, 44]: a HAM-D score of 7 cannot be considered a priori a sign of true *remission*, and, for example, a lower score (<5) appears to be in some studies a more objective cut-off point [45]. Another controversial issue is the duration threshold for remission and recovery [46]; in the original proposal of operational criteria by Frank and colleagues [2], full remission required ≥2 weeks and less than 6 months asymptomatic, while recovery ≥6 months asymptomatic. Other authors considered a threshold of ≥8 weeks to define symptomatic remission [33, 47]. These duration thresholds have been found not to be empirically supported [48], so that the duration criteria for declaring remission and recovery seem unnecessary to date.

Moreover, results showing that a significant proportion of patients do not reach full psychosocial *recovery* even when they reach symptomatic "affective" *remission* indicate how non-affective symptoms are relevant for functional outcome [10, 49, 50].

Considering that cognitive dysfunctions (i.e. impairments in psychomotor speed, attention, verbal memory, executive functions) are among the most frequently encountered residual symptoms [51, 52], constitute a substantial risk for relapse in depression [53] and are strongly related to impaired psychosocial functioning, some authors have proposed the term *cognitive remission* as a new main objective in the treatment of MDD [54–56]. Cognitive dysfunctions may constitute a different dimension of major depressive symptomatology, responding differently (to different strategies) and in a non-synchronous way with respect to affective symptoms [56, 57]; thus, evaluating cognitive remission may be of clinical utility. Although different instruments have been proposed for evaluating cognitive dysfunctions in MDD and proved to be sensitive to changes during treatment (e.g. Digit Symbol Substitution Test—DSST; Trails Making Test B—TMT-B; or the THINC-it tool, a freely available, patient-administered, computerized screening tool integrating subjective and objective measures of cognitive function in adults with major depressive disorder) [58–60], no operationalized criteria for cognitive remission have been proposed.

Other authors pointed out that remission from depression as it is currently conceptualized (and defined with the HAM-D or MADRS cut-offs) is probably adequate for remitting negative mood, but not good enough for recovering positive mood, hedonic tone, functioning, or meaningfulness of life [61]; the focus is too much on the decrease of negative affect (i.e. depressive and anxiety symptoms) instead of on restoring positive affect or hedonic tone, despite the fact that loss of interest and pleasure is a core criterion for the diagnosis of MDD.

In this regard, *remission* is substantially different from *recovery*, also considering that even subthreshold depressive symptoms may be associated with substantial psychosocial impairment and that the number of residual symptoms correlates to the likelihood of subsequent relapse [47, 62]. Depressed individuals experience not only mood symptoms, but impairments in physical, occupational, and social functioning too [63, 64]. It is also worth mentioning that impaired functioning is a predictor of subsequent relapse of MDD; moreover, although measures of psychosocial functioning generally move in parallel with depressive symptoms (as depressive symptoms increase in severity, psychosocial disability worsen), improvements in affective symptoms and functionality do not always resolve in tandem [23]. In light of this, some authors have proposed *functional recovery* as a more adequate endpoint/outcome for the MDD treatment [10]. Research shows, in fact, that the prioritized therapeutic objective in MDD is the return to premorbid functioning, positive mental health, over the extinction of depressive symptomatology. Several functional outcome assessment tools have been proposed, such as the Global Assessment of Functioning (GAF) scale, the Quality of Life Enjoyment and Satisfaction Questionnaire (Q-LES-Q), the Sheehan Disability Scale (SDS), the Social Adjustment Scale-Self Report (SAS-SR), the WHO Disability Assessment Schedule (DAS 2.0), the Work and Social Adjustment Scale (WSAS), among others. Most of these instruments represent patient-reported outcomes that measure subjective perception of functioning, quality of life enjoyment and satisfaction, adjustment. Functional capacity is a more objective outcome; it may be measured with the University of California San Diego Performance-based Skills Assessment (UPSA), which assesses the capacity of an individual to perform specific skills required for independent living in a controlled situation. *Functional remission or recovery* in MDD has been proposed to be operationalized as having a GAF disability score ≥ 61, or a Sheehan Disability Scale score <5 on the three subscales, or as having an improvement on the University of California San Diego Performance-based Skills Assessment (UPSA) ≥ 7 or ≥ 9 points [65, 66].

Ongoing functional impairment may negatively impact on return back into daily life and in turn delay *full functional recovery*. *Full functional recovery* can be defined as a condition in which the patient starts to enjoy his/her usual activities again, returns to work and is able to take care of him/herself [3, 58]. Although full functional recovery has not been operationalized, it may be conceptualized as made of both clinical/symptomatic remission and functional remission/recovery.

Despite the evidence-based effective treatments available to date for MDD (both pharmacological and psychosocial), the achievement of full symptomatic and functional *recovery* persists to be an open challenge in psychiatry. The return to previous functioning levels may also have a slower trajectory with respect to symptomatic *response* or *remission* [67–70]. Among several clinical trials, rates of *remission* are low for any antidepressant drug (approximately 33%) [71, 72] and may be worse in clinical practice [73, 74]. Even more challenging is the achievement of both symptoms *remission* and *functional recovery* after a trial of an antidepressant treatment [75]; moreover, *functional remission* does not always move in tandem with *symptoms remission* and it may take longer to reach *functional recovery* [23]. In a pooled analysis of three randomized, double blind, short-term (8-weeks) treatment studies in MDD Sheehan et al. [76] reported that only 23% of subjects achieved combined symptomatic *remission* and *functional recovery*. *Full functional recovery* (symptomatic remission + functional recovery) remains a difficult-to-reach target of the long-term treatment of MDD: post hoc analysis from a 24-week prospective, observational study that involved 1549 MDD patients found that *clinical* and *functional remission* was achieved in 70.6% and 56.1% of the MDD patients, respectively, but only 52.1% of them reached *full functional recovery* at the end of the 6-month trial [77].

This historical shift from symptomatic remission to full functional recovery as the treatment target in clinical trials is reflected by a similar trend in identifying more holistic objectives of mood disorders management by recent practice guidelines for mood disorders. The CANMAT 2016 clinical guidelines for the management of the adults with MDD, for example, state that the goals of the acute treatment (8–12 weeks) are the remission of symptoms and the restoration of functioning, while the goals of the maintenance phase (6–24 months) are the return to full functioning and quality of life and the prevention of recurrence [78]. The more recent 2020 Royal Australian and New Zealand College of Psychiatrists clinical practice guidelines for mood disorders [79] explicitly recommend that "the aims of mood disorder treatment should go beyond symptom relief to include resilience and improve well-being"; this is particularly recommended in the context of chronic and relapsing mood disorders, where an episode of care is viewed also as an opportunity to develop the patient's resilience against the future illness. Resilience is here defined as the "ability to adapt to, and recover from, stress; not simply the absence of vulnerability". Guidelines identify *personal recovery* as the ultimate goal of treatment, as the "process of adaptation to serious mental illness", and encourage clinicians to have a more active engagement with patients [79]. The development of resilience "focuses on instituting new strategies, embedding new resources and addressing vulnerabilities".

As one can see, the term personal recovery appears for the first time as the goal of treatment in MDD.

13.3 Dimensions of Personal Recovery in Severe Mental Disorders

Different definitions of personal recovery in SMD have been proposed and several determinants of personal recovery identified. However, all definitions of personal recovery include components such as accepting mental illness, finding hope for the future, re-establishing a positive identity, developing meaning in life, taking control of one's life through individual responsibility, spirituality, empowerment, overcoming stigma, and having supportive relationships [6]. Probably, a higher consensus definition of personal recovery has not been achieved yet due to the complexity of the recovery construct. The complexity is increased by the evidence that there are at least five stages of recovery [12]: (1) moratorium (i.e. denial, confusion, hopelessness, identity confusion and self-protective withdrawal); (2) awareness (i.e. the initial appraisal that recovery is possible, with the possibility of a better life, including the development of the awareness of a possible self, other than that of being a patient with a SMD); (3) preparation (i.e. person start to working on recovery, by learning about mental illness and available services, by becoming involved in groups, and connecting with others who are in other stage of recovery); (4) rebuilding (the hardest phase of the recovery process, which involves a change to a more positive identity, by reassessing old values and moving towards a new way of living, taking responsibility for managing illness and for control of life, and showing tenacity by takings risks and suffering setbacks); (5) growth (i.e. gaining new skills on how to manage symptoms and disabilities).

One of the most comprehensive definitions of personal recovery has been provided by Leamy et al. [80], who developed a framework to understand the concept of personal recovery, through a systematic review and narrative synthesis: the CHIME Framework. It consists of three interlinked superordinate categories of recovery, including the characteristics of recovery journey, the recovery processes and recovery stages. The acronym CHIME derives from the recovery process identified by the framework: Connectedness (i.e. peer support and support from social groups, good social relationships, supports from others, being part of the community), Hope and optimism (i.e. belief in the possibility to recover, motivation to change, hope-inspiring relationships, positive thinking and valuing success, having dreams and aspirations), Identity (i.e. dimensions of identity, ability to rebuild or redefining a positive sense of identity and to overcome stigma), Meaning in life (i.e. meaning of mental illness experiences, spirituality, quality of life, meaningful life and social roles and goals, ability to rebuilding life), Empowerment (i.e. personal responsibility, control over life, focusing upon strengths). In particular, empowerment is a core concept of the World Health Organization vision of mental health promotion [81] and it plays a key role in the concept of personal recovery. Empowerment is the core component of the UK movement "no decision about me without me", a user-led movement which aimed to transform the English National Health System to a recovery-oriented service system [82]. Empowerment refers to people's ability to become stronger and more confident, particularly in controlling their own life and claiming for their rights. Empowerment helps to adopt autonomy and self-determination and to influence the decision-making process, thus impacting self-esteem and self-efficacy [83].

The process of personal recovery is defined by three main dimensions: the inner experience, the contribution from others and the participation in social activities [5]. The first category refers to patients' inner experiences of the disease and to their ability to accept themselves as persons rather than as patients, and to identify themselves as responsible to build up an independent life. In this sense, recovery refers to the ability to accept the disability. Acceptance, which should not be considered a synonym of giving up and surrendering to symptoms, is the most difficult stage of the whole recovery process, but also the most essential [84]. Acceptance includes hope, spirituality, empowerment, connection, purpose, self-identity, symptom management and stigma [85].

The second category refers to the support from relevant others in the recovery process, including professionals, family members and other caregivers, friends, other patients. As regards the professional support, several therapeutic approaches have shown to be effective in fostering the process of personal recovery, including cognitive remediation, psychoeducational interventions, and cognitive-behavioural approaches [86]. Independently from the therapeutic approach, a key element of professional support, strongly linked with personal recovery, is the provision of a guide to patients through symptoms, and of instruments to help them to overcome the crises. Mental health professionals' characteristics associated with a better personal recovery are empathy and respect, being active and carefully listening and showing interest to patients' problems [5, 87]. The role of mental health professionals and of the organization of mental health services has become a key topic in the promotion of personal recovery in the last years. In fact, many countries have adopted national mental health policies shifting towards recovery-oriented mental health services and interventions [88]. The recovery-oriented approaches offer a transformative conceptual framework for practice, culture and service delivery in mental health service provision [89]. Several studies have highlighted that spirituality is a relevant factor in the personal recovery, since religion can motivate and inspire patients to live their lives with greater acceptance [90]. Moreover, being part of a faith community and having a religious affiliation is seen as an important component of an individual's recovery [80].

The third component of personal recovery includes patients' participation in social activities. Being active on a daily basis and staying in contact with the real world allows patients to avoid isolation and reduces detachment from reality [91]. Moreover, having a stable employment helps keeping the feeling of being able to give something back to the society, feeling competent and appreciated by colleagues [87], while reducing at the same time the stigma and building a sense of independence from others. Moreover, the participation in leisure activities is a major contributing factor to the recovery process. Participating in leisure activities allows people to being distracted from mental health problems, to meet new people and to create social networks, thus enriching their social life [5].

An integrated dimensional model of recovery has been proposed by Whitley and Drake [92]. It defines recovery on the basis of five dimensions: (1) clinical—reduction in symptoms; (2) existential—better sense of hope, empowerment, and spiritual well-being; (3) functional—recovering meaningful role; (4) physical—promoting physical health; and (5) social—consolidating relationships with others and feeling that one is part of society. One of the advantages of this framework is to provide an integrated approach with both a focus on clinical and personal aspects of recovery (including a focus on physical health—and thus strategies implementing physical health) and may provide clinicians with a useful framework for identifying and promoting strategies to foster recovery.

13.4 Personal Recovery in Major Depression

The recovery process from MDD is still understudied. In fact, recovery has been mainly investigated in patients with schizophrenia, other psychoses and/or bipolar disorders. Patients with major depression are underrepresented in the consumers' movements, where the concept of personal recovery has been developed and conceptualized [10, 15]. Despite personal recovery is conceptualized as a process which can occur independently from patients' symptoms, several studies have highlighted that the type and the severity of psychiatric symptoms can have a different impact on personal recovery [93]. In fact, the core symptoms of schizophrenia, such as delusions and hallucinations, have a reduced influence on patient's experience of recovery, while affective symptoms are considered a barrier in the process of recovery of patients with schizophrenia [94]. In particular, authors reported that personal recovery was predicted mainly by affective symptoms, while the negative and positive ones were not associated with personal recovery in a sample of 105 patients with schizophrenia and bipolar disorder. Moreover, the severity of affective symptoms was more strongly related to personal recovery in patients with non-psychotic disorders than in those with schizophrenia.

Only a few studies have assessed personal recovery in major depression. Available evidence suggests that the recovery journey in MDD can be considered a complex, personalized and multifaceted process. Complexity arises from the fact that several social, clinical and contextual factors are potentially implicated in the process of recovery [15].

Social support, measured as the size of social network, subjective feeling to be supported by relatives or friends and the number of close relationships and satisfaction with received support, is one of the most influential factors that can impede or foster the process of recovery in MDD [95, 96]. In particular, Gladstone et al. [97] reported that more than 50% of patients with MDD feel that recovery is made difficult by lack of perceived social support. Interventions targeting the development and maintenance of supportive relationships may then prove to be effective approaches to foster personal recovery. The relationship between perceived poor social support and depression, leading to a delay in the recovery process is, however, complex: it is possible that the depressive state is associated with a negative perception of social support while this is not true, but also that chronicity of depression or multiple recurrences of depression trigger erosion of social support networks over time (a sort of social scar of recurrent or chronic MDD).

It is then essential to carefully assess this dimension in the real life of the patient. This also implies that clinicians should promptly recognize, diagnose and appropriately treat MDD since its onset; an early personalized and optimized treatment is essential in terms of a) pharmacologic compound or psychotherapeutic intervention, b) appropriate dose (drug) or frequency (psychotherapeutic intervention), c) right choice of the specific intervention according to the clinical subtype/predominant symptom dimension of MDD, and d) quick adoption of alternative strategies when at least a partial response is not evident within the first weeks of treatment [3, 98]. The duration of untreated illness and the lack of an early improvement in depressive symptoms (e.g. $\geq$20% decrease in HAM-D score after 2 weeks) have been consistently found to be associated with non-remission and/or relapses/recurrences, thus interfering with the personal recovery journey [99–101].

It is also imperative, in order to promote recovery from depression, to aggressively treat the full spectrum of symptoms accompanying the episode, including residual symptoms and dysfunctions eventually associated with drug side effects (e.g. sexual dysfunctions). Integrating multiple treatment approaches (sequentially) may prove to be the optimal way of fostering personal recovery.

If we refer to the integrated model of recovery proposed by Whitley and Drake [92], these may be conceptualized as strategies fostering clinical recovery and

13 Dimensions and Predictors of Personal Recovery in Major Depression

contributing, at a later time, to personal recovery. Other strategies that patients themselves can implement together with healthcare providers include, for example, analysing and changing dysfunctional beliefs (cognitive-behavioural treatments) and/or learning how to pay attention to mood changes (e.g. regularly taking notes on mood changes) in order to recognize early signs of a relapse and thus implement appropriate strategies as soon as they became aware that symptoms are becoming more intense [102].

As regards contextual factors, it should be noted that patients and clinicians hold different perspectives regarding what constitutes recovery from major depression and what they consider important for recovery from MDD [103–105]. In fact, most physicians consider the reduction of the number and severity of depressive symptoms, as well as the improvement of patients' functioning, the focus of their treatment goals, while patients focus mainly on restoration of positive affect, including having a meaningful life, satisfaction with personal relationships, improving their ability to concentrate and their personal strengths [106]. Moreover, perceptions of MDD symptoms and the associations between these symptoms and functioning differ significantly between patients and healthcare providers across all phases of the disorder (acute, post-acute and remission) [107]. The findings of this latter study highlight the need for improved communication between patients and healthcare providers in order to set appropriate treatment goals. Different priorities in treatment outcomes between patients and clinicians can lead clinicians to systematically ignore all the components of personal recovery as an outcome to be achieved, thus reducing the possibility that patients will recover.

An interesting study found that discordance between what patients and physicians consider important in the definition of cure from depression significantly influences clinical outcomes at 6 months: the subgroup with a poor physician–patient agreement on expectations had a worse clinical outcome than the subgroup with an excellent physician–patient agreement, with differences in response rate between these groups ranging from 9 to 27% [108].

Again, the clinical complexity and heterogeneity of MDD in terms of predominant symptom dimensions, perceived different relevance of each symptom dimension according to patients and healthcare providers perspectives, subtype, chronicity, etc. highlights the need of a personalized, individually tailored approach to the person living with MDD [109].

MDD patients consider four elements as the main factors that can impede their recovery journey; the first one is the lack of consensus on the nature of depression: having no personalized treatment, receiving insufficient information about proposed treatments and lack of discussion concerning medications (e.g. mechanisms of action, potential side effects, time to response) are reported as major impeding elements in the patient-clinician relationship [30]. In this regard, psychoeducational consensus checklists may be used by practitioners in order to promote a better relationship and improve shared decision-making in MDD [110]. Other elements that are seen by patients with MDD as potentially interfering with the recovery journey are: (1) a precarious relationship with the clinician, including lack of trust in clinicians' abilities to treat depression, lack of continuity in treatment due to frequent changes in treating clinicians, inappropriate professional attitudes, and lack of professional guidance; (2) the unavailability of mental healthcare when needed, particularly in case of emergencies (long waiting lists, unavailability of treating clinician and lack of care after symptom resolution are the most relevant factors in this category), and (3) insufficient involvement of significant others, preventing full use of support networks [30].

In order to promote recovery from depression, several approaches have been proposed in the last few years [111]. One of the most promising is the self-management approach, which increases individualism, empowerment, and participation in social activities [102]. Self-management includes both professional- and user-led strategies. Among the former, booklets, books and e-health programmes have been proposed [112, 113]. Promising suggestions come from patients' perspectives on how they recovered from depression; an interesting study [102] explored strategies used by people recovering from depressive and anxiety disorders, classifying them according to the model proposed by Whitley and Drake [92]: these strategies may be implemented in clinical practice to foster recovery. Having a proactive role towards depression and its treatments (e.g. seeking information from mental health professionals about depressive symptoms and gaining insight into illness, taking your medication), managing daily symptoms (e.g. analysing and changing your thoughts/emotions and behaviours) and remaining vigilant to signs and symptoms of potential relapses are among the self-management strategies used to foster *clinical recovery*. Among strategies fostering *existential recovery,* patients reported having a positive outlook, e.g. taking inspiration from someone who has previously recovered—well-known public personalities with the same disorder, or people in a support groups, having spiritual beliefs, using humour, developing a balanced sense of self (e.g. distinguishing the illness from your personality), finding meaning (e.g. finding a project, a goal, a dream), among others. Self-managed strategies fostering *functional recovery* included creating a routine (e.g. following a schedule, having and respecting regular rhythms—going to bed at a regular time) and proactively taking activities (e.g. engaging in pleasant activities and engaging in activities in which you can feel competent); again, the usefulness of this approach is that psychosocial interventions (led by healthcare providers but also led by peers) may be implemented in order to train patients to adopt these strategies. Regaining and promoting physical health is another important dimension of recovery; strategies fostering *physical recovery* include engaging in sport activities, adopting sleep hygiene, eating at regular times and well, reducing consumption of alcohol, smoking and other substances. In this regard, it has to be borne in mind that physical health is compromised in mood disorders because of different contributors, some of them not modifiable such as genetic predisposition, other modifiable such as dysregulations in social rhythms, substance abuse, poor sleep hygiene, or side-effects of medications. Both individuals living with the disorder and their healthcare providers can intervene to prevent physical complications and foster physical recovery. Lastly but not least, self-management strategies fostering *social recovery* reported by patients with depressive disorders consisted of surrounding myself with people who make me feel better and avoiding negative people, and taking care of others such as family members or friends [102].

13.5 The Way Forward

Despite the recent interest of the scientific community, much work has still to be done in order to define a clear and internationally recognized conceptualization of personal recovery for individuals living with major depression and its dimensions. There are still too many unanswered questions, such as whether the process of personal recovery from depression is similar or distinct from that of personal recovery from other severe mental disorders. The methodology adopted in the different studies is very heterogeneous, and different instruments have been used to assess personal recovery, hindering cross-studies' comparisons. Differently from what happened in studies on personal recovery of patients with schizophrenia or bipolar disorders, the paucity of data does not allow to identify which aspects should be considered as the most important in recovery from major depression. This information is essential in order to provide clinicians with useful information to guide patients in their "journey to recovery". It is not a case that one of the most important factors slowing the process of recovery is the lack of professional support perceived by patients. Patients with major depression often perceive the clinician as an authority who makes decisions about treatments on their behalf with a low level of encouragement to obtain autonomy, motivation and self-management [30]. Several authors have highlighted that the way in which decisions are made during the clinical encounter affect patients' recovery, and that the identification of treatment priorities should be always shared with patients, according to the shared decision-making model, which is associated with better outcomes in terms of symptom reduction and improvement of psychosocial functioning, empowerment and satisfaction with received care [83, 114].

Different views have been reported between clinicians and patients about dimensions of personal recovery for patients with major depression, but only a few studies exploring the impact of these differences have been carried out [103–106].

Lastly, available studies on recovery from depression, and from other severe mental disorders, show that a shift in the provision of psychiatric care is needed [115]. In fact, there is the need to move away from a "treat-and-recover" approach, in which priority is given to the provision of treatments with the aim to make people re-engage with their life [116]. For decades, mental health services have been organized around a clinical version of recovery, where professionals diagnose and treat patients, with the aim of reducing their symptoms, and where they do not consider the possibility to recover from severe mental disorders beyond symptoms' reduction [117]. Many interventions are now available to promote users' personal recovery, including the "Wellness Recovery Action Planning (WRAP)" [118], the "Illness

Management and Recovery Program (IMR)" [119], and the "REFOCUS" intervention [120]. All these approaches have shown their efficacy in promoting personal recovery in patients with severe mental disorders in randomized controlled trials.

13.6 Conclusions

Over the course of recent years, the focus of interest of clinicians and individuals living with MDD shifted from just achieving symptomatic remission to clinical recovery, functional recovery and ultimately personal recovery. Personal recovery is an idiographic process, that is each persons' recovery is unique. Personal recovery is not a dichotomous outcome of interventions but rather a journey, a dynamic process, that requires a shared decision-making approach. Living well despite depressive residual symptoms and despite the scars of an often chronic, recurrent, long-lasting condition such as MDD (e.g. cognitive scars, social scars, physical scars) is not only possible, but should become the main objective of the management of MDD, as recently acknowledged by international clinical guidelines [79].

The journey towards personal recovery in MDD may be viewed as a sequential, multi-dimensional route where several individuals contribute to the final outcome; it starts with strategies aimed at fostering clinical recovery in order to quickly move at implementing strategies to promote existential, functional, physical and social recovery. Healthcare providers, individuals living with the condition, peers and family members/caregivers can contribute each in its own way to this final outcome.

Personal recovery in MDD is still understudied as compared to personal recovery as an outcome in other severe mental disorders; it is necessary and urgent that future studies can be funded and performed in order to achieve a better understanding of dimensions and predictors of clinical and personal recovery in MDD.

References

1. Collard RM, Wassink-Vossen S, Schene AH, et al. Symptomatic and functional recovery in depression in later life. Soc Psychiatry Psychiatr Epidemiol. 2018;53:1071–9.
2. Frank E, Prien RF, Jarrett RB, Keller MB, Kupfer DJ, Lavori PW, Rush AJ, Weissman MM. Conceptualization and rationale for consensus definitions of terms in major depressive disorder. Remission, recovery, relapse, and recurrence. Arch Gen Psychiatry. 1991;48(9):851–5.
3. Habert J, Katzman MA, Oluboka OJ, McIntyre RS, McIntosh D, MacQueen GM, Khullar A, Milev RV, Kjernisted KD, Chokka PR, Kennedy SH. Functional recovery in major depressive disorder: focus on early optimized treatment. Prim Care Companion CNS Disord. 2016;18(5).
4. Anthony WA. Recovery from mental illness: the guiding vision of the mental health system in the 1990s. Innov Res. 1993;2:17–24.
5. Salzmann-Erikson M. An integrative review of what contributes to personal recovery in psychiatric disabilities. Issues Ment Health Nurs. 2013;34:185–91.
6. Cavelti M, Kvrgic S, Beck EM, et al. Assessing recovery from schizophrenia as an individual process. A review of self-report instruments. Eur Psychiatry. 2011;27:19–32.
7. Libermann RP, Kopelowicz A. Recovery from schizophrenia: a challenge for the 21st century. Int Rev Psychiatry. 2002;14:242–55.

8. Slade M, Longden E. Empirical evidence about recovery and mental health. BMC Psychiatry. 2015;14(15):285.
9. Bejerholm U, Roe D. Personal recovery within positive psychiatry. Nord J Psychiatry. 2018;72:420–30.
10. Stotland NL. Recovery from depression. Psychiatr Clin North Am. 2012;35:37–49.
11. Lim MW, Remington G, Lee J. Personal recovery in serious mental illness: making sense of the concept. Ann Acad Med Singap. 2017;46:29–31.
12. Andresen R, Oades L, Caputi P. The experience of recovery from schizophrenia: towards an empirically-validated stage model. Aust N Z J Psychiatry. 2003;37:586–94.
13. Macpherson R, Pesola F, Leamy M, Bird V, Le Boutillier C, Williams J, Slade M. The relationship between clinical and recovery dimensions of outcome in mental health. Schizophr Res. 2016;175:142–7.
14. Law H, Morrison AP. Recovery in psychosis: a Delphi study with experts by experience. Schizophr Bull. 2014;40:1347–55.
15. Richardson K, Barkham M. Recovery from depression: a systematic review of perceptions and associated factors. J Ment Health. 2017;6:1–13.
16. Judd LL, Akiskal HS, Maser JD, Zeller PJ, Endicott J, Coryell W, Paulus MP, Kunovac JL, Leon AC, Mueller TI, Rice JA, Keller MB. A prospective 12-year study of subsyndromal and syndromal depressive symptoms in unipolar major depressive disorders. Arch Gen Psychiatry. 1998a Aug;55(8):694–700.
17. Eaton WW, Shao H, Nestadt G, Lee HB, Bienvenu OJ, Zandi P. Population-based study of first onset and chronicity in major depressive disorder. Arch Gen Psychiatry. 2008;65(5): 513–20.
18. Ten Have M, de Graaf R, van Dorsselaer S, Tuithof M, Kleinjan M, Penninx BWJH. Recurrence and chronicity of major depressive disorder and their risk indicators in a population cohort. Acta Psychiatr Scand. 2018;137(6):503–15.
19. Judd LL, Akiskal HS, Maser JD, Zeller PJ, Endicott J, Coryell W, Paulus MP, Kunovac JL, Leon AC, Mueller TI, Rice JA, Keller MB. Major depressive disorder: a prospective study of residual subthreshold depressive symptoms as predictor of rapid relapse. J Affect Disord. 1998b Sep;50(2–3):97–108.
20. Nil R, Lütolf S, Seifritz E. Residual symptoms and functionality in depressed outpatients: a one-year observational study in Switzerland with escitalopram. J Affect Disord. 2016;197:245–50.
21. Verhoeven FEA, Wardenaar KJ, Ruhé HGE, Conradi HJ, de Jonge P. Seeing the signs: using the course of residual depressive symptomatology to predict patterns of relapse and recurrence of major depressive disorder. Depress Anxiety. 2018;35(2):148–59.
22. Moussavi S, Chatterji S, Verdes E, Tandon A, Patel V, Ustun B. Depression, chronic diseases, and decrements in health: results from the World Health Surveys. Lancet. 2007;370(9590):851–8.
23. Sheehan DV, Nakagome K, Asami Y, Pappadopulos EA, Boucher M. Restoring function in major depressive disorder: a systematic review. J Affect Disord. 2017;215:299–313.
24. Gorwood P, Richard-Devantoy S, Baylé F, Cléry-Melin ML. Psychomotor retardation is a scar of past depressive episodes, revealed by simple cognitive tests. Eur Neuropsychopharmacol. 2014;24(10):1630–40.
25. Gorwood P, Corruble E, Falissard B, Goodwin GM. Toxic effects of depression on brain function: impairment of delayed recall and the cumulative length of depressive disorder in a large sample of depressed outpatients. Am J Psychiatry. 2008;165(6):731–9.
26. GBD 2017 Disease and Injury Incidence and Prevalence Collaborators. Global, regional, and national incidence, prevalence, and years lived with disability for 354 diseases and injuries for 195 countries and territories, 1990-2017: a systematic analysis for the Global Burden of Disease Study 2017. Lancet. 2018;392(10159):1789–858.
27. van Grieken RA, Kirkenier AC, Koeter MW, et al. Patients' perspective on self-management in the recovery from depression. Health Expect. 2015;18:1339–48.
28. Solomon DA, Keller MB, Leon AC, Mueller TI, Lavori PW, Shea MT, Coryell W, Warshaw M, Turvey C, Maser JD, Endicott J. Multiple recurrences of major depressive disorder. Am J Psychiatry. 2000;157(2):229–33.

29. Rush AJ, Trivedi MH, Wisniewski SR, Nierenberg AA, Stewart JW, Warden D, Niederehe G, Thase ME, Lavori PW, Lebowitz BD, McGrath PJ, Rosenbaum JF, Sackeim HA, Kupfer DJ, Luther J, Fava M. Acute and longer-term outcomes in depressed outpatients requiring one or several treatment steps: a STAR*D report. Am J Psychiatry. 2006;163(11):1905–17.
30. van Grieken RA, Beune EJ, Kirkenier AC, et al. Patients' perspectives on how treatment can impede their recovery from depression. J Affect Disord. 2014;167:153–9.
31. van Randenborgh A, Hüffmeier J, Victor D, et al. Contrasting chronic with episodic depression: an analysis of distorted socio-emotional information processing in chronic depression. J Affect Disord. 2012;141:77–84.
32. Keller MB. Remission versus response: the new gold standard of antidepressant care. J Clin Psychiatry. 2004;65(Suppl 4):53–9.
33. Keller MB. Past, present, and future directions for defining optimal treatment outcome in depression: remission and beyond. JAMA. 2003;289(23):3152–60.
34. Nierenberg AA, DeCecco LM. Definitions of antidepressant treatment response, remission, nonresponse, partial response, and other relevant outcomes: a focus on treatment-resistant depression. J Clin Psychiatry. 2001;62(Suppl 16):5–9.
35. Wisniewski SR, Rush AJ, Nierenberg AA, Gaynes BN, Warden D, Luther JF, McGrath PJ, Lavori PW, Thase ME, Fava M, Trivedi MH. Can phase III trial results of antidepressant medications be generalized to clinical practice? A STAR*D report. Am J Psychiatry. 2009;166(5):599–607.
36. McIntyre RS, Fallu A, Konarski JZ. Measurable outcomes in psychiatric disorders: remission as a marker of wellness. Clin Ther. 2006;28(11):1882–91.
37. Bakish D. New standard of depression treatment: remission and full recovery. J Clin Psychiatry. 2001;62(Suppl 26):5–9.
38. Kelsey JE. Clinician perspective on achieving and maintaining remission in depression. J Clin Psychiatry. 2001;62(Suppl 26):16–21. Review.
39. Nierenberg AA, Wright EC. Evolution of remission as the new standard in the treatment of depression. J Clin Psychiatry. 1999;60(Suppl 22):7–11.
40. Berk M, du Plessis AD, Birkett M, Richardt D. An open-label study of duloxetine hydrochloride, a mixed serotonin and noradrenaline reuptake inhibitor, in patients with DSM-III-R major depressive disorder. Lilly Duloxetine Depression Study Group. Int Clin Psychopharmacol. 1997;12(3):137–40.
41. Schweizer E, Rynn M, Mandos LA, Demartinis N, García-España F, Rickels K. The antidepressant effect of sertraline is not enhanced by dose titration: results from an outpatient clinical trial. Int Clin Psychopharmacol. 2001;16(3):137–43.
42. Trivedi MH, Rush AJ, Pan JY, Carmody TJ. Which depressed patients respond to nefazodone and when? J Clin Psychiatry. 2001;62(3):158–63.
43. Østergaard SD, Bech P, Miskowiak KW. Fewer study participants needed to demonstrate superior antidepressant efficacy when using the Hamilton melancholia subscale (HAM-D$_6$) as outcome measure. J Affect Disord. 2016;190:842–5. https://doi.org/10.1016/j.jad.2014.10.047.
44. Fountoulakis KN, Möller HJ. Antidepressant drugs and the response in the placebo group: the real problem lies in our understanding of the issue. J Psychopharmacol. 2012;26(5):744–50. https://doi.org/10.1177/0269881111421969.
45. Berk M, Ng F, Wang WV, Calabrese JR, Mitchell PB, Malhi GS, Tohen M. The empirical redefinition of the psychometric criteria for remission in bipolar disorder. J Affect Disord. 2008;106(1–2):153–8. Epub 2007 Jul 26.
46. Slofstra C, Booij SH, Rogier Hoenders HJ, Castelein S. Redefining therapeutic outcomes of depression treatment. J Pers Oriented Res. 2019;5(2):1–8.
47. Judd LL, Schettler PJ, Rush AJ, Coryell WH, Fiedorowicz JG, Solomon DA. A new empirical definition of major depressive episode recovery and its positive impact on future course of illness. J Clin Psychiatry. 2016;77(8):1065–73.
48. de Zwart PL, Jeronimus BF, de Jonge P. Empirical evidence for definitions of episode, remission, recovery, relapse and recurrence in depression: a systematic review. Epidemiol Psychiatr Sci. 2019;28(5):544–62.

13 Dimensions and Predictors of Personal Recovery in Major Depression

49. Carvalho AF, Miskowiak KK, Hyphantis TN, Kohler CA, Alves GS, Bortolato B, et al. Cognitive dysfunction in depression—pathophysiology and novel targets. CNS Neurol Disord Drug Targets. 2014;13(10):1819–35.
50. McIntyre RS. Using measurement strategies to identify and monitor residual symptoms. J Clin Psychiatry. 2013;74(Suppl 2):14–8.
51. Conradi HJ, Ormel J, de Jonge P. Presence of individual (residual) symptoms during depressive episodes and periods of remission: a 3-year prospective study. Psychol Med. 2011;41(6):1165–74.
52. Lee RS, Hermens DF, Porter MA, Redoblado-Hodge MA. A meta-analysis of cognitive deficits in first-episode Major Depressive Disorder. J Affect Disord. 2012;140(2): 113–24.
53. Saragoussi D, Touya M, Haro JM, Jönsson B, Knapp M, Botrel B, Florea I, Loft H, Rive B. Factors associated with failure to achieve remission and with relapse after remission in patients with major depressive disorder in the PERFORM study. Neuropsychiatr Dis Treat. 2017;13:2151–65.
54. McIntyre RS, Cha DS, Soczynska JK, Woldeyohannes HO, Gallaugher LA, Kudlow P, et al. Cognitive deficits and functional outcomes in major depressive disorder: determinants, substrates, and treatment interventions. Depress Anxiety. 2013;30(6):515–27.
55. Trivedi MH, Greer TL. Cognitive dysfunction in unipolar depression: implications for treatment. J Affect Disord. 2014;152-154:19–27. https://doi.org/10.1016/j.jad.2013.09.012.
56. Bortolato B, Miskowiak KW, Köhler CA, Maes M, Fernandes BS, Berk M, Carvalho AF. Cognitive remission: a novel objective for the treatment of major depression? BMC Med. 2016;14:9.
57. Rock PL, Roiser JP, Riedel WJ, Blackwell AD. Cognitive impairment in depression: a systematic review and meta-analysis. Psychol Med. 2014;44(10):2029–40.
58. Fiorillo A, Carpiniello B, De Giorgi S, La Pia S, Maina G, Sampogna G, Spina E, Tortorella A, Vita A. Assessment and management of cognitive and psychosocial dysfunctions in patients with major depressive disorder: a clinical review. Front Psych. 2018;9:493.
59. McIntyre RS, Best MW, Bowie CR, Carmona NE, Cha DS, Lee Y, Subramaniapillai M, Mansur RB, Barry H, Baune BT, Culpepper L, Fossati P, Greer TL, Harmer C, Klag E, Lam RW, Wittchen HU, Harrison J. The THINC-Integrated Tool (THINC-it) screening assessment for cognitive dysfunction: validation in patients with major depressive disorder. J Clin Psychiatry. 2017;78(7):873–81.
60. McIntyre RS, Subramaniapillai M, Park C, Zuckerman H, Cao B, Lee Y, Iacobucci M, Nasri F, Fus D, Bowie CR, Tran T, Rosenblat JD, Mansur RB. The THINC-it tool for cognitive assessment and measurement in major depressive disorder: sensitivity to change. Front Psych. 2020;11:546.
61. Demyttenaere K, Kiekens G, Bruffaerts R, Mortier P, Gorwood P, Martin L, Di Giannantonio M. Outcome in depression (I): why symptomatic remission is not good enough. CNS Spectr. 2020;19:1–7.
62. Sakurai H, Suzuki T, Yoshimura K, Mimura M, Uchida H. Predicting relapse with individual residual symptoms in major depressive disorder: a reanalysis of the STAR*D data. Psychopharmacology. 2017;234(16):2453–61.
63. American Psychiatric Association. Diagnostic and statistical manual of mental disorders. 5th ed. Arlington, VA: American Psychiatric Publishing; 2013.
64. Kessler RC, Berglund P, Demler O, Jin R, Koretz D, Merikangas KR, Rush AJ, Walters EE, Wang PS, National Comorbidity Survey Replication. The epidemiology of major depressive disorder: results from the National Comorbidity Survey Replication (NCS-R). JAMA. 2003;289(23):3095–105.
65. Sheehan KH, Sheehan DV. Assessing treatment effects in clinical trials with the discan metric of the Sheehan Disability Scale. Int Clin Psychopharmacol. 2008;23(2):70–83.
66. Christensen MC, Loft H, McIntyre RS. Vortioxetine improves symptomatic and functional outcomes in major depressive disorder: a novel dual outcome measure in depressive disorders. J Affect Disord. 2018;227:787–94.

67. Miller IW, Keitner GI, Schatzberg AF, Klein DN, Thase ME, Rush AJ, Markowitz JC, Schlager DS, Kornstein SG, Davis SM, Harrison WM, Keller MB. The treatment of chronic depression, part 3: psychosocial functioning before and after treatment with sertraline or imipramine. J Clin Psychiatry. 1998;59(11):608–19.
68. Bech P. Social functioning: should it become an endpoint in trials of antidepressants? CNS Drugs. 2005;19(4):313–24. Review.
69. Papakostas GI. Major depressive disorder: psychosocial impairment and key considerations in functional improvement. Am J Manag Care. 2009;15(11 Suppl):S316–21.
70. IsHak WW, Greenberg JM, Balayan K, Kapitanski N, Jeffrey J, Fathy H, Fakhry H, Rapaport MH. Quality of life: the ultimate outcome measure of interventions in major depressive disorder. Harv Rev Psychiatry. 2011;19(5):229–39. https://doi.org/10.3109/10673229.2011.61409 9. Review.
71. Thase ME. Bipolar depression: issues in diagnosis and treatment. Harv Rev Psychiatry. 2005;13(5):257–71. Review.
72. Machado M, Iskedjian M, Ruiz I, Einarson TR. Remission, dropouts, and adverse drug reaction rates in major depressive disorder: a meta-analysis of head-to-head trials. Curr Med Res Opin. 2006;22(9):1825–37.
73. Trivedi MH, Rush AJ, Wisniewski SR, Nierenberg AA, Warden D, Ritz L, Norquist G, Howland RH, Lebowitz B, McGrath PJ, Shores-Wilson K, Biggs MM, Balasubramani GK, Fava M, STAR*D Study Team. Evaluation of outcomes with citalopram for depression using measurement-based care in STAR*D: implications for clinical practice. Am J Psychiatry. 2006;163(1):28–40.
74. Möller HJ. Outcomes in major depressive disorder: the evolving concept of remission and its implications for treatment. World J Biol Psychiatry. 2008;9(2):102–14. https://doi.org/10.1080/15622970801981606.
75. Soares CN, Endicott J, Boucher M, Fayyad RS, Guico-Pabia CJ. Predictors of functional response and remission with desvenlafaxine 50 mg/d in patients with major depressive disorder. CNS Spectr. 2014;19(6):519–27. https://doi.org/10.1017/S1092852914000066.
76. Sheehan DV, Harnett-Sheehan K, Spann ME, Thompson HF, Prakash A. Assessing remission in major depressive disorder and generalized anxiety disorder clinical trials with the discan metric of the Sheehan disability scale. Int Clin Psychopharmacol. 2011;26:75–83.
77. Novick D, Montgomery W, Vorstenbosch E, Moneta MV, Dueñas H, Haro JM. Recovery in patients with major depressive disorder (MDD): results of a 6-month, multinational, observational study. Patient Prefer Adherence. 2017;11:1859–68.
78. Lam RW, McIntosh D, Wang J, Enns MW, Kolivakis T, Michalak EE, Sareen J, Song WY, Kennedy SH, MacQueen GM, Milev RV, Parikh SV, Ravindran AV, CANMAT Depression Work Group. Canadian Network for Mood and Anxiety Treatments (CANMAT) 2016 clinical guidelines for the management of adults with major depressive disorder: section 1. Disease burden and principles of care. Can J Psychiatr. 2016;61(9):510–23.
79. Malhi GS, Bell E, Bassett D, Boyce P, Bryant R, Hazell P, Hopwood M, Lyndon B, Mulder R, Porter R, Singh AB, Murray G. The 2020 Royal Australian and New Zealand College of Psychiatrists clinical practice guidelines for mood disorders. Aust N Z J Psychiatry. 2021;55(1):7–117.
80. Leamy M, Bird V, Le Boutillier C, Williams J, Slade M. Conceptual framework for personal recovery in mental health: systematic review and narrative synthesis. Br J Psychiatry. 2011;199:445–52.
81. World Health Organization. User empowerment in mental health—a statement by the WHO Regional Office for Europe. 2010. http://www.euro.who.int/__data/assets/pdf_file/0020/113834/E93430.pdf.
82. National Health System (NHS), Department of Health. Liberating the NHS: no decision about me without me. Government response. 2012. https://assets.publishing.service.gov.uk/government/uploads/system/uploads/attachment_data/file/216980/Liberating-the-NHS-No-decision-about-me-without-me-Government-response.pdf.

83. Luciano M, Sampogna G, Del Vecchio V, Loos S, Slade M, Clarke E, Nagy M, Kovacs A, Munk-Jørgensen P, Krogsgaard Bording M, Kawohl W, Rössler W, Puschner B, Fiorillo A, CEDAR Study Group. When does shared decision making is adopted in psychiatric clinical practice? Results from a European multicentric study. Eur Arch Psychiatry Clin Neurosci. 2020;270(6):645–53.
84. Llewellyn-Beardsley J, Rennick-Egglestone S, Bradstreet S, et al. Not the story you want? Assessing the fit of a conceptual framework characterising mental health recovery narratives. Soc Psychiatry Psychiatr Epidemiol. 2020;55:295–308.
85. Schrank B, Slade M. Recovery in psychiatry. Psychiatr Bull. 2007;31:321–5.
86. Morin L, Franck N. Rehabilitation interventions to promote recovery from schizophrenia: a systematic review. Front Psych. 2017;8:100.
87. Happell B. Who cares for whom? Re-examining the nurse—patient relationship. Int J Ment Health Nurs. 2008;17:381–2.
88. Burgess P, Pirkis J, Coombs T, et al. Assessing the value of existing recovery measures for routine use in Australian mental health services. Aust N Z J Psychiatry. 2011;45:267–80.
89. Leamy M, Clarke E, Le Boutillier C, et al. Recovery practice in community mental health teams: national survey. Br J Psychiatry. 2016;209:340–6.
90. Sells DJ, Stayner DA, Davidson L. Recovering the self in schizophrenia: an integrative review of qualitative studies. Psychiatry Q. 2004;75:87–97.
91. Dunn EC, Wewiorski NJ, Rogers ES. The meaning and importance of employment to people in recovery from serious mental illness: results of a qualitative study. Psychiatr Rehabil J. 2008;32:59–62.
92. Whitley R, Drake RE. Recovery: a dimensional approach. Psychiatr Serv. 2010;61(12):1248–50.
93. Van Eck RM, Burger TJ, Schenkelaars M, et al. The impact of affective symptoms on personal recovery of patients with severe mental illness. Int J Soc Psychiatry. 2018;64:521–7.
94. Van Eck RM, Burger TJ, Vellinga A, et al. The relationship between clinical and personal recovery in patients with schizophrenia spectrum disorders: a systematic review and meta-analysis. Schizophr Bull. 2018;44:631–42.
95. George LK, Blazer DG, Hughes DC, et al. Social support and the outcome of major depression. Br J Psychiatry. 1989;154:478–85.
96. Brugha TS, Bebbington PE, Sturt E, et al. The relation between life events and social support networks in a clinically depressed cohort. Soc Psychiatry Psychiatr Epidemiol. 1990;25:308–13.
97. Gladstone GL, Parker GB, Malhi GS, et al. Feeling unsupported? An investigation of depressed patients' perceptions. J Affect Disord. 2007;103:147–54.
98. Oluboka OJ, Katzman MA, Habert J, McIntosh D, MacQueen GM, Milev RV, McIntyre RS, Blier P. Functional recovery in major depressive disorder: providing early optimal treatment for the individual patient. Int J Neuropsychopharmacol. 2018;21(2):128–44.
99. Okuda A, Suzuki T, Kishi T, Yamanouchi Y, Umeda K, Haitoh H, Hashimoto S, Ozaki N, Iwata N. Duration of untreated illness and antidepressant fluvoxamine response in major depressive disorder. Psychiatry Clin Neurosci. 2010;64(3):268–73.
100. Bukh JD, Bock C, Vinberg M, Kessing LV. The effect of prolonged duration of untreated depression on antidepressant treatment outcome. J Affect Disord. 2013;145(1):42–8.
101. Szegedi A, Jansen WT, van Willigenburg AP, van der Meulen E, Stassen HH, Thase ME. Early improvement in the first 2 weeks as a predictor of treatment outcome in patients with major depressive disorder: a meta-analysis including 6562 patients. J Clin Psychiatry. 2009;70(3):344–53.
102. Villaggi B, Provencher H, Coulombe S, Meunier S, Radziszewski S, Hudon C, Roberge P, Provencher MD, Houle J. Self-management strategies in recovery from mood and anxiety disorders. Glob Qual Nurs Res. 2015;2:2333393615606092.
103. Battle CL, Uebelacker L, Friedman MA, Cardemil EV, Beevers CG, Miller IW. Treatment goals of depressed outpatients: a qualitative investigation of goals identified by participants in a depression treatment trial. J Psychiatr Pract. 2010;16(6):425–30.

104. Baune BT, Christensen MC. Differences in perceptions of major depressive disorder symptoms and treatment priorities between patients and health care providers across the acute, post-acute, and remission phases of depression. Front Psych. 2019;10:335.
105. Zimmerman M. Discordance between researchers and patients in defining remission from depression. J Clin Psychiatry. 2012;73(9):1262–3.
106. Demyttenaere K, Donneau AF, Albert A, et al. What is important in being cured from depression? Discordance between physicians and patients. J Affect Disord. 2015a;174:390–6.
107. Christensen MC, Wong CMJ, Baune BT. Symptoms of major depressive disorder and their impact on psychosocial functioning in the different phases of the disease: do the perspectives of patients and healthcare providers differ? Front Psych. 2020;11:280.
108. Demyttenaere K, Donneau AF, Albert A, Ansseau M, Constant E, van Heeringen K. What is important in being cured from: does discordance between physicians and patients matter? (2). J Affect Disord. 2015b;174:372–7.
109. Maj M, Stein DJ, Parker G, Zimmerman M, Fava GA, De Hert M, Demyttenaere K, McIntyre RS, Widiger T, Wittchen HU. The clinical characterization of the adult patient with depression aimed at personalization of management. World Psychiatry. 2020;19(3):269–93.
110. Dell'Osso B, Albert U, Carrà G, Pompili M, Nanni MG, Pasquini M, Poloni N, Raballo A, Sambataro F, Serafini G, Viganò C, Demyttenaere K, McIntyre RS, Fiorillo A. How to improve adherence to antidepressant treatments in patients with major depression: a psycho-educational consensus checklist. Ann General Psychiatry. 2020;19:61.
111. Rush AJ. Distinguishing functional from syndromal recovery: implications for clinical care and research. J Clin Psychiatry. 2015;76:e832–4.
112. Salkovskis P, Rimes K, Stephenson D, et al. A randomized controlled trial of the use of self-help materials in addition to standard general practice treatment of depression compared to standard treatment alone. Psychol Med. 2006;36:325–33.
113. Cuijpers P. Prevention of depressive disorders: towards a further reduction of the disease burden of mental disorders. Early Interv Psychiatry. 2011;5:179–80.
114. Loos S, Clarke E, Jordan H, et al. Recovery and decision-making involvement in people with severe mental illness from six countries: a prospective observational study. BMC Psychiatry. 2017;17:38.
115. Slade M. Implementing shared decision making in routine mental health care. World Psychiatry. 2017;16:146–53.
116. Slade M, Amering M, Oades L. Recovery: an international perspective. Epidemiol Psichiatr Soc. 2008;17:128–37.
117. Whitley R, Shepherd G, Slade M. Recovery colleges as a mental health innovation. World Psychiatry. 2019;18(2):141–2.
118. Doughty C, Tse S, Duncan N, McIntyre L. The Wellness Recovery Action Plan (WRAP): workshop evaluation. Australas Psychiatry. 2008;16(6):450–6.
119. Mueser KT, Corrigan PW, Hilton DW, Tanzman B, Schaub A, Gingerich S, Essock SM, Tarrier N, Morey B, Vogel-Scibilia S, Herz MI. Illness management and recovery: a review of the research. Psychiatr Serv. 2002;53(10):1272–84.
120. Slade M, Bird V, Le Boutillier C, Williams J, McCrone P, Leamy M. REFOCUS trial: protocol for a cluster randomised controlled trial of a pro-recovery intervention within community based mental health teams. BMC Psychiatry. 2011;11:185.

Recovery-Oriented Treatments in Major Depressive Disorder

14

Gaia Sampogna, Matteo Di Vincenzo, Vincenzo Giallonardo, Mario Luciano, and Andrea Fiorillo

14.1 Toward a Recovery-Oriented Model of Major Depression

Major depressive disorder (MDD) is a common, often chronic, and recurring severe mental disorder affecting more than 264 million people worldwide [1, 2]. By the year 2030, MDD is expected to be the leading cause of diseases burden around the world, accounting now for 2.5% of global disability-adjusted life years lost (DALYs). It is estimated that about 30 million of people suffer from MDD in Europe, and that one in five US adults reports symptoms of depression in the lifetime [3]. MDD is associated with a very high mortality risk, mainly due to suicide and physical diseases such as cardiovascular diseases (CVD).

Historically, major depression has been considered an affective syndrome only, and until 1980s no attention was paid to other symptom clusters. At that time, clinicians had to distinguish between endogenous vs. exogenous depression, with the former being basically considered a biological disorder (and therefore being responsive to pharmacological treatment) and the latter being due to external causes (and therefore being sensible to psychotherapies). The reality is much different, and several biological, clinical, and social studies have found that MDD should be conceptualized as a systemic syndrome characterized by different affective, physical, and cognitive symptom domains, and that immune, neuroendocrine, and inflammatory systems are involved in the pathogenesis of the disorder [4, 5]. This theory has led to the discovery of a third generation of antidepressant agents that act at different levels, and to the conceptualization of full functional recovery as

G. Sampogna (✉) · M. Di Vincenzo · V. Giallonardo · M. Luciano · A. Fiorillo
Department of Psychiatry, University of Campania "L. Vanvitelli", Naples, Italy
e-mail: gaia.sampogna@gmail.com; dr.matteodivincenzo@gmail.com; enzogiallo86@gmail.com; mario.luciano@unicampania.it; andrea.fiorillo@unicampania.it

© The Author(s), under exclusive license to Springer Nature Switzerland AG 2022
B. Carpiniello et al. (eds.), *Recovery and Major Mental Disorders*, Comprehensive Approach to Psychiatry 2, https://doi.org/10.1007/978-3-030-98301-7_14

the final aim of treatment of MDD patients. In fact, while in the past the aim of therapy was response (i.e., reduction of symptoms' severity by, e.g., $\geq 50\%$ assessed by Montgomery–Åsberg Depression Rating Scale - MADRS or Hamilton Rating Scale for Depression - HAM-D scale) or remission (i.e., defined as MADRS score of ≤ 10 or HAM-D17 score ≤ 7), more recently it became clear that this goal was not satisfying anymore, and that the patients' perspective should be taken into account [6, 7]. All this has led to the recovery-oriented movement, according to which MDD treatment should be personalized, individualized, and shared with the patient [8]. This new paradigm of care for major depression is described and discussed in the next paragraphs.

14.2 Toward Full Functional Recovery: How to Improve Patients' Outcome with Personalized and Precision Interventions

Full functional recovery can be defined as a condition in which the patient starts to enjoy again his/her usual activities, returns to work, and is able to take care of him/herself [9, 10]. This is a continuing and evolving clinical process, and several patient, illness, and contextual factors can influence it. The response rate for an initial antidepressant treatment is between 50 and 75% [8]. This will lead to treatment failure, multiple trials, poor treatment response, and patient frustration. Therefore, when choosing a treatment for MDD, clinicians should do it according to a series of factors, including patient's age, pre-morbid level of functioning, educational level, working condition, social network, cognitive schemas, presence of comorbidities, severity and type of symptoms, duration of illness, clinical staging, previous treatments, time to remission, patient's social network, family ties, and environmental exposures (Table 14.1). This process is now known as personalized medicine, which can help to identify a priori which patients will best respond to the different therapeutic approaches.

In fact, the current symptoms of MDD are not predictive of response to any antidepressant or psychotherapy or psychosocial intervention. We still choose the

Table 14.1 Factors predicting recovery in patients with MDD

Patient-related factors	Illness-related factors	Contextual-related factors
Age	Symptoms	Access to care
Personal history	Neurocognition	Neighborhoods
Family history	Severity	Social network
Antecedent environmental factors	Clinical staging	Therapeutic relationship
Recent environmental factors	Physical comorbidities	
Personality traits and coping strategies	Duration of illness and duration of untreated illness	
Cognitive schemas	Number of episodes	
Social functioning		

"best" treatment on the basis of a clinical diagnosis, and not taking into account the different clinical and personal characteristics of the patient. We still rely on clinical algorithms and guidelines, while in many cases they have proved to be far away from clinical practice [11]. What we really need now is an individualized approach aiming to treat the "person" with depression and not the "depressive illness" [2].

All the abovementioned factors should be taken into account by clinicians when selecting the appropriate treatment in order to fulfill the goal of full functional recovery.

In fact, a systematic review on 21 antidepressants showed that these drugs have a similar efficacy and tolerability [12], and the same happens with psychotherapies and psychosocial interventions [13]. Therefore, what is most important in the selection of the "right" treatment is the assessment of patients' individual characteristics, needs, and desires. For example, a young patient affected by MDD will most probably benefit from an antidepressant which is different from the one effective in a person with a late-life depression. Unfortunately, the basic general assumption is that the illness "depression" can be treated with the same "antidepressant" and that all antidepressants are equally effective. This has led to an increased use of antidepressants of 5% in the last decade [14], with about 25% of individuals taking antidepressants for more than 10 years.

However, clinicians are unable to predict what drug works more or less in a given patient for the treatment of MDD symptoms. In the absence of validated biomarkers and genetic data, the personalized approach of major depression will include patients' personal account and the shared decision-making approach [15–17]. In some patients, the adoption of the shared clinical decision-making approach is hampered by anhedonia, lethargy, amotivation, physical and cognitive symptoms, as well as by patient's feelings of vulnerability and self-stigma [18, 19], thus making more difficult a personalized approach.

14.3   Recovery-Oriented Pharmacological Treatments

When antidepressant agents had been developed in the late 1950s, the only aim of clinicians was symptoms' remission. And in fact, the discovery of antidepressants along the years has followed three different lines. The first antidepressants were discovered by "serendipity" searching for the treatment of tuberculosis. These drugs include the tricyclic and I-MAO antidepressants [20], which have been used as first-line treatment for patients with major depression, regardless of their side effect profile [21].

Following the introduction of the Selective Serotonin Reuptake Inhibitors (SSRIs) in 1974, with the fluoxetine being the first antidepressant of that class, the paradigm of care started to change. Clinicians began to consider the profile of side effects when choosing the "appropriate" medication, and the "refinement" era started [22, 23]. In the last 20 years, with the introduction of several other antidepressants with very different pharmacological profiles, clinicians can finally "tailor" their treatment approach. Although the new antidepressants have less side effects compared to I-MAOs and tricyclics, the tolerability of these compounds remains an unsolved issue, with many patients still reporting side effects such as headache, gastrointestinal problems, obesity, insomnia, nausea, and sexual dysfunctions. Therefore, many patients have a low treatment adherence and remission rates are still not satisfying, being approximately ≤50% for any given drug in clinical trials [24], and even lower in everyday clinical practice. This may be due to the fact that the choice of antidepressants in clinical practice is largely based on clinicians' preferences, drugs' availability, and costs. In fact, antidepressants are frequently chosen through "trial-and-error" steps, paying little or no attention to the individual characteristics of the patient and to his/her clinical history [2]. This may be one of the reasons why the majority of patients with a diagnosis of major depression do not achieve a full remission after the first treatment, and at least 30% of them do not respond to two consecutive evidence-based treatments and are classified as treatment-resistant.

Therefore, since the profile of efficacy of antidepressant drugs varies significantly, a personalized approach in drug selection can help in identifying a priori which group of patients will respond better to the different medications [25].

Moreover, in order to have a better response, the treatment should be initiated as soon as possible, since inadequate or delayed interventions are correlated with brain damage and altered morphometry, in terms of hippocampal loss of volume, probably due to chronic neuronal losses, suppressed neurogenesis and disruption of neural connections in mood-related circuits [26, 27].

Finally, even those patients who have responded well to antidepressants may present persistent residual symptoms, such as lack of energy, sleep disturbances, and cognitive deficits. Recently, new drugs targeting the altered domains in MDD have been developed. In particular, since cognitive deficits represent the missing link between symptomatic remission and functional recovery, drugs addressing cognitive symptoms are welcome.

These novel targets for pharmacological drugs have a focus on the glutamatergic, GABAergic, opioidergic, and inflammatory systems, which are implicated in the pathophysiology of MDD. In particular, among the new drugs, ketamine, esketamine, and rapastinel are effective on the glutamatergic system; brexanolone and SAGE-217 act through the GABAergic system; minocycline influences the inflammatory system; the combinatory agent buprenorphine + samidorphan works through the opioidergic system.

The glutamate represents the main excitatory neurotransmitter in the central nervous system; it binds the presynaptic and postsynaptic receptors, and those on astrocytes. Ketamine, a non-competitive N-methyl-D-aspartate (NMDA) antagonist (channel blocker), gives rapid and prolonged antidepressant effects [28]. Ketamine is a dissociative anesthetic drug with hallucinogenic features, approved by the U.S. Food and Drug Administration (FDA) in 1970 as short-acting anesthetic. During mid-1990s, it became a drug of recreational abuse, also known as "Special K". At subanesthetic or emergency use from anesthetic doses, ketamine may produce altered perceptions, depersonalization and derealization lasting from 30 to 60 min. The use of ketamine as antidepressant has been tested in several preclinical and clinical studies, supporting the idea of a complex and multistep cascade of events on different targets: antagonism of NMDA receptors, reduction of nitric-oxide production, increase of glutamate release, increased activation of

14 Recovery-Oriented Treatments in Major Depressive Disorder

α-Ammino-3-idrossi-5-Metil-4-isossazol-Propionic Acid (AMPA) receptors, activation of mTOR, and increased signaling of neurotrophic factors [29]. Due to the potential risk of addiction, ketamine has not been approved for use in clinical practice as antidepressant, but in 2019, the U.S. FDA approved esketamine, the s-enantiomer of ketamine, for the treatment of adults with treatment-resistant depression, i.e., patients who have not responded adequately to at least two different trials with antidepressants at adequate dose and duration [30]. This innovative drug provides a rapid response, with reduction of depressive symptoms within 24 h, as opposed to weeks noted with conventional antidepressants.

14.4 Psychotherapies and the Role of Combination Therapies

The individual response to treatments depends on biological, clinical, psychological, and environmental factors. Therefore, interventions addressing the different factors implicated in the etiopathogenesis of MDD should be used and coordinated. For the most severe cases of depression, psychotherapy is recommended as add-on treatment in combination with pharmacotherapy, while for the less severe cases it may be provided alone [31]. Cognitive behavioral therapy (CBT), interpersonal therapy (IPT), psychodynamic therapy, and Internet-based therapy are among the most effective psychotherapeutic approaches in MDD (Table 14.2).

However, other psychotherapeutic approaches are being studied and look promising, such as mindfulness and problem-solving therapy.

Patients receiving psychotherapies consistently show brain activation changes with a decreased activation in specific brain areas, with peak coordinates in the left anterior cingulate cortex, inferior frontal gyrus (bilaterally), and in left insula [32–34]. These changes seem to be independent from the type of psychotherapy and outline the importance of nonspecific factors in psychiatric treatments. Combination therapy is more effective than psychotherapy or pharmacotherapy alone in achieving full recovery [13]. Moreover, acceptability is significantly better in patients treated with a combined therapy compared with those receiving pharmacotherapy alone.

Psychotherapeutic approaches have been recently adapted to be provided through tele-medicine. Most of Internet-delivered treatments are based on the cognitive behavior therapy (CBT). iCBT is now considered a valid option for the treatment of patients with major depression at a distance [35–38].

Table 14.2 Psychotherapies in patients with major depressive disorder

Type of intervention	Acronym	Description
Cognitive behavioral therapy	CBT	It is focused on cognitive distortions and behaviors, aims to improve emotional regulation, and to develop personal coping strategies
Internet-based CBT	i-CBT	CBT delivered through Internet
Interpersonal therapy	IPT	A brief, attachment-focused psychotherapy focusing on solving interpersonal problems and symptomatic recovery
Psychodynamic therapy	PT	It focuses on the interpretation of individual's mental and emotional processes rather than on behavior

14.5 Psychosocial Interventions

In the last 20 years, several studies have highlighted the role of psychosocial interventions in the treatment of patients with MDD (Table 14.3).

Individual, group, or family psychoeducation aims to: (a) increase the levels of knowledge of patients and families about the illness; (b) improve the recognition of early warning signs of relapses and the identification of patient's dysfunctional cognitive schemas; and (c) improve communication skills and problem-solving strategies [39, 40].

The cognitive remediation techniques are effective in the treatment of cognitive impairments in verbal fluence, visual-spatial ability, verbal learning, and executive functioning in patients with MDD [41–43].

Stress, fatigue, unbalanced diet, heavy tobacco smoking, disturbed sleep hygiene, and low physical activity are among the altered lifestyle behaviors in patients with MDD. Recently, psychosocial interventions aimed to improve patients' lifestyle have been developed and found to be effective [44]. Most international guidelines suggest including these interventions in the recovery-oriented management plan of MDD patients [45–47]. Physical activity and healthy diet have in fact a protective factor by increasing the neurogenesis in the hippocampus. Exercise interventions are the ones with the most robust evidence from clinical trials.

Some psychosocial interventions can be provided through the Internet [35–38]. These approaches have demonstrated their efficacy as an initial intervention for mild depression in the stepped managed care of mood disorders in primary care [46]. Many models of online delivery have been explored, from simple information to self-help strategies and supported time-limited structured therapies. Another opportunity to improve the recovery process of patients with depression is the use of smartphone apps. Other psychosocial interventions successfully used in MDD include art therapies and behavioral activation (Table 14.3).

Table 14.3 Psychosocial interventions for patients with major depressive disorder

Type of intervention	Main features
Psychoeducation	A structured intervention to be delivered in an individual, group or family format; trained professionals provide participants with information on the illness, possible causes and risk factors, possible treatments
Lifestyle intervention	A structured intervention aiming to provide information on healthy lifestyle behaviors, physical activity and treatment adherence
Cognitive remediation	A computerized or paper-and-pencil intervention aiming to improve patient's cognitive functioning (verbal fluence, visual-spatial ability, verbal learning, and executive functioning)
Internet-based/ smartphone-based intervention	A variety of interventions provided through Internet or using dedicated applications for smartphones aiming to provide practical strategies on how to deal with (mild) depressive symptoms

14.6 Conclusions

Depression is a heterogeneous, complex, and multidimensional syndrome, representing the leading cause of disability worldwide. The final aim of the management plan of MDD patients has shifted from symptom remission to full recovery. The need for personalized recovery-oriented interventions is confirmed. The treatment plan for MDD patients should be tailored on patients' preferences according to the shared decision-making approach. An active involvement of patients in their therapeutic plan is associated with an improvement in long-term outcome [48–50].

The recovery-oriented management of patients with MDD starts with the clinical characterization of the individual patient, even considering that there is "no one size that fits for all," and that the concept of interchangeability of treatments is very far from clinical reality. The comparisons between antidepressant medications and psychotherapies, and between different psychotherapeutic techniques, have suffered from this limitation, supporting the idea that all treatments for depression are "equivalent" and interchangeable. Of course, this paradigm has proven to be false, and it has had detrimental effects on education, research, and clinical practice. We do believe that all patients with major depression are treatable, but the treatment will have to be differentiated on the basis of several clinical, personal, and contextual factors.

References

1. World Health Organization. Depression and other common mental disorders: global health estimates. Geneva: World Health Organization; 2017.
2. Maj M, Stein DJ, Parker G, Zimmerman M, Fava GA, De Hert M, et al. The clinical characterization of the adult patient with depression aimed at personalization of management. World Psychiatry. 2020;19(3):269–93.
3. Weinberger AH, Gbedemah M, Martinez AM, Nash D, Galea S, Goodwin RD. Trends in depression prevalence in the USA from 2005 to 2015: widening disparities in vulnerable groups. Psychol Med. 2018;48(8):1308–15.
4. Cramer AO, van Borkulo CD, Giltay EJ, van der Maas HL, Kendler KS, Scheffer M, Borsboom D. Major depression as a complex dynamic system. PLoS One. 2016;11(12):e0167490.
5. Maj M. The need for a conceptual framework in psychiatry acknowledging complexity while avoiding defeatism. World Psychiatry. 2016;15(1):1–2.
6. Möller HJ. Outcomes in major depressive disorder: the evolving concept of remission and its implications for treatment. World J Biol Psychiatry. 2008;9(2):102–14.
7. Thase ME, Haight BR, Richard N, Rockett CB, Mitton M, Modell JG, et al. Remission rates following antidepressant therapy with bupropion or selective serotonin reuptake inhibitors: a meta-analysis of original data from 7 randomized controlled trials. J Clin Psychiatry. 2005;66(8):974–81.
8. McIntyre R, Gill H. The unmet needs for major depressive disorder. In: Pompili M, McIntyre R, Fiorillo A, Sartorius N, editors. New directions in psychiatry. Springer; 2020. p. 27–38.

9. Oluboka OJ, Katzman MA, Habert J, McIntosh D, MacQueen GM, Milev RV, et al. Functional recovery in major depressive disorder: providing early optimal treatment for the individual patient. Int J Neuropsychopharmacol. 2018;21(2):128–44.
10. Fiorillo A, Carpiniello B, De Giorgi S, La Pia S, Maina G, Sampogna G, et al. Assessment and management of cognitive and psychosocial dysfunctions in patients with major depressive disorder: a clinical review. Front Psych. 2018;11(9):493.
11. Kan K, Feenstra TL, de Vries SO, Visser E, Schoevers RA, Jörg F. The clinical effectiveness of an algorithm-guided treatment program for depression in specialized mental healthcare: a comparison with efficacy trials. J Affect Disord. 2020;275:216–23.
12. Cipriani A, Furukawa TA, Salanti G, Chaimani A, Atkinson LZ, Ogawa Y, Leucht S, Ruhe HG, Turner EH, Higgins JPT, Egger M, Takeshima N, Hayasaka Y, Imai H, Shinohara K, Tajika A, Ioannidis JPA, Geddes JR. Comparative efficacy and acceptability of 21 antidepressant drugs for the acute treatment of adults with major depressive disorder: a systematic review and network meta-analysis. Lancet. 2018;391(10128):1357–66.
13. Cuijpers P, Noma H, Karyotaki E, Vinkers CH, Cipriani A, Furukawa TA. A network meta-analysis of the effects of psychotherapies, pharmacotherapies and their combination in the treatment of adult depression. World Psychiatry. 2020;19(1):92–107.
14. Pratt LA, Brody DJ, Gu Q. Antidepressant use among persons aged 12 and over: United States, 2011–2014. NCHS Data Brief. Number 283. National Center for Health Statistics. 2017.
15. Slade M. Implementing shared decision making in routine mental health care. World Psychiatry. 2017;16(2):146–53.
16. Fiorillo A, Luciano M, Del Vecchio V, Sampogna G, Obradors-Tarragó C, Maj M, et al. Priorities for mental health research in Europe: a survey among national stakeholders' associations within the ROAMER project. World Psychiatry. 2013;12(2):165–70.
17. Fiorillo A, Barlati S, Bellomo A, Corrivetti G, Nicolò G, Sampogna G, et al. The role of shared decision-making in improving adherence to pharmacological treatments in patients with schizophrenia: a clinical review. Ann General Psychiatry. 2020;19:43.
18. Demyttenaere K. Taking the depressed "person" into account before moving into personalized or precision medicine. World Psychiatry. 2016;15(3):236–7.
19. Habert J, Katzman MA, Oluboka OJ, McIntyre RS, McIntosh D, MacQueen GM et al. Functional recovery in major depressive disorder: focus on early optimized treatment. Prim Care Companion CNS Disord. 2016;18(5).
20. Pereira VS, Hiroaki-Sato VA. A brief history of antidepressant drug development: from tricyclics to beyond ketamine. Acta Neuropsychiatr. 2018;30(6):307–22.
21. Kessler RC, Petukhova M, Sampson NA, Zaslavsky AM, Wittchen HU. Twelve-month and lifetime prevalence and lifetime morbid risk of anxiety and mood disorders in the United States. Int J Methods Psychiatr Res. 2012;21(3):169–84.
22. McIntyre RS, Lee Y, Mansur RB. Treating to target in major depressive disorder: response to remission to functional recovery. CNS Spectr. 2015;20:20–30.
23. Zimmerman M, Martinez JA, Attiullah N, Friedman M, Toba C, Boerescu DA, Rahgeb M. Why do some depressed outpatients who are in remission according to the Hamilton Depression Rating Scale not consider themselves to be in remission? J Clin Psychiatry. 2012;73(6):790–5.
24. Galling B, Ferrer AC, Daou MAZ, Sangroula D, Hagi K, Correll CU. Safety and tolerability of antidepressant co-treatment in acute major depressive disorder: results from a systematic review and exploratory meta-analysis. Expert Opin Drug Saf. 2015;14:1587–608.
25. Ragguett RM, Tamura JK, McIntyre RS. Keeping up with the clinical advances: depression. CNS Spectr. 2019;24(S1):25–37.
26. Fu CH, Steiner H, Costafreda SG. Predictive neural biomarkers of clinical response in depression: a meta-analysis of functional and structural neuroimaging studies of pharmacological and psychological therapies. Neurobiol Dis. 2013;52:75–83.
27. Wise T, Cleare AJ, Herane A, Young AH, Arnone D. Diagnostic and therapeutic utility of neuroimaging in depression: an overview. Neuropsychiatr Dis Treat. 2014;19(10):1509–22.
28. Siegel AN, Di Vincenzo JD. Brietzke E, Gill H, Rodrigues NB, Lui LMW, Teopiz KM, Ng J, Ho R, McIntyre RS, Rosenblat JD. Antisuicidal and antidepressant effects of ketamine

and esketamine in patients with baseline suicidality: a systematic review. J Psychiatr Res. 2021;137:426–36.

29. Sanders B, Brula AQ. Intranasal esketamine: from origins to future implications in treatment-resistant depression. J Psychiatr Res. 2021;137:29–35.

30. Food and Drug Administration. FDA approves new nasal spray medication for treatment-resistant depression; available only at a certified doctor's office or clinic. Maryland: Silver Spring; 2019. https://www.fda.gov/news-events/press-announcements/fda-approves-new-nasal-spray-medication-treatment-resistant-depression-available-only-certified.

31. Cuijpers P, Reynolds CF 3rd, Donker T, Li J, Andersson G, Beekman A. Personalized treatment of adult depression: medication, psychotherapy, or both? A systematic review. Depress Anxiety. 2012;29(10):855–64.

32. Sheline YI, Gado MH, Kraemer HC. Untreated depression and hippocampal volume loss. Am J Psychiatry. 2003;160(8):1516–8.

33. Arnone D, McKie S, Elliott R, Juhasz G, Thomas EJ, Downey D, et al. State-dependent changes in hippocampal grey matter in depression. Mol Psychiatry. 2013;18(12):1265–72.

34. Nugent AC, Davis RM, Zarate CA Jr, Drevets WC. Reduced thalamic volumes in major depressive disorder. Psychia Psychiatry Res. 2013;213(3):179–85.

35. Andersson G, Titov N, Dear BF, Rozental A, Carlbring P. Internet-delivered psychological treatments: from innovation to implementation. World Psychiatry. 2019;18(1):20–8.

36. Andrews G. We can manage depression better with technology. Aust Fam Physician. 2014;43(12):838–41.

37. Batterham PJ, Sunderland M, Calear AL, Davey CG, Christensen H, Teesson M, et al. Developing a roadmap for the translation of e-mental health services for depression. Aust N Z J Psychiatry. 2015;49(9):776–84.

38. Firth J, Torous J, Nicholas J, Carney R, Rosembaum S, Sarris J. Can smartphone mental health interventions reduce symptoms of anxiety? A meta-analysis of randomized controlled trials. Affect Disord. 2017;218:15–22.

39. Luciano M, Del Vecchio V, Giacco D, De Rosa C, Malangone C, Fiorillo A. A 'family affair'? The impact of family psychoeducational interventions on depression. Expert Rev Neurother. 2012;12(1):83–91.

40. Brady P, Kangas M, McGill K. "Family matters": a systematic review of the evidence for family psychoeducation for major depressive disorder. J Marital Fam Ther. 2017;43(2):245–63.

41. Bowie CR, Gupta M, Holshausen K, Jozik R, Best M, Milev R. Cognitive remediation for treatment-resistant depression: effects on cognition and functioning and the role of online homework. J Nerv Ment Dis. 2013;201(8):680–5.

42. Jahnshan C, Rassovsky Y, Green MF. Enhancing neuroplasticity to augment cognitive remediation in schizophrenia. Front Psych. 2017;8:191.

43. Listunova L, Kienzle J, Bartolovic M, Jaehn A, Grützner TM, Wolf RC, et al. Cognitive remediation therapy for partially remitted unipolar depression: a single-blind randomized controlled trial. J Affect Disord. 2020;276:316–26.

44. De Rosa C, Sampogna G, Luciano M, Del Vecchio V, Pocai B, Borriello G, et al. Improving physical health of patients with severe mental disorders: a critical review of lifestyle psychosocial interventions. Expert Rev Neurother. 2017;17(7):667–81.

45. Lam RW, McIntosh D, Wang JL, Enns MW, Koliwakis T, Michalak EE, et al. Canadian Network for Mood and Anxiety Treatments (CANMAT) 2016 clinical guidelines for the management of adults with major depressive disorder. Can J Psychiatr. 2016;61(9):510–23.

46. Malhi GS, Bassett D, Boyce P, Bryant R, Fitzgerald PB, Fritz K, et al. Royal Australian and New Zealand College of Psychiatrists clinical practice guidelines for mood disorders. Aust N Z J Psychiatry. 2015;49(12):1087–206.

47. Kennedy SH, Lam RW, McIntyre RS, Tourjman SV, Bhat V, Blier P, Hasnain M, Jollant F, Levitt AJ, MacQueen GM, McInerney SJ, McIntosh D, Milev RV, Muller DJ, Parikh SV, Pearson NL, Ravindran AV, Uher R. Canadian Network for Mood and Anxiety Treatments (CANMAT) 2016 clinical guidelines for the management of adults with major depressive disorder: Section 3. Pharmacological treatments. Can J Psychiatr. 2016;61:540–60.

48. Demyttenaere K, Donneau AF, Albert A, Ansseau M, Constant E, van Heeringen K. What is important in being cured from depression? Discordance between physicians and patients. J Affect Disord. 2015;174:390–6.
49. Boschloo L, Bekhuis E, Weitz ES, Reijnders M, DeRubeis RJ, Dimidjian S, Dunner DL, Dunlop BW, Hegerl U, Hollon SD, Jarrett RB, Kennedy SH, Miranda J, Mohr DC, Simons AD, Parker G, Petrak F, Herpertz S, Quilty LC, John Rush A, Segal ZV, Vittengl JR, Schoevers RA, Cuijpers P. The symptom-specific efficacy of antidepressant medication vs. cognitive behavioral therapy in the treatment of depression: results from an individual patient data meta-analysis. World Psychiatry. 2019;18(2):183–91.
50. Fiorillo A, Barlati S, Bellomo A, Corrivetti G, Nicolò G, Sampogna G, Stanga V, Veltro F, Maina G, Vita A. The role of shared decision-making in improving adherence to pharmacological treatments in patients with schizophrenia: a clinical review. Ann General Psychiatry. 2020;19:43.

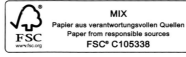

Printed by Books on Demand, Germany